For Margaret,

With warm regards

&

thanks for a great deal

Anne

SALMONELLA INFECTIONS, NETWORKS OF KNOWLEDGE, AND PUBLIC HEALTH IN BRITAIN, 1880–1975

Salmonella Infections, Networks of Knowledge, and Public Health in Britain, 1880–1975

ANNE HARDY

OXFORD
UNIVERSITY PRESS

OXFORD
UNIVERSITY PRESS

Great Clarendon Street, Oxford, OX2 6DP,
United Kingdom

Oxford University Press is a department of the University of Oxford.
It furthers the University's objective of excellence in research, scholarship,
and education by publishing worldwide. Oxford is a registered trade mark of
Oxford University Press in the UK and in certain other countries

First Edition published in 2015

Impression: 1

Published in the United States of America by Oxford University Press
198 Madison Avenue, New York, NY 10016, United States of America

British Library Cataloguing in Publication Data
Data available

Library of Congress Control Number: 2014940798

ISBN 978–0–19–870497–3

Printed and bound by
CPI Group (UK) Ltd, Croydon, CR0 4YY

Preface

The subject of this book has kept me company for more years than I care to count. Admittedly, other projects intervened, and some six years of community service as an academic administrator proved a significant distraction. In parting from this research I do, however, wish to record the fun I have had in doing it, and my continuing fascination with *Salmonella* and their history.

In the course of time I have accumulated many debts, not all of which can be acknowledged here. Spending 20-odd years as a member of staff at the Academic Unit of the Wellcome Institute, and its successor the Wellcome Trust Centre for the History of Medicine at UCL—experiencing the diverse intellectual approaches offered by my colleagues and our many academic visitors—greatly enriched my appreciation of history as a discipline. I am grateful to W. F. Bynum, who facilitated my admission to this world and encouraged me to undertake this project, and to the journal editors who published the related articles which marked the progress of my research. I owe a particular debt to Astri Andresen, of the Department of Archaeology, History, Classics, and Religion at the University of Bergen, Norway, who for ten years from 2003 organized an annual workshop on the history of health and medicine whose every meeting I was privileged to attend, and where several papers based in this project were aired. I am everlastingly grateful to my Norwegian colleagues in Bergen and Oslo for their patience in listening to me, for their critiques and encouragement, and for the enjoyable times we have spent together in their delightful cities. I am grateful to Amy Fairchild, Alfredo Morabia, and especially Gerald Oppenheimer for arranging for me to visit the Center for History and Ethics in Public Health at Columbia University, New York, in spring 2011, a sojourn which allowed me to explore the American aspects of my story. I am doubly indebted to Astri Andresen for inviting me to spend a month at her Department in spring 2012, during which I was able finally to get my head around the completion of this project. I am more than grateful to the late Nils Rosdahl for drawing the writings of Fritz Kauffmann to my attention, and to Harold J. Cook for opening my mind to the possibilities of transnational history. A number of people formally and informally provided invaluable research assistance: Mary Dobson, Jennifer Holmes, William Hubbard, Sharon Messenger, Caroline Overy, and Carole Reeves. Hal Cook and Stephen Casper provided valuable commentary on an earlier version of Chapter 6; William Hubbard, Michael Neve, Ros Stanwell-Smith, and Keir Waddington gallantly undertook the task of reviewing the penultimate version of the manuscript. I am grateful to all, and to the referees of Oxford University Press for comments, suggestions, and support. The book would have been the poorer without their help. Several people most kindly contributed towards the project: Pratik Chakrabati solved the mystery identity of S. S. Bhatnagar; Tom Humphrey conducted a retrospective analysis of food-poisoning outbreaks detailed in 1890 and 1925; Lars Ole Andersen provided valuable material relating to the Danish State Serum Institute; Donald Jerne supplied biographical information on Fritz Kauffmann; Roger Feldman provided me with a CD-Rom copy of the CDC's *Atlas of Salmonella in the United States 1968–1998*; and Gordon Dougan outlined the principal problems of salmonellosis in the twenty-first century. I am indebted to them all for their generosity. The staffs of the Bodleian Library, the British Library, the Royal Society of Medicine Library, and the Wellcome Library have been unfailingly courteous and helpful. Christopher Wheeler and Cathryn Steele of Oxford University Press demonstrated exemplary editorial patience with authorial worries. I have greatly appreciated their support, and that of Robert Faber and the Delegates of Oxford University Press.

As is often the case with long-standing projects, earlier versions of several chapters have appeared elsewhere. I am grateful to Mark Pollard of Chatto and Pickering for permission to use material taken from 'An Oyster Odyssey', published in *Health and Citizenship*, edited by Frank Huisman and Harry Oosterhuis (2013), and to Olav Røsset of Novus Forlag, for permission to use material from 'Us and Them: Bacterial Invasion and Colonisation in the Twentieth Century', published in *International and Local Approaches to Health and Health Care*, edited by Astri Andresen, William Hubbard, and Teemu Ryymin (2011). Material from Chapters 2 and 6 has also appeared in conference proceedings edited by Astri Andresen and her colleagues and published by the Stein Rokkan Centre for Social Studies, Bergen University. Some material from Chapter 4 appeared in 'Food, hygiene, and the laboratory: a short history of food poisoning in Britain, circa 1850–1950', *Social History of Medicine* 12 (1999): pp. 293–311; similarly, material in Chapters 5 and 7 appeared in 'Scientific strategy and ad hoc response: The problem of typhoid in America and England, c. 1910–1950', in *The Journal of the History of Medicine and Allied Sciences*, 69 (2014): pp. 1–37.

This book was completed during the most difficult period of my life, and I am immensely grateful to the friends and colleagues who supported me through it. Special mention must go to Astri Andresen, Virginia Berridge, Nandini Bhattacharya, Caroline and Guy Bodger, Michael Crawford and Ulrike Roth, Anne Crowther, Mary and Christopher Dobson, Marguerite Dupree and Rick Trainor, Helen Fraser and Grant MacIntyre, Veronica Gosling, Christoph Gradmann, Jim and Pam Hardy, John Hardy, William Hubbard and Berit Henriksen, Frank Huisman, Margaret Humphreys, John Landers and Diana Parker, Vivienne Lo, Kate Mackenzie and Martin Brown, Nicola Miller and John North, the late Dick Millsom, Serena Moore, Michael Neve, Malcolm Nicolson, Jim Pancott, David Robey, Barbara and Patrick Roche, Helga Satzinger, Julia Sheppard, Susanne Stirling, Mads and Lis Strandgaard, Andrea Tanner, Marie Claire Thorsen, Keir Waddington, and the late Patricia Utechin. I am especially grateful to Virginia Berridge and the London School of Hygiene and Tropical Medicine for providing me with a professional home since 2010. Andrea, Barbara, Julia, and Mary have been my Graces. Pernille and Bob and Jens and Marianne have been stalwart, and Ellen, Michael, and Romola make it all worthwhile.

Anne Hardy

Gloucestershire, 2014

Contents

Abbreviations

BSE	Bovine spongiform encephalopathy
BMB	*British Medical Bulletin*
BMJ	*British Medical Journal*
BPP	British Parliamentary Papers
BVA	British Veterinary Association
CCHE	Central Council for Health Education
CMO	Chief Medical Officer
CMOAR	Chief Medical Officer's Annual Report
CDC	Communicable Disease Center
DSSI	Danish State Serum Institute
EPHLS	Emergency Public Health Laboratory Service
Epi and Inf	*Epidemiology and Infection*
EEC	European Economic Community
EU	European Union
FTG	*Fish Trades Gazette*
FERG	Foodborne Infections Epidemiology Reference Group
Jnl Hyg	*Journal of Hygiene*
Jnl Inf Dis	*Journal of Infectious Diseases*
Jnl Path and Bact	*Journal of Pathology and Bacteriology*
Jnl State Med	*Journal of State Medicine*
JAPHA	*Journal of the American Public Health Association*
JRAMC	*Journal of the Royal Army Medical Corps*
Jnl Roy Inst PH	*Journal of the Royal Institute of Public Health*
Jnl Roy San Inst	*Journal of the Royal Sanitary Institute*
Jnl San Inst	*Journal of the Sanitary Institute*
LGB	Local Government Board
LCC	London County Council
MO	*Medical Officer*
MOH	Medical Officer of Health
MOAR	Medical Officer's Annual Report
MRC	Medical Research Council
MAFF	Ministry of Agriculture, Fisheries and Food
MBEPHLS	*Monthly Bulletin of EPHLS*
MBMH	*Monthly Bulletin of the Ministry of Health*
MDR	Multi Drug Resistant
NIMR	National Institute for Medical Research
PRSM	*Proceedings of the Royal Society of Medicine*
PH	*Public Health*
PHLS	Public Health Laboratory Service
Reps on PH	*Reports on Public Health and Medical Matters*
Reps on PH	*Reports on Public Health and Medical Subjects*
Roy San Inst Jnl	*Royal Sanitary Institute Journal*

Roy Soc Hlth Jnl	*Royal Society of Health Journal*
RSM	Royal Society of Medicine
VIC	Veterinary Investigation Centre
VIS	Veterinary Investigation Service
Vet Rec	*Veterinary Record*
WHO	World Health Organization

Introduction

Food poisoning is generally regarded as little more than an unpleasant and inconvenient episode. On a national and global scale, however, it constitutes a public health problem of major significance. In 2007 the World Health Organization (WHO) established the Foodborne Disease Burden Epidemiology Reference Group (FERG) with a view to providing reliable estimates of the global impact of all food-borne diseases, and by November 2009 the 'shocking' level of the problem was clear.[1] While no data were available for China, Latin America, and the Middle East, more than 5 billion episodes of diarrhoea were recorded annually among the under-5s, with an estimated 1.15 million deaths a year in South East Asia and Africa in that age group. Nor was this simply a problem of children or of poverty: 419 million episodes of diarrhoea were recorded annually in Europe and 455 million in North America, with under-reporting known to be a difficulty.[2] FERG's project is still in progress: the WHO plans to present a first global estimate in 2014.[3] The inference is, however, already clear: foodborne disease constitutes a significant economic and social cost for developed as well as developing states.[4] In England in 2003 the average cost per case of *Salmonella* infection was £606, of *Campylobacter* £315, and of rotavirus £176. The estimated cost of all intestinal infections was £743 million, expressed in 1994/5 prices.[5] The Food Standards Agency has recently estimated some one million food poisoning cases a year in Britain, costing nearly £1.5 billion annually.[6]

These shocking statistics of food poisoning sit within a complex global context. If the problem of food infections can be associated with poor hygiene and defective sanitary infrastructures in poorer areas of the world, its prevalence in the developed world originates in modern intensive farming systems, industrial food processing practices, and the internationalization of food sourcing. Human travel and migration,

[1] Susan Jones, 'Counting the global burden of foodborne disease': <http://blogs.plos.org/speakingof medicine/2009/11/02/counting-the-global-burden-of-foodborne-disease/>, accessed 18 August 2013.

[2] Jones, 'Counting the burden'.

[3] A. H. Havelaar et al., 'WHO initiative to estimate the global burden of foodborne disease', *The Lancet*, 381 (2013): p. 559.

[4] See also Anon, 'Estimating the global burden of foodborne disease', *The Lancet Infectious Diseases*, 9 (2009): pp. 80–1.

[5] J. A. Roberts et al., 'The study of infectious intestinal disease in England: Socio-economic impact', *Epidemiology and Infection*, 130 (2003): p. 1.

[6] Foodborne Disease Strategy 2010–15: <http://www.food.gov.uk/multimedia/pdfs/fds2015.pdf>.

sanitary habits, and lack of state and municipal action also contribute.[7] But food infections are not merely a human problem. Many food poisoning pathogens, including *Salmonella, Escherichia coli* (*E. coli*), and *Campylobacter*, link the human and animal worlds. Their natural habitat is in the guts of birds and animals, and sometimes humans, where they are carried—temporarily or permanently—and enter the wider environment in the creatures' excreta to contaminate items consumed by other animals and humans. Meat and milk may also carry several of these infections. In the twenty-first century, major pathogenic players in this game are *E. coli*, brucellosis, dysentery, cholera, *Campylobacter*, and *Salmonella*.[8] Although norovirus has in recent years acquired public notoriety as the 'winter vomiting bug' and a scourge of cruise liners and expensive restaurants, the bacterial pathogens cause misery to many more people, some still cause problems among populations of domestic animals, and in all they come with severe economic costs.

FOOD POISONING IN HISTORY

The modern history of food poisoning begins with the recognition of bacterial pathogens as the causal agent in the late nineteenth century.[9] Outbreaks were linked to *Salmonella* from 1888, to *Clostridium botulinum* from 1897, and to staphylococcal infections from *circa* 1930. For much of the twentieth century, however, the *Salmonella* family of bacteria were considered to be the main cause of food poisoning in the world.[10] This book takes the history of *Salmonella* since 1880 to explore the processes by which food poisoning became recognized as a serious public health problem, and as a significant and persistent economic problem in the modern world. It is a history which shows that despite accumulating scientific knowledge, recognition of core public health issues, and continued public health endeavour across a century and more, certain problems and behaviours persist in nature. Three distinct, somewhat overlapping, phases in the realization of the food poisoning problem shape the structure of the book: the discovery of pathways of transmission *circa* 1880–1940, the scientific elucidation of the family and its natural history from around 1900 onwards, and the recognition of the complex problem presented by their control (1940–75). Although *Salmonella* were, and are, a world problem, much of their scientific elucidation took place in Europe, with

[7] For example, BBC News, 'Typhoid making a comeback in UK', 23 August 2007; BBC News, 'Health risk from bad food hygiene', 11 June 2006; accessed 12 September 2013.

[8] Anon, 'Estimating the global burden'.

[9] For the wider history of food poisoning see Elliot B. Dewberry, *Food Poisoning. Food-borne Infections and Intoxication*, 4th edn (1959), chapters 1 and 2.

[10] The situation is not fully clear but see Public Health Laboratory Service report, 'Food poisoning in England and Wales', *Monthly Bulletin of the Ministry of Health*, 18 (1959): p. 177: 'It becomes clearer each year that food poisoning in England and Wales is largely a matter of salmonellosis'; Anon, 'Epidemiology of salmonellosis', *Medical Officer* (*MO*), 111 (1964): pp. 236–7. See also the 13 regional essays in Eugène van Oye, ed, *The World Problem of Salmonellosis* (1964), covering Europe (two essays), Israel, Africa (three essays), Canada, the United States, Mexico, South America, Japan, Indochina and China (one essay), and Australia.

British researchers playing a key role. The wider story is therefore both national and transnational: British *Salmonella* scientists were central to the formation of a transnational community.

Beyond the part played by scientists lies the question of attempts at control on the ground—public health approaches to the problem of food poisoning—where a case-study approach is indicated. England and Wales furnish a good unit for examining approaches to the problems of salmonellosis because, as a geographically small state with an established and integrated public health administration and a tradition of outbreak investigation by epidemiological methods, its surveillance and response systems were broadly effective. Moreover this administration early established a strong tradition of cutting-edge research. Unlike North America and most European states, the countries comprising Britain each possessed at the end of the nineteenth century a central public health department under a Chief Medical Officer, and a public health administration headed at local level by Medical Officers of Health (MOHs) with specific responsibility for investigating and resolving infectious disease outbreaks and incidence in their areas. This administration was backed by the General Register Offices, which collected data on cause of death, and from *circa* 1890 by systems for notification, of cases (as opposed to deaths) from specific infectious diseases. The preventive medical personnel of Scotland and Ireland shared identity, community, and professional journals with their English and Welsh colleagues. Although this study is largely based on sources from England and Wales, material on Scotland and Ireland has not been excluded.

The discovery of food poisoning as a public health problem was closely related to the practices of local observation and local knowledge of disease incidence contained within this public health organization. By the early 1900s, it possessed a generally well-trained and dedicated cadre of local MOHs, who made use of two specialist journals, *Public Health* (from 1888) and *Medical Officer* (1908–72), to communicate local events and discuss and comment on mutual problems. Field surveillance and investigation were undertaken both by staff of the Medical Department of the Local Government Board (1872–1919) and the Ministry of Health (1919–68), and by local MOHs. As bacteriology came to be recognized as providing essential support to outbreak investigation and knowledge accumulation, the central medical authority provided a certain measure of laboratory support, and a variety of other laboratories became involved to a greater or lesser degree in bacteriological research and provision of such services as identifying the bacteria responsible for disease outbreaks. The food-poisoning *Salmonella* were initially considered not to be an American problem, but from the mid-1930s in the USA and after World War II in Britain, veterinarians were increasingly drawn into the world of *Salmonella* identification and prevention as the bacteria became a problem in intensive farming systems. During the interwar period, an international community of *Salmonella* researchers became established, and American veterinary bacteriologists were drawn into the networks of *Salmonella* researchers by reason of the cutting-edge research being done outside America. Their integration into the international *Salmonella* community meant that they played an important part in the post-war establishment of a major *Salmonella* surveillance and research programme in America.

Through the work of this international *Salmonella* community, the bacteria of the *Salmonella* family were found to be variously pathogenic. Many cause a human illness simply termed 'food poisoning', but one, *Salmonella typhi*, is responsible for a distinct disease entity: typhoid. The identification of typhoid as a disease of human beings took place in the early nineteenth century, and was achieved by clinical observation and the meticulous recording and synthesis of clinical symptoms and anatomical effects.[11] Its transmission by faecally contaminated drinking water and milk was known by the 1870s, and measures were being taken for its control in England and Wales well before the identification of the typhoid bacillus by Karl Eberth and Georg Theodor Gaffky between 1880 and 1884.[12] As Andrew Cunningham has noted of plague, before the laboratory identification of the specific micro-organism of a particular disease was possible, diseases were defined by symptom. Subsequently they were defined by the isolation of the causal organism.[13] In the case of *Salmonella*, laboratory identification of the causal organism created a new disease category. August Gärtner's discovery of the bacillus now known as *Salmonella enteritidis* in 1888 alerted microbiologists to the existence of bacterial food poisoning.[14] In identifying food poisoning as a result of bacterial infection, microbiology created a new public health problem, as practitioners of preventive medicine began to realize in the years that followed. Although the notification of infectious diseases was introduced into England and Wales *circa* 1890, food poisoning, in its status as a relatively very minor infection, was not made notifiable until 1939. While notification statistics for salmonellosis come with all kinds of qualifications (food poisoning cases frequently escape medical attention and do not get notified), the general trend of dramatically falling reports of typhoid cases as against rapidly rising reports of *Salmonella* food poisoning are evident from data recorded in England and Wales and in America in the mid-twentieth century.[15]

[11] A. Lafontaine, 'Introduction', in *World Problem*, edited by van Oye, p. 7.

[12] Anne Hardy, *The Epidemic Streets: Infectious Disease and the Rise of Preventive Medicine 1856–1900* (1993), chapter 6. Eberth described the typhoid bacillus in 1880; Gaffky isolated it four years later. See Guido Ghyssels, 'Les salmonelloses: 80 ans d'histoire', in *World Problem*, edited by van Oye, pp. 10–11. It may be noted here that the words 'bacterium' and 'bacteria' denote a certain type of micro-organism, whereas the words 'bacillus' and 'bacilli' denote pathogenic bacteria (*Oxford English Dictionary*).

[13] Andrew Cunningham, 'Transforming plague: The laboratory and the identity of infectious disease', in *The Laboratory Revolution in Medicine* (1992), edited by Andrew Cunningham and Perry Williams, pp. 209–44.

[14] The scientific history of the genus *Salmonella* is set out in William D. Foster, *A History of Medical Bacteriology and Immunology* (1970), pp. 177–84, 189–95. See also Ghyssels, 'Les salmonelloses'.

[15] For enteric fever in England and Wales 1870–1923 see Chief Medical Officer's Annual Report, England and Wales (1925), p. 19; for data on *Salmonella* food poisoning in England and Wales 1923–44 see H. P. R. Seeliger and A. E. Maya, 'Epidemiologie der salmonellosen in Europa 1850–1960' in *World Problem*, edited by van Oye, p. 270; for typhoid and other salmonelloses reported in the USA 1951–61 see Mildred M. Galton et al., 'Epidemiology of salmonellosis in the United States' in *World Problem*, edited by van Oye, p. 423.

The chronology of the *Salmonella* story thus begins in 1880, with Karl Eberth's description of *Salmonella typhi*, while the lesser strains of *Salmonella* began to be identified from 1885. 1880 was also the year in which the first recorded major food poisoning outbreak in England was investigated by the public health authorities, and in which food poisoning entered the domain of public health concern.[16] I have chosen effectively to end my account in the mid-1970s for four reasons. First, the English public health administration underwent the first major re-organization since its creation (1848–72) in 1974, with the replacement of the MOHs, whose duties specifically included epidemiology, by community physicians who practised community medicine.[17] Second, Britain joined the European Economic Community in 1973, after which its food and farming industries, technically at least, became subject to EEC regulations. Third, the first reports of antibiotic drug-resistant typhoid came in 1975, presaging ominous future developments.[18] Finally, *Campylobacter* emerged as a major food poisoner in the late 1970s, and quickly displaced *Salmonella* as the leading cause of food poisoning in many European countries, including England, while the emergence of bovine spongiform encephalopathy in the 1980s added a new dimension to British food concerns.[19] Although the rise of modern investigative journalism in the 1970s meant *Salmonella* achieved greatly heightened public notice in the 1980s following well-publicized incidents associated with Italian chocolate, powdered baby food, and an outbreak at the Stanley Royd Hospital, Wakefield, in 1987,[20] the later 1970s saw a paradigm shift in Britain's public health regime which effectively opened a new chapter in its history of food-borne disease.

SALMONELLA: BETWEEN SCIENCE AND SANITATION

For most of this history, two distinct strands of pre-occupation with *Salmonella* run side by side. On the one hand, the natural history and family relationships of *Salmonella* have fascinated public health specialists and microbiologists alike. The eminent Belgian scientist, Jules Bordet, once declared them to be 'one of the most fascinating subjects in pure microbiology, in bacteriology in the service of epidemiology, in pathology and in hygiene'.[21] Named for Daniel Salmon, the senior of the

[16] See Anne Hardy, 'Food, hygiene and the laboratory: A brief history of food poisoning, circa 1850–1950', *Social History of Medicine*, 12 (1999): pp. 293–311.

[17] See Michael Warren and Huw Francis, eds, *Recalling the Medical Officer of Health. Writings by Sidney Chave* (1987), pp. 144–51.

[18] E. S. Anderson, 'The problem and implications of chloramphenicol resistance in the typhoid bacillus', *Journal of Hygiene*, 74 (1975): pp. 289–99.

[19] For *Campylobacter* see CMOAR (1978), p. 46; on bovine spongiform encephalitis, see Maxime Schwarz, *How the Cows Turned Mad: Unlocking the Mysteries of Mad Cow Disease* (2003).

[20] For this outbreak see Hugh Pennington, *When Food Kills. BSE, E. coli and Disaster Science* (2003), pp. 45–55. An illuminating paper on the Stanley Royd outbreak was delivered by Jennifer Wallis at the European Association for the History of Health and Medicine conference, Lisbon, September 2013.

[21] Lafontaine, 'Introduction', p. 8. Author's translation of the quotation. Lafontaine was director of the Institute for Hygiene and Epidemiology, Brussels, Belgium.

two American microbiologists who first isolated a member of the family from pigs in 1885,[22] the taxonomic variety of *Salmonella* has intrigued microbiologists while simultaneously exasperating public health personnel: one expert study group described it in 1977 as 'a large family . . . with a beautiful name but most unpleasant habits'.[23] It is these unpleasant habits that have made *Salmonella* such an intractable problem in public health. In the case of *Salmonella* food poisoning, laboratory science and public health activity did not always travel companionably together. During the interwar period, when the British public health community was beginning to realize the dimensions of the food poisoning problem, many microbiologists were absorbed in taxonomy, which did not appear to be serving the wider cause of public health.

The inter-war activities of medical and veterinary microbiologists in Britain and America would eventually pay off in the discovery of the vastness of the *Salmonella* family, its diffusion through the animal kingdom, and its affinity for inter-continental travel, which became clear during World War II and has since been repeatedly confirmed. There are currently some 2,600 known zoonotic serotypes of *Salmonella*, almost all of which are thought may cause illness in humans.[24] *Salmonella typhi*, which seems to be exclusive to humans, is the most virulent, but others may cause serious illness in certain birds and animals, and *Salmonella* are variously carried by many species of animals, birds, and reptiles, from mice, geckoes, and tortoises through mink and foxes to domestic poultry, pigs, and cattle. Their ability to survive for long periods of time, sometimes indefinitely, in soil, water, and alimentary tracts, makes them very difficult to manage, let alone control, and healthy carriers both animal and human may shed large numbers of bacteria in their excreta. In certain circumstances cows' milk, birds' eggs, and the meat of cattle, pigs, and poultry may also carry infection. Infection in all living creatures is generally caused by the ingestion of food or drink contaminated by human or animal excreta carrying the bacteria, and such discharges may also in favourable circumstances cause widespread infection of natural environments.[25] Such are the deplorable habits of *Salmonella* uncovered by science, and one strand of this book is concerned with the gradual realization of the relationship between human and animal infection and its environmental consequences.

Balancing between microbiology and public health, this book sets out to explore the ways in which epidemiological investigation—which in the nineteenth century meant field observation—influenced public health action, how the expanding science of microbiology contributed to the understanding and control of the causal

[22] For the complex story of this attribution, see Claude E. Dolman and Richard J. Wolfe, *Suppressing the Diseases of Animals and Man. Theobald Smith, Microbiologist* (2003), chapter 5.

[23] British Association for the Advancement of Science, *Salmonella: The Food Poisoner* (1977), p. 1.

[24] European Food Safety Authority, *European Union Summary Report on Trends in Zoonoses*: <http://www.efsa.europa.eu/en/efsa/efsajournal/doc/3547.pdf>, p. 20, accessed 24 June 2014; T. A. Cogan and T. J. Humphrey, 'The rise and fall of *Salmonella* Enteritidis in the UK', *Journal of Applied Microbiology*, 94 (2003): p. 114S.

[25] The degree of illness suffered is largely determined by the number of bacteria ingested—the greater the intake, the worse the symptoms; slight infections may not generate recognizable clinical disease.

organisms of disease, and how the focus of preventive attention came to shift from the wider environment to sites identified as critical to the entry of *Salmonella* into the human food chain. A central feature of *Salmonella* history and a core theme of this book is environmental pollution by faecal matter, human or animal, whether 'environment' is defined as land or water, outdoors or indoors, spaces industrial, domestic, or minute (machines, worktops), or other people. In the early days of urban history, Richard Schoenwald wrote a persuasive essay on the training of urban man.[26] Schoenwald noted that water closets and sewers, although they bring order, 'do not ensure the disappearance of crime, or laziness, or untidiness'.[27] All three of these underpin the continuing problem of food infections. Training humans is more than a matter of teaching them to build sewers, use lavatories, and drink clean water. Training is also required in scrupulous personal hygiene and a sense of responsibility towards the well-being of others. Unpleasant habits are not just a characteristic of the *Salmonella* family but also of the human family.

The tensions in the relationship between science and sanitation can also be seen in negotiations around public health strategies. One striking feature of *Salmonella* history is the range of still significant public health issues which it illustrates and which are explored in this book. These include the political and administrative difficulties of public health administration; the management of individuals who represent a public health risk; the regulation of noxious trades and food trades; the construction of perceptions of risk (food scares and personal habits); the impact of expert disagreement and of vested economic and political interests on public health action; the operation of scientific elites; the reluctance of government to legislate in the face of powerful industries; the impact of complex food chains; the failure under normal circumstances of education as a preventive strategy; and the variable effectiveness of major food scares in changing consumer behaviours and producer responses. The relationship between epidemiology and public health practice, and between public health practice and laboratory findings are themes that run through the book. Yet the knowledge generated by research in the field and laboratory was not always successfully translated into policy and practice. Knowledge and policy intentions can be defeated by crime, laziness, and untidiness and by socio-economic interests, as several case studies in this book show. In all, the *Salmonella* story demonstrates how human behaviours operate to create public health problems and to complicate their resolution.

SALMONELLA AND HISTORY

In spanning the years between 1880 and the mid-1970s, this history of *Salmonella* ventures into ground as yet sparsely explored by historians of medicine, public

[26] Richard L. Schoenwald, 'Training urban man. A hypothesis about the sanitary movement', in *The Victorian City: Images and Realities*, vol 2 (1973), edited by H. J. Dyos and Michael Wolff, pp. 669–92.

[27] Schoenwald, 'Training urban man', p. 683.

health, and science. Although the histories of bacteriology and of germ theory have been well served in recent years, these accounts generally end at 1914.[28] Histories of specific diseases are a recognized genre of historical writing, and in recent years have come to be written as much as a means of exploring social, economic, political, intellectual, and other contexts of their occurrence as for the charting of epidemic outbreaks, demographic impact, or the accumulation of scientific knowledge.[29] This book is, however, less a history of food poisoning as a disease than of *Salmonella* as an important family of food infections. The agents that cause disease are less commonly the subject of historical inquiry, although, as new medical problems, both prions and the HIV virus have attracted attention.[30] Adding an older problem to this literature contributes a further dimension to our understanding of the complex world which surrounds disease phenomena.

Situating this study within existing historical work on public health administration, epidemiology, bacteriology, laboratories, veterinary medicine, knowledge networks, hygiene, and environment is not easy, at least in part because relatively little exists for the years after 1914. Since this book examines salmonellosis as a health problem in the British context, it seems as well to consider the public health administration which formed the front line of observation and such control as was possible. The story of Victorian public health reform has been told from several different perspectives but that of twentieth-century British public health practice has received relatively little attention.[31] John Eyler's study of Arthur Newsholme's work as MOH at Brighton, and later as Chief Medical Officer, bridges the worlds of Victorian and Edwardian public health, and shows that the Victorian impetus in public health held up until World War I.[32] Charles Webster and Jane Lewis have argued for a falling off in mission and method among local government health officers after 1918.[33] More recent research, including my own, suggests that MOHs continued generally to serve their local communities with diligence and effectiveness, in a world where the nature of their responsibilities, perceptions of what constituted public health, and disease patterns had entered a process of

[28] Rosemary Wall, *Bacteria in Britain, 1880–1939* (2013) has begun to extend this reach.

[29] See for example Ilana Löwy, *Virus, Moustiques et Modernité: La Fièvre Jaune au Brésil, entre Science et Politique* (2001); Peter Baldwin, *Disease and Democracy: The Industrialised World Faces AIDS* (2005); Emily K. Abel, *Tuberculosis and the Politics of Exclusion: A History of Public Health and Migration in Los Angles* (2007); Christopher Hamlin, *Cholera: The Biography of a Disease* (2009); James M. Stark, *The Making of Modern Anthrax, 1875–1920: Uniting Local, National and Global Histories of Disease* (2013).

[30] See Eve Seguin, ed, *Infectious Processes: Knowledge, Discourse and the Politics of Prions* (2004); Jacques Pepin, *The Origins of AIDS* (2012).

[31] On Victorian sanitary reform see Royston Lambert, *Sir John Simon, 1816–1904, and English Social Administration* (1965); Anthony S. Wohl, *Endangered Lives: Public Health in Victorian Britain* (1984); Christopher Hamlin, *Public Health and Social Justice in the Age of Chadwick: Britain 1800–1854* (1998). On medical administration see Jeanne Brand, *Doctors and the State: The British Medical Profession and Government Action in Public Health* (1965).

[32] John M. Eyler, *Sir Arthur Newsholme and State Medicine, 1885–1935* (1997).

[33] Charles Webster, 'Medical officers of health—for the record', *Radical Community Medicine*, 8 (1996): pp. 10–14; Jane Lewis, *What Price Community Medicine? The Philosophy, Practice and Politics of Public Health since 1919* (1986), pp. 30–49.

continuous change.[34] While the current volume is not a formal study of public health practice, or of government action in public health, both MOHs and the central departments were concerned by problems of food poisoning by the inter-war period, as they became aware of a vast underlying problem of minor illness. Local MOH responses to food poisoning episodes were generally subdued because of the difficulties around identification and management, but the evidence does suggest ongoing concerns to improve public hygiene and food-handling practices, especially in the years after 1920. Responses to typhoid outbreaks were rather more substantial, often involving investigators from the central Medical Department or Ministry of Health, but by 1920 this was largely fire-fighting, increasingly turning on the identification and management of local carriers.

Despite a long interest in the history of epidemics, the history of epidemiology remains largely unexplored, even by epidemiologists, still less by historians. The recent work of Jacob Steere-Williams on typhoid and epidemiology in later nineteenth-century England sets something of the scene for this project in its examination of the methods used by Victorian outbreak investigators.[35] Studies of early twentieth-century epidemiology, by Andrew Mendelsohn and the late Olga Amsterdamska, focus on academic and theoretical epidemiology rather than outbreak investigation.[36] While this academic epidemiology was important for the intellectual development of the discipline, for practitioners of public health in the period to 1940, the word 'epidemiology' carried the double-meaning of disease behaviour in the field and of outbreak investigation. The term 'field', describing a physical area of epidemiological enterprise as distinct from the laboratory and from 'the haze of luminous modern speculative epidemiology',[37] became current from the mid-1920s in the context of the expansion of theoretical laboratory-based epidemiology as practised by W. W. C. Topley and his team at the London School of Hygiene and Tropical Medicine and by Rockefeller-funded researchers in the USA.[38] It is in this latter sense of outbreak investigation and observed knowledge of disease behaviour that epidemiology is considered in this book.

[34] See John Welshman, *Municipal Medicine: Public Health in Twentieth Century Britain* (2000), p. 39; John Welshman, 'The Medical Officer of Health in England, 1900–1974: Watchdog or lapdog?', *Journal of Public Health*, 19 (1997): pp. 443–50.

[35] Jacob Steere-Williams, 'The perfect food and the filth disease: Milk-borne typhoid and epidemiological practice in late Victorian Britain', *Journal of the History of Medicine and Allied Sciences*, 65 (2010): pp. 514–45. See also William Coleman, *Yellow Fever in the North: The Methods of Early Epidemiology* (1987).

[36] Andrew Mendelsohn, 'From eradication to equilibrium: How epidemics became complex after World War I', in *Greater Than the Parts: Holism in Biomedicine 1920–1950* (1998), edited by Christopher Lawrence and George Weisz, pp. 303–31; Olga Amsterdamska, 'Demarcating Epidemiology', *Science, Technology and Human* Values, 30 (2005): pp. 17–51; Olga Amsterdamska, 'Standardising epidemic: Infection, inheritance and environment in pre-war experimental epidemiology', in *Heredity and Infection: The History of Disease Transmission* (2001), edited by Jean-Paul Gaudillière and Ilana Löwy, pp. 135–79.

[37] Editorial, 'Typhus fever in Ireland', *MO*, 38 (1927): p. 277. The term 'field investigation' had been used of outbreak investigation by George Buchanan already in 1890: Medical Officer's Annual Report Local Government Board, British Parliamentary Papers, 1890–91, xxxiv, p. x.

[38] For this research see Amsterdamska, 'Standardising epidemic infection'.

The nineteenth-century history of bacteriology and germ theory has been well served in recent years by Christoph Gradmann, in examining Robert Koch's key role in establishing the norms of bacteriological laboratory practice, and by Christopher Hamlin and Michael Worboys, whose demonstration of the uncertainties of bacteriology and the nuances of bacteriological understandings of germs provides essential background for the starting point of this study.[39] Worboys's questioning of the event of a 'bacteriological revolution' in the 1880s is pertinent here, since this *Salmonella* history suggests that shifts in ideas and practices only began to occur in the mid- to late 1890s.[40] Beyond a few classic textbooks such as Foster's *History of Medical Bacteriology* and institutional histories such as that of Britain's Public Health Laboratory Service, however, the twentieth-century history of bacteriology has been largely unexplored.[41] Worboys has recently called for historians to realize the potential of exploring the practice of science in medicine,[42] and this project has had much that object in its attempt to trace the relationship between field epidemiology, disease prevention, and the laboratory. More recently Rosemary Wall has initiated exploration of the underbelly of bacteriology—of the ways in which it was understood and adapted by the general public in situations of perceived epidemic emergency.[43] For the twentieth century, Olga Amsterdamska's essay on early research on variation in bacteriology illuminates the discussions of and differences in approach to the *Salmonella* group of bacteria in the 1900s and 1910s (Chapter 5).[44] Keith Vernon has examined the institutionalization of microbe studies in Britain between 1870 and 1940, concluding that it was in the inter-war period that medical microbiology became established as an independent discipline.[45] Vernon's study of the crystallization of medical microbiology as a discipline provides a useful background to the formation of the specialist *Salmonella* community here described (Chapter 6), in which the taxonomic preoccupation of the research microbiologists became dominant in the 1920s at the expense of public health practice but a decade later was brought back into the fold of public health by scientific discovery and institutional change.

[39] Christoph Gradmann, *Laboratory Disease: Robert Koch's Medical Bacteriology* (2009), translated by Elborg Forster; Christopher Hamlin, *A Science of Impurity: Water Analysis in Nineteenth-century England* (1990); Michael Worboys, *Spreading Germs: Disease Theories and Medical Practice in Britain, 1865–1900* (2000).

[40] Michael Worboys, 'Was there a bacteriological revolution in late-nineteenth-century medicine?', *Studies in the History and Philosophy of Biology and Biomedical Sciences*, 38 (2007): pp. 20–42.

[41] William D. Foster, *A History of Medical Bacteriology and Immunology* (1970); Robert E. O. Williams, *Microbiology for the Public Health. The Evolution of the Public Health Laboratory Service, 1939–1980* (1985). Wall, *Bacteria*, explores popular understandings and uses of bacteriology before World War II.

[42] Michael Worboys, 'Practice and the science of medicine in the nineteenth century', *Isis* 102 (2011): p. 119.

[43] Wall, *Bacteria*, chapters 3, 5, 6.

[44] Olga Amsterdamska, 'Medical and biological constraints: Early research on variation in bacteriology', *Social Studies of Science*, 17 (1987): pp. 657–87.

[45] Keith Vernon, 'Pus, sewage, beer and milk: Microbiology in Britain, 1870–1840', *History of Science*, 28 (1990): pp. 289–325.

The discovery of the family of *Salmonella* bacteria and the emergence of a community of *Salmonella* specialists was, of course, dependent on the developments in laboratory research practice which underpinned the rise of bacteriology. Despite the interest in germ theory and scientific practice, the history of the laboratory itself has been strangely neglected. Although we know the outline of the emergence of a patchwork of university, hospital, municipal, commercial, and independent research laboratories in Britain before the establishment of the Emergency Public Health Laboratory Service in 1939, the details have been given no systematic historical attention.[46] Insider accounts of the work of the Lister Institute and of the PHLS provide an entry point to this world,[47] but for the most part the world and work of the pre-1945 laboratory in its many incarnations remains to be explored.[48] Although I have begun the attempt to uncover something of the work performed in the service of public health in some of these laboratories (Chapter 5), I have little more than scratched the surface of a much larger enterprise.

It is, however, clear from the material presented in Chapters 5 and 6 that research laboratories provided focal points for the construction of scientific networks.[49] Elucidation of the ways and means of construction of international networks is an emerging field, with international conferences rightly identified as a prime locus for network activity.[50] Later nineteenth-century international congresses, it has been argued, helped to create a 'congress elite' of individuals whose construction of extensive professional and personal relationships at such meetings enabled them to influence social reform in their own countries.[51] While this 'congress elite' is not so apparent in *Salmonella* science, at least in the inter-war period and in respect of influencing social policy, the *Salmonella* story shows that research publications,

[46] One attempt at such a reconstruction was abandoned: see E. P. Hennock, 'The urban sanitary movement in England and Germany, 1838–1914: A comparison', *Continuity and Change*, 15 (2000): p. 269. For broader discussions of the laboratory in late nineteenth-century medicine see Keir Waddington, 'More like cooking than science', *Journal of Literature and Science*, 3 (2010): pp. 50–70; Graeme Gooday, 'Placing the laboratory in the history of science', *Isis*, 99 (2008): pp. 783–95; Bruno Latour, 'The costly ghastly kitchen', in *The Laboratory Revolution in Medicine*, edited by Cunningham and Williams, pp. 295–302; Bruno Latour and Steve Woolgar, *Laboratory Life: The Construction of the Scientific* (1986).

[47] Harriette Chick et al., *War on Disease. A History of the Lister Institute* (1971); Leslie H. Collier, *The Lister Institute of Preventive Medicine. A Concise History* (2000); Williams, *Microbiology for the Public Health*. Vernon has briefly discussed the Lister: see his 'Pus, sewage, milk and beer'.

[48] But see Steve Sturdy, 'The political economy of scientific medicine: science, education and the transformation of medical practice in Sheffield, 1890–1922', *Medical History*, 36 (1992): pp. 125–59.

[49] This is also apparent in the history of the Danish State Serum Institute and its personnel: see C. Julius Salomonsen, 'Reminiscences of a summer semester, 1877, at Breslau', edited by Clarice L Temkin, *Bulletin of the History of Medicine*, 24 (1950): pp. 333–51; Anne Hardy, 'Questions of quality: The Danish State Serum Institute, Thorvald Madsen and biological standardization', in *Evaluating and Standardizing Therapeutic Agents, 1890–1950*, edited by Christoph Gradmann and Jonathan Simon (2010): pp. 139–52.

[50] See for example, Deborah J. Neill, *Networks in Tropical Medicine: Internationalism, Colonialism and the Rise of the Medical Specialty, 1890–1930* (2012): pp. 38–40.

[51] Chris Leonards and Nico Randeraad, 'Transnational experts and social reform, 1840-1900', *International Review of Social History*, 55 (2010): pp. 215–39. For the role of international networks in economic integration see Gary B. Magee and Andrew S. Thompson, *Empire and Globalisation: Networks of People, Goods and Capital in the British World, c. 1850–1914* (2010).

personal contact by letter, positive responses to the work of others, exchange of specimens, and laboratory visiting played important roles in establishing scientific friendships and networks; a collective activity that led to accumulating knowledge about the *Salmonella* family. Here we see knowledge in transit in line with the processes of movement, translation, and transmission described by James Secord.[52] Similarly, the importance of just a handful of research laboratories in this story is suggestive of the importance of place. While David Livingstone's work has shown the influence of location on knowledge creation and reception to be important, and Olga Amsterdamska has demonstrated the influence of institutional histories and disciplinary relations on thought styles in microbiology,[53] an extended analysis of the five laboratories important here is beyond the scope of this work. The importance of non-human salmonellosis may lie behind the interest in Kentucky and Copenhagen, given the important livestock interests in both places; the British Ministry of Health's determination to ensure safety of food supplies may have been important to London, as may the experience of non-typhoid diarrheal disease in World War I. Equally, the fascination which these bacteria exercised over individual research scientists located in particular laboratories was important. As James Stark has shown, locality matters not just for historical enquiry, but also for the historical actors themselves.[54] And as Chapter 6 also shows, changes in laboratory personnel and allegiance to particular ways of understanding science—even to particular laboratory methods—could make or break scientific networks.

Public health, epidemiology, and bacteriology define the fields of medical knowledge and practice within the purview of this project. The related knowledge systems of veterinary medicine and bacteriology, and human and animal hygiene are associated rather with a strand of environmental history in which human activity or human practices generate pathological sites and pathological landscapes, with impacts both on humans and on other animals. This is a rare strand in environmental history as currently practised,[55] while Virginia Berridge and Martin Gorsky have drawn attention to the divergence of health and the environment as subjects of interest between *circa* 1880 and the 1960s.[56] The current study shows that the environmental impact of human activity on both human and animal health may repay further study. Veterinary medicine and bacteriology and veterinary public health, more particularly for the twentieth century, have been largely

[52] James A. Secord, 'Knowledge in transit', *Isis*, 95 (2004): pp. 654–72.

[53] David N. Livingstone, *Putting Science in its Place: Geographies of Scientific Knowledge* (2003); *Geographies of Nineteenth-Century Science* (2011), edited by David N. Livingstone and Charles W. J. Withers; Olga Amsterdamska, 'Achieving disbelief: thought styles, microbial variation, and American and British epidemiology, 1900–1949', *Studies in the History and Philosophy of the Biological and Biomedical Sciences*, 35 (2004): pp. 483–507.

[54] Stark, *Modern Anthrax*, p. 8.

[55] But see innovative studies by Mary J. Dobson, *Contours of Death and Disease in Early Modern England* (1997), and Linda L. Nash, *Inescapable Ecologies: A History of Environment, Disease and Knowledge* (2006).

[56] Virginia Berridge and Martin Gorsky, 'Introduction', in *Environment, Health and History* (2010), edited by Virginia Berridge and Martin Gorsky, pp. 4–19.

neglected as areas of historical study.[57] Yet these are topics of considerable historical importance, given the role which food and companion animals played in the social, economic, and disease history of that century. The environmental and health impacts of the modernization of the farming and food supply industries in the course of the century remain unexplored. The chequered histories of bovine tuberculosis, brucellosis, and BSE in twentieth-century Britain and elsewhere merit closer scrutiny than they have so far been given. Farming practices from manuring to methods of feed production as well as the processing of raw animal protein can all result in contaminated environments affecting live animals and their products in ways potentially harmful to both humans and animals. Business historians have begun to explore this world of industrial agricultural development,[58] but there is room also for other historical approaches to the production history of modern food supplies. Kate Soper's concern with the tensions between ecological discourses of destruction, waste, and pollution, and the appeal to nature based on relations with the animal world constructed through ideas of human difference and identity, seem applicable here.[59]

If histories of industrial food and farm hygiene are scarce, histories of human hygiene tend, perhaps not surprisingly, to present a history of progress.[60] Nancy Tomes has shown how popular understandings of germs and their role in generating disease became engrained in American culture, but the evidence suggests that this understanding was not complete in certain respects, was not equally disseminated in the developed world, and was achieved, if consciously pursued at all, with less success in some other countries, including Britain.[61] Given the imperfect human acceptance of hygiene, even in advanced cultures, the processes of human food production and consumption remain fraught with potential for the transmission of *Salmonella* and other food-poisoning organisms.[62] Contamination through

[57] But see Abigail Woods, 'A historical synopsis of animal diseases and public policy in twentieth century Britain', *Philosophical Transactions of the Royal Society*, series B, 366 (2011), doi: 10.1098/rstb.2010.0388; Anne Hardy, 'Professional advantage and public health: British veterinarians and state veterinary services, 1865–1939', *Twentieth Century British History*, 14 (2003): pp. 1–23; Anne Hardy, 'John Bull's beef: Meat hygiene and veterinary public health in England in the twentieth century', *Review of Agricultural and Environmental Studies*, 91 (2010): pp. 369–92.

[58] Andrew C. Godley and Bridget Williams, 'The chicken, the factory farm and the supermarket: The emergence of the modern poultry industry in Britain', in *Food Chains: From Farmyard to Shopping Cart* (2009), pp. 47–61, edited by Warren Belasco and Richard Horowitz, pp. 47–61; Andrew C. Godley and Bridget Williams, 'Demarcating luxury and the contentious "invention of the technological chicken" in Britain', *Business History Review*, 83 (2009): pp. 267–90.

[59] Kate Soper, *What is Nature? Culture, Politics and the Non-human* (1995).

[60] Alain Corbin, *The Foul and the Fragrant: Odor and the Social Imagination* (1986); Suellen Hoy, *Chasing Dirt: The American Pursuit of Cleanliness* (1995); Virginia Smith, *Clean: A History of Personal Hygiene and Purity* (2007), especially pp. 307–8; Victoria Kelley, *Soap and Water: Cleanliness, Dirt and the Working Classes in Victorian and Edwardian Britain* (2010).

[61] Nancy Tomes, *The Gospel of Germs: Men, Women and the Microbe in American Life* (1998). For the popularization of germ theory in Britain, and progress in cleanliness see Kelley, *Soap and Water*, pp. 22–3, 189–95. But contrasts between America and Britain are flagged in, for example, Thomas Stuttaford, 'Americans come clean on how to avoid tummy trouble', *The Times*, 28 January 1999, p. 11.

[62] See for example, Nichols Fox, *Spoiled: The Dangerous Truth about a Food Chain Gone Haywire* (1997); <http://www.food.gov.uk/news_updates/news/2013/aug/campylobacter>, accessed 1 September 2013. The first week of October 2012 saw reporting of a *Salmonella* outbreak due to smoked salmon in

ignorance or carelessness is not the only issue. Throughout the period covered by this book, socio-economic interests concerned with food production and the food industries repeatedly deflected attempts by public health professionals to reform unsatisfactory practices.

Yet despite the role which human activity has played in disseminating many different *Salmonella* serotypes across the world, their wide natural distribution in the animal kingdom, for example in reptiles, and the existence of species-specific serotypes, suggests that the history of their evolution is an ancient one, and that it is not exclusively associated with humans and their activities. Although a number of studies of animal disease have appeared in recent years,[63] the general lack of historical interest in veterinary bacteriology and veterinary public health, indeed in veterinary history more broadly, is regrettable when we come to consider the importance of animal infections to human disease, and their environmental connections. In the story of *Salmonella* this underdevelopment is especially regrettable, for animals broadly defined play a critical part, whether as intrinsic agents of infection or as passive transmitters carrying infection only because their natural habitats have been polluted by the excreta of others.

These various historiographic strands are threaded through much of this text. To some extent, the book represents a series of explorations rather than a conventional linear history. These explorations fall into three parts. Part I, 'Pathways in Nature', examines the discovery of the natural pathways by which *Salmonella* have travelled from their source of origin through the environment into the human food chain, and the attempts made to disrupt these paths of transmission before World War II. Attention is focused on six major areas of public health concern. Chapter 1, 'Human Animals', looks at preventive approaches to typhoid before and after recognition of the healthy human carrier in the first decade of the twentieth century. Chapter 2, 'The Hygiene of the Sea', explores the food scare that erupted around oysters sourced from sewage contaminated waters in the years around 1900. Chapter 3, 'Things with Wings,' contrasts the preventive focus on the transmission of gastro-enteritis by flies, despite shaky bacteriological evidence, with lack of interest in transmission via duck eggs in the face of clear bacteriological confirmation for this source of infection. Chapter 4, 'Other Animals', traces the realization

the Netherlands and the United States; of *E. coli* cases linked to factory processed beef in Canada; and gastro-enteritis due to contaminated strawberries (imported from China) affecting more than 11,000 children in Germany. On 18 July 2013, the *New York Times* reported that bacterial counts of *Campylobacter* and *Salmonella* were found to be higher in farmers' market chickens than in birds sourced from grocery stores: Nicholas Bakalar, 'Farmers' market chickens higher in bacteria', <well.blogs.nytimes.com/2013/07/18/farmers-market-chickens-higher-in-bacteria/?_php=true&_type=blogs&_r=0>, accessed 20 July 2013.

63 See for example, Abigail Woods, *A Manufactured Plague? The History of Foot and Mouth Disease in Britain* (2004); Keir Waddington, *The Bovine Scourge: Meat, Tuberculosis and Public Health, 1850–1914* (2006); Neil Pemberton and Michael Worboys, *Mad Dogs and Englishmen: Rabies in Britain, 1830–2000* (2007); Susan D. Jones, *Death in a Small Package: A Short History of Anthrax* (2010); Peter J. Atkins, *Animal Cities: Beastly Urban Histories* (2012). On the history of veterinary public health see Hardy, 'Professional advantage and public health', pp. 1–23; Hardy, 'John Bull's beef', pp. 369–92.

that the flesh and milk of infected domestic animals can cause salmonellosis in humans. The core themes of this section lie in the relationship between epidemiology, public health action, and the laboratory, and in the contamination of different environments by human and animal faeces.

Part II, 'Laboratory Pursuits', shifts focus to the world of the laboratory. The laboratory was not in my original plan, but it became evident that the creation of an international *Salmonella* community and the research it undertook in the inter-war years was crucially important to the preventive reaction to the upswing in *Salmonella* infections that began during World War II. Chapter 5, 'Pursuing Parasites', describes the laboratory landscape of the interwar period, and the emergence in the 1920s of two separate strands of concern with *Salmonella*, one preventive, one taxonomic. Chapter 6, 'Network and Knowledge', examines the emergence of a dominant faction within the international *Salmonella* community and the processes of network-building, knowledge transmission, and scientific power-play. Chapter 7, 'Names and Places', charts the realization by this community of the connection between farming practices, manufacturing processes, the international trade in food products, and the global spread of *Salmonella* infections during and after World War II. A core theme of this section is how the re-convergence of the two *Salmonella* interest groups transformed preventive understandings of how typhoid and the food poisoning *Salmonella* are disseminated in the years after 1940.

Part III, 'Sites of Infection', returns to the theme of environmental contamination, and preventive attempts at damage limitation. It considers how epidemiological and laboratory findings helped to shape the efforts made to contain *Salmonella* after 1945, the difficulties encountered in these attempts, and how these problems helped to focus attention on specific sites where critical forms of transmission were considered to occur. Chapter 8, 'Field and Farm', examines the veterinary realization of the importance of modernizing farming practices in generating infection in animals and how such infections created risks for both animals and humans. Chapter 9, 'Ghastly Kitchens—the Borgia Tradition', traces the processes by which certain places—such as commercial and domestic kitchens—were identified as critical sites for the transmission of *Salmonella* onwards through the human and animal food chains, and discusses the failure of attempts at public education in hygiene. The core theme of this section is the expansion of bacterial opportunity created by the modernization of farming and food production systems, and the ongoing struggle to educate producers and consumers in elementary personal and kitchen hygiene.[64]

Finally, three different caveats must be entered here. First, readers will become aware that I omit detailed consideration of developments during the two World Wars from my account. This has been done partly in the interests of word length, but also because both wars brought significant disruption to normal scientific and public health activity. John Eyler, for example, has noted of the Great War that it made 'continuance of even routine duties extremely difficult' in the public

[64] For ongoing problems in this area see Pennington, *When Food Kills.*

health service.[65] Official reports shrank to a fraction of their former size; the number of the Local Government Board's *Reports on Public Health*, published annually, fell away from 13 in 1914 to an average of under three a year between 1915 and 1919. By November 1915 the public health community, initially positive in its support for the war, was on the defensive, calling for the Local Government Board to make clear to the military authorities that 'the public health service is essential for the defence of the realm, and that . . . it must not be drawn on too far for military purposes'.[66] On the other hand, the war fostered some important work in *Salmonella* science. Individuals who did not serve in the military, such as Frederick Andrewes and Harry Schütze, spent the war working on dysentery, *Salmonella*, and bacterial variation, relating to problems with gastro-enteritis in the war zones. Wartime experience set others, such as Philip Bruce White and Arthur Felix, on the way to careers in microbiology.[67] As is well known, World War II was foreseen and prepared for in Britain: it led to the creation of the Emergency Public Health Laboratory Service (EPHLS), where consolidation of microbiological expertise proved the nursery for post-war challenge to the pre-war *Salmonella* orthodoxy. The 'catastrophic' effect of the German occupation of Denmark on work at the State Serum Institute after 31 May 1940[68] may also have contributed to later shifts in the locus of power in *Salmonella* microbiology. While British food-poisoning outbreaks continued to be locally reported during both wars, the need to conserve scarce food supplies ensured that developments which might undermine public trust in any valued nationwide food source were suppressed. The EPHLS and the Ministry of Health were aware of problems with *Salmonella* in imported American dried egg by February 1944, but the details were not made public, since conditions were 'not favourable'.[69] The war-time chapters in the history of microbiology and public health deserve fuller treatment than they could possibly be given here.

Second, the scientific understanding and language of description of *Salmonella* has changed since the 1970s, with increasingly sophisticated laboratory methods and understandings.[70] From considerations of fidelity to the accounts of my protagonists, I have retained the scientific names and usages employed by my sources. Varieties of *Salmonella* are referred to as serotypes, and are designated by the names generally used in the pre-1980 literature.[71] The practice of microbiologists

[65] Eyler, *Newsholme*, p. 265.

[66] Editorial, 'Depletion of the public health service', *MO*, 14 (1915): p. 201.

[67] Bruce White worked under Schütze and J. A. Arkwright at the Lister for some months; Felix served with a mobile bacteriological unit.

[68] E. Schelde Møller, *Thorvald Madsen* (1970), p. 172.

[69] T. V. Cooper, 'Case of fever due to *Bact. Oranienburg*', *Monthly Bulletin of the Ministry of Health*, 3 (1944): pp. 40–1.

[70] See E. J. Threlfall, 'Salmonella', in *Topley and Wilson's Microbiology and Microbial Infections*, 10th edn (2005), vol 2, edited by S. P. Borriello et al., pp. 1398–9. In the general literature, four terms exist for the illnesses brought about in humans by organisms of the *Salmonella* family: typhoid (*Salmonella typhi* infection), enteric fever (typhoid, paratyphoid, severe food poisoning), food poisoning, and salmonellosis (illness caused by *Salmonella* in humans and animals).

[71] For the most recent usages, see Threlfall, 'Salmonella'.

past and present in italicization of the 'original' *Salmonella* serotypes (eg *typhi, typhimurium*) varies; I have used the italic form in line with present usage.[72]

Finally, I have tried in writing this book to emphasize the respective roles of field epidemiology and the laboratory in the process of constructing knowledge of the *Salmonella*, their natural habitats, and means and pathways of transmission. I have also taken the opportunity to explore such social, economic, and political contexts as seemed appropriate to the various chapters, and to select stories that illustrate the power of socio-economic interests. My approach to this work derives from my background in social, economic, and urban history. I am not a historian of science and only by adoption a historian of medicine. There has been a recent call in this latter subdiscipline to emphasize the value of historiography and theory at the expense of history.[73] This book is in part an attempt to re-assert the importance of historical methodologies which engage in primary research and the telling of stories, the importance of what Keir Waddington has called a 'richer, complex world'.[74] When I began this project, I had very little idea of the riches which my sources would reveal, and the wonderful stories and complex histories which they would contain. The working epidemiologists of the late nineteenth century and of the first half of the twentieth were trained in a tradition which prized the art of story-telling. Reviewing Harold Scott's *Some Notable Epidemics* in 1935, the journal *Medical Officer* noted that students of epidemiology should learn the lesson that 'the history of an outbreak should read like a detective story, but it must also be written like one, with the exception that the data must be sought in the field and not sought in the imagination'.[75] It was a precept that several generations of outbreak investigators from the 1870s to the 1950s followed with relish, and which historians might with advantage consider.

[72] Contrary to current practice, D. C. Old and E. J. Threlfall, 'Salmonella', in *Topley and Wilson's Microbiology and Microbial Infections*, 9th edn (1998), edited by Leslie H. Collier et al., p. 970, advise that 'serotype names should be given in Roman (*not* italic) type'. I am indebted to Ros Stanwell-Smith for clarification here.

[73] Roger Cooter, 'After death/after-"life": The social history of medicine in post-postmodernity', *Social History of Medicine* 20 (2007): pp. 441–64.

[74] Keir Waddington, *A History of Medicine in Europe since 1500* (2011), p. 15. There are other exponents of medical history as story-telling, a notable example being Jacalyn Duffin, *Medical Miracles: Doctors, Saints and Healing in the Modern World* (2009).

[75] Notes and Comments, 'Field epidemiology', *MO*, 53 (1935): p. 2. The relationship between science and detective fiction is explored in Lawrence Frank, *Victorian Detective Fiction and the Nature of Evidence* (2003).

PART I

PATHWAYS IN NATURE

1

Human Animals

Late in November 1890, in grey, wet weather, Frederick William Barry set out from the market town of Darlington to follow the course of the river Tees toward its source. On his journey, during which he crossed and re-crossed the river, he explored numerous hamlets, villages, and farmsteads before reaching the pretty market town of Barnard Castle, an inland watering place much favoured by the inhabitants of the East Coast towns. Barnard Castle lies on the Durham side of the river, facing the villages of High and Low Stainsforth on the Yorkshire side. The area was already popular with holiday-makers during the summer months, but Barry's eyes were not for the grandeur of the scenery. He was on a mission to discover one particular feature of this natural environment—the extent to which it was polluted by human sewage. As he tracked the drainage condition of houses, farms, and settlements, and the fall of drains, sewers, and open ditches into the river, his concern mounted. On reaching Barnard Castle, he was appalled: public and private drains discharged directly onto the river banks, and privies, urinals, and water closets emptied their contents onto the foreshore. House and retaining walls fronting the river contained many openings which discharged liquid filth, and layers of solid sewage lay deep on the foreshore. Never in his whole experience, wrote Barry, had he seen 'such a mass of stinking abominations' as lay alongside the Tees at Barnard Castle at the time of his visit. Nor were things much better on the Yorkshire side: here the Swan Inn's privy shoot, urinal, water closet, and stables all voided themselves onto the foreshore, while a projecting privy, common to four houses and supported on 'corbels of some architectural pretensions', dropped its contents in full public view.[1]

Barry was in search of the causes of an outbreak of typhoid which had occurred over a wide area north and south of the Tees in the six weeks from 7 September to 18 October. As a Medical Inspector for the Medical Department of the Local Government Board, his job was to investigate unusual disease prevalences and to discover their cause if possible. Sanitary improvements having considerably reduced typhoid incidence in urban areas by the 1890s, public health investigators were increasingly paying attention to rural conditions as sources of urban pollution and disease, and Barry was seeking to explain the circumstances which had enabled typhoid to invade ten registration districts, including the urban sanitary districts of

[1] Frederick W Barry, 'Report to the Local Government Board on the epidemic prevalence of enteric fever during 1890–91 in certain sanitary districts situate in the valley of the river Tees in South Durham and North Yorkshire', British Parliamentary Papers, 1893–94 xlii, Appendix C, p. 425.

Darlington, Stockton, and Middlesborough. Before he could finish his investigations, however, the area was hit by a second outbreak, which lasted from 28 December 1890 until 7 February 1891. Some 2,769 cases were reported to have occurred in the combined outbreaks.[2] As a result of the second outbreak, Barry's report on the causes of the epidemic was so delayed that he was able to make use of the 1891 population census data in constructing his final analysis. His conclusions were stark: pollution of the Tees, aggravated by heavy rainfall and flooding, which had washed the filthy foreshores clean, and consumption of the polluted Tees water by local residents had generated both outbreaks. During those two periods, 15 typhoid cases had occurred among Tees water drinkers for every one among those who did not drink Tees water.[3]

The evidence for Barry's indictment of the Tees water supply was circumstantial, but was nonetheless accepted by his contemporaries. The investigation was a classic of late Victorian observational epidemiology: a broad and detailed survey of the terrain in which the unwonted typhoid had occurred. The report gave a detailed statistical analysis of the outbreaks and of their incidence in the ten registration districts involved. According to usual practice, the sanitary circumstances of the districts were described: their geographical size, population size, occupational and class structure, number of houses with their rateable value and sanitary condition, the state of the roads, the nature of the local economy, and the distribution of disease. Barry detailed the local arrangements for the disposal of human excrement and refuse (privies of one kind or another were almost universal, the midden privy being the commonest), as well as sewerage and drainage provision and water supply. Drinking water provision, supplied by the Darlington Corporation Waterworks, received particular attention: it was for this purpose that Barry undertook his up-river journey toward the source of the Tees. He gave the history of the local corporation water undertakings since 1870 in full, concluding that their deficiencies were responsible for the outbreaks. In all these respects, Barry's report was a model of many undertaken by himself and his colleagues during the 1890s.[4]

More than 20 unusual prevalences of typhoid were investigated by the inspectors of the Medical Department in the last decades of the nineteenth century. Not all were reported in as much as detail as the Tees epidemic, whose size and geographical spread made it a special case, but the principle underlying each remained constant: a thorough-going inquiry into the environmental circumstances of the afflicted district. Collectively and thematically, the dominant feature of these reports was man's treatment of, and relationship to, the urban and rural landscapes which he inhabited, and the ways in which his unthinking abuse of those environments contributed to human illness and death. Typhoid was brought to Rotherham in Yorkshire and Camborne in Cornwall through the human pollution of

[2] Barry, 'Report', p. 278.

[3] Richard Thorne Thorne, 'Introduction' in Barry, 'Report', p. 267.

[4] Pollution of the Tees with crude sewage and industrial effluent was still causing health problems into the 1940s: T. L. Hughes and W. Goldie, 'River Tees shellfish', *Monthly Bulletin of the Ministry of Health*, 5 (1946): pp. 71–4.

upland gathering grounds; the back-garden pit privies of houses along the Gaywood river contaminated the water supply of King's Lynn; the use of Leeds 'town manure', highly prized by farmers, brought typhoid to the villages of Ryedale in North Yorkshire.[5] A strong sense of environmental consciousness runs through most of these reports. Images of the natural and built environments are vividly evoked: the black slick of ancient sewage which stained the Tees for a hundred yards below Gainsford; the privy on its corbels above the river at Startforth; the rain-soaked gardens of Gaywood onto which householders emptied their box privies; the river Trent, 'almost from its source polluted with sewage', in which dismayed riverside fishermen viewed human faeces floating down the tide.[6] Human activity stood at the intersection between disease and the environment.

UNDERSTANDING TYPHOID

Typhoid was the first of the food poisoning *Salmonella* to attract medical and preventive attention in the nineteenth century. Concerted scientific attempts to understand its epidemiology brought realization of the concept of the healthy carrier in 1906–7. At first applied only to typhoid and to humans, it was later found that animals too could be carriers of lesser *Salmonella*. Human and animal carriers are the instruments through which these gastro-enteric infections are perpetuated, and by which they gain access to wider environmental means of distribution. The carrier state remains an ongoing problem in modern public health, involving issues of detection, of personal liberty and responsibility, and of economy, environment, personal habits, and food safety. The extent and complexity of the *Salmonella* problem was just beginning to be understood in the years before World War I.

In the 1890s, medical understanding of its causes involved both human and environmental factors. That the disease was caused by a specific infection carried in the stools of the sick, as first suggested by William Budd in 1836, had been generally accepted since the 1870s, and its ability to travel in water and milk was recognized.[7] The existence of 'ambulatory' and unrecognized cases of the disease was also known, and known to be a cause of further infection: typhoid is very variable in symptom and severity, and clinical diagnosis can be difficult. Nonetheless, one of the central problems of nineteenth-century epidemiology was the way

[5] Theodore Thomson, 'An outbreak of enteric fever in Rotherham, Rawmarsh and Greasborough', Medical Officer's Annual Report, Local Government Board, BPP, 1894 xxxix, Appendix A no 7, pp. 45–66; Robert Bruce Low, 'An outbreak of enteric fever in the urban district of Camborne and in portions of the adjoining districts of Redruth and Helston', MOAR LGB, BPP, 1899 xxxviii, Appendix A no 10, pp. 159–78; Robert Bruce Low, 'An outbreak of typhoid fever in King's Lynn', MOAR LGB, BPP, 1894 xxxix, Appendix A no 8, 67–82; Robert Bruce Low, 'An outbreak of enteric fever in certain villages situated on the river Rye in North Yorkshire; and on the water supply of Malton Sanitary District', MOAR LGB, BPP 1894 xl Appendix A no 8, pp. 595–602.

[6] Robert Bruce Low, 'The circumstances of the river Tent in Lincolnshire and part of Nottinghamshire', MOAR LGB, BPP 1894, xl, Appendix A no 9, p. 552.

[7] Medical Officer's Annual Report to the Privy Council, BPP, 1867–68 xxxvi, p. 421.

in which infectious disease—and typhoid was no exception—could suddenly appear apparently from nowhere. This phenomenon had originally been explained by the theory of spontaneous generation: the great English fever specialist Charles Murchison, for example, was a staunch adherent of this explanation.[8] When Louis Pasteur discredited spontaneous generation in the 1860s, other explanations were sought: it came to be thought that the 'germ' of typhoid could live a saprophytic existence in sewage-contaminated water and soil, where it could survive for months or even years, and that its virulence increased with prolonged immersion in 'filth', to constitute a focus of fresh infection if disturbed.[9]

The description of the specific organism of typhoid by Karl Eberth in 1880 did not resolve the etiological problems surrounding typhoid.[10] Although the existence of the bacillus initially suggested a relatively simple model of causation, the picture rapidly clouded. In the ferment of bacteriological research that gripped Europe and America after 1880, investigators began to develop a more complex picture. The path to secure scientific knowledge was far from smooth. Bacteriology was a young science, wrestling with new and often clumsy tools, and haunted, too, by the shadows of past beliefs. Many researchers doubted the causal role of the bacillus, because it could not be found in the blood of typhoid patients; others argued the behaviour of the disease suggested that, like anthrax, it must exist in a spore state in nature.[11] In 1892, Edmond McWeeney, professor of pathology at Cork University, Ireland, noted wryly that within the preceding two years, the subject of the causation of typhoid had developed into 'as complicated a network of confusing possibilities and probabilities as is to be met with in the whole range of scientific medicine'.[12] The question of the life of the bacillus in the external world was gradually resolved by extensive laboratory experiment during the 1890s; members of the Medical Department were deeply engaged in this project.[13] The process was not without confusion and dissent. The bacillus itself was an elusive laboratory specimen (as many were), bacteriological techniques were still largely experimental,

[8] Charles Murchison, *Continued Fevers of Great Britain*, 2nd edn (1873), pp. 470–97.

[9] Robert Koch [summary], 'The crusade against typhoid fever', *British Medical Journal*, 1903, i: p. 503.

[10] Eberth described the typhoid bacillus, which he observed in the spleen and mesenteric glands of patients dead of typhoid in 1880; in 1884 Georg Gaffky isolated the bacillus and obtained it in pure culture. For the complexities of nineteenth-century germ theory, and for germ theory and typhoid in particular, see Michael Worboys, *Spreading Germs: Disease Theories and Medical Practice in Britain 1865–1900* (2000), pp. 265–71.

[11] Edward Klein, 'On the etiology of typhoid fever', MOAR LGB, BPP, 1894 xl, Appendix B no 1, p. 345.

[12] Edmond J. McWeeney, 'On some points in the aetiology of typhoid fever', *Journal of State Medicine*, 1 (1892): p. 65.

[13] See, for example, Edward Klein, 'On the behaviour of the bacillus of enteric fever and of Koch's vibrio in sewage', MOAR LGB, BPP, 1895, li, Appendix B no 2, pp. 885–8; Sidney Martin, 'Preliminary report on the growth of typhoid bacilli in soil', MOAR LGB, BPP 1897, xxxvii: Appendix B no 2, pp. 291–302; Sidney Martin, 'On the nature of antagonism of soil to the typhoid bacillus', MOAR LGB, BPP, 1901 xxvi, Appendix B no 5, pp. 487–510. See also Worboys, *Spreading Germs*, p. 267, especially the references in chapter note 138.

and the independent duplication of results—essential for establishing scientific fact—was not always easy to achieve.[14]

AGENT AND ENVIRONMENT

The history of typhoid in later nineteenth-century Britain reflected efforts of state medicine and the sanitary movement at environmental reform. John Simon, the great instigator of the English programme of state medicine, had, from his appointment as Principal Medical Officer in 1858, waged a vigorous campaign against 'filth in general and filthy water in particular'.[15] The passing of the Public Health Act 1875 marked a watershed: most local authorities found themselves sooner or later obliged to do something about the quality of water provided for drinking.[16] The years between 1870 and 1885 saw a rapid decline in the national typhoid death rates, followed by over a decade of virtual stagnation. From 1900 a steady fall resumed (Table 1.1). A similar pattern was observed in Scotland.[17] Writing in the 1930s, the epidemiologist Major Greenwood associated this later fall with the discovery of the human carrier, 'and the consequent importance of personal as distinct from communal cleanliness'.[18] Other explanations were offered: there was some consensus that the discovery of typhoid transmission in shell-fish initiated this second decline; others pointed to the increasing proportion of typhoid cases being hospitalized.[19] The chlorination of domestic water supplies after around 1918 also

Table 1.1. Annual Enteric Fever Death Rates per 100,000, England and Wales

1871–75	1876–80	1881–85	1886–90	1891–95	1896–1900
37	28	22	18	18	18
1901–05	**1906–10**	**1911–15**	**1916–20**	**1921–25**	**1926–30**
11	7	5	2	1	0.9

Source: Forbes, 'Fragment', p. 55.

[14] On the difficulty of retrieving the typhoid bacillus even from human excreta, see Edward Klein and Alexander C. Houston, 'Report on the identification of the bacillus typhosus in stools', MOAR LGB, BPP, 1904, xxvi, Appendix B no 8, pp. 622–46. Similar difficulties attended contemporary investigations of the tuberculosis bacillus: see Keir Waddington, *The Bovine Scourge: Meat, Tuberculosis and Public Health, 1850–1914* (2006), pp. 118–24.

[15] Major Greenwood, *Epidemics and Crowd Diseases* (1935), p. 157. For the details of Simon's career and work see Royston Lambert, *Sir John Simon (1816–1904) and English Social Administration* (1965); for the enterprise of state medicine, Elisabeth Fee and Dorothy Porter, 'Public health, preventive medicine and professionalisation: England and America in the nineteenth century', in Andrew Wear, ed, *Medicine in Society* (1992), pp. 249–75.

[16] For the problems this could cause see Nigel Richardson, *Typhoid at Uppingham: Analysis of a Victorian Town and School in Crisis 1875–1877* (2008).

[17] Archibald K. Chalmers, *The Health of Glasgow 1818–1925* (1930), pp. 301–10.

[18] Greenwood, *Epidemics*, p. 158.

[19] Duncan Forbes, 'A fragment of epidemiological history: shell-fish and typhoid fever', *MO*, 55 (1933): p. 55.

played a part, but the pattern of local introduction was uneven, with some consumers and scientists being strongly opposed to its introduction.[20] In terms of chronology, the shell-fish contingent may have had a point: the association with shell-fish was highly publicized in the years 1895–1903, whereas knowledge of the existence of healthy human carriers only began to percolate through the British medical community from mid-1907, and even then continued to have at least one powerful English detractor.[21]

Whatever the reasons for the fall in typhoid deaths from 1900, the introduction of the concept of the healthy carrier wrought a change of perspective on the nature of the typhoid problem, and on the means of controlling it. Although healthy carriers are the crucial originators and transmitters of typhoid infection, and still constitute an important problem of management in public health, their discovery did not immediately transform public health practice. The carrier concept was most influential in America, where the supervision and monitoring of individual carriers became an integral part of public health practice in many states.[22] In Germany, practical control measures based on carrier management proved highly problematic.[23] In Britain—at least in part because of the national political tradition of individual liberty, but also because of a holistic medical tradition which valued a 'generalist' approach to medicine—the concept of the healthy carrier never came to carry such weight.[24] British public health specialists—the medical inspectors, medical officers of health, and the few academic epidemiologists who existed before 1940—for the most part retained a generally environmentalist approach to typhoid prevention, even while seeking to defuse the dangers represented by known typhoid carriers. This is not to say that the epidemiological focus did not narrow: it did. Investigations began with an environmental survey which would illuminate the means of transmission, but ideally narrowed to one end point: the detection of the carrier.

The concept of the carrier, as distinct from that of the ambulatory, mild, or sub-clinical undiagnosed case, emerged in the years around 1900. Animal experiments

[20] For improvements in the purity of supply see John Hassan, *A History of Water in Modern England and Wales* (1998), pp. 53–4.

[21] On shellfish see Chapter 2; Anne Hardy, 'Exorcising Molly Malone: typhoid and shellfish consumption in urban Britain 1860–1960', *History Workshop Journal*, 55 (2003): pp. 73–90. William Hamer, Chief Medical Officer to the London County Council 1911–26, remained vocally opposed to the healthy carrier concept for the rest of his life. See William H. Hamer, 'Typhoid carriers and contact infections. Some difficulties . . . ', *Proceedings of the Royal Society of Medicine*, 4(2) (1910–11): p. 146; Anon, 'Sir William Hamer', *Lancet* (1936), ii: p. 161.

[22] See C. H. Browning et al., 'Chronic enteric carriers and their treatment', Medical Research Council, *Special Report Series*, no 179 (1933): p. 27; Judith Walzer Leavitt, *Typhoid Mary: Captive to the Public's Health* (1996); Berton Rouché, *Eleven Blue Men* (1947), pp. 32–3.

[23] See John C. G. Ledingham, 'The carrier problem in relation to enteric fever and diphtheria' (The Harben Lectures 1925. Lecture II), *Jnl State Med*, 34 (1926): pp. 65–82.

[24] For the concept of liberty and medical intervention see Roy M. Macleod, 'Law, medicine and public opinion: The resistance to compulsory health legislation, 1870–1907', *Public Law*, Summer 1967: pp. 106–26, 188–211; Anne Hardy, '"Straight back to barbarism": Anti typhoid inoculation and the Great War, 1914', *Bulletin of the History of Medicine*, 74 (2000): p. 267; on the holistic tradition see Christopher Lawrence and George Weisz, eds, *Greater Than the Parts: Holism in Biomedicine 1920–1950* (1999).

had demonstrated the persistence of typhoid bacilli in bile for up to four months, and several investigators had recovered bacilli from abscesses and gall bladders months and years after patients had recovered from the disease. By 1900, Percival Horton-Smith, assistant physician at the Brompton and Metropolitan hospitals, was asking, 'How long might the bacillus remain in the body?' and suggesting that, contrary to William Budd's teachings, faeces were only one means by which typhoid infection could be spread.[25] In the United States, meanwhile, the outbreak of typhoid among troops engaged in the Spanish–American War of 1898 offered new opportunities for field observation and bacterial investigation. In 1900 Walter Reed and his colleagues published their report on the origins and spread of typhoid in the military camps.[26] Their conclusions were very specific: that healthy carriers of the typhoid bacillus existed, and both faeces and urine were capable of transmitting the organism. 'We desire to emphasise the fact', they recorded, 'that the typhoid bacillus may grow in the intestines of an individual and pass from the same without causing typhoid fever . . . in the human body . . . the Eberth bacillus may continue to grow and reproduce its kind quite indefinitely'.[27] It was perhaps an indication of English insularity that these findings went unremarked in the British medical literature.[28]

Despite the premonitory rumblings which preceded this as so many other significant scientific 'discoveries', active realization of the healthy carrier concept came with European research. Even in America, practical recognition of the carrier concept as applied to typhoid seems only to have begun with George Soper's publication of the story of Typhoid Mary Mallon in 1907, and with knowledge of German anti-typhoid practices. The practical and political difficulties of healthy carrier identification and monitoring were clearly a deterrent factor.[29] In this regard, the work of Robert Koch seems to have been more influential than that of the Reed Commission. Koch was the first specifically to call attention to the

[25] Percival Horton-Smith, 'The Goulstonian Lectures on the typhoid bacillus and typhoid fever', *BMJ*, 1900, i: pp. 827–34. See also Percival Horton-Smith, 'On the respective parts taken by the urine and the faeces in the dissemination of typhoid fever', *BMJ* (1899), i: pp. 1346–51. Horton-Smith's core interest was, however, in diseases of the chest: Anon, 'Sir Percival Horton-Smith-Hartley', *BMJ* (1952), ii: p. 99.

[26] W. Reed et al., *Abstract of Report on the Origin and Spread of Typhoid Fever in U.S. Military Camps during the Spanish War of 1898* (1900).

[27] Reed, *Abstract*, pp. 202, 204.

[28] The New York correspondent of the *Lancet* mentioned publication of the report but not the findings on healthy carriers: From Our Own Correspondent, 'New York', *Lancet* (1900), i: pp. 1915–16. The copy of the report in the Bodleian Library, Oxford, was donated from the library of the (Canadian) physician Sir William Osler, then Regius Professor of Medicine, in 1925.

[29] Typhoid carriers were briefly mentioned, but only in relation to nurses and those closely nursing patients, by the bacteriologist Theobald Smith in 1904. See Theobald Smith, 'Some of the ways in which infection is disseminated', *Journal of the Massachusetts Board of Health*, 14(1) (1904): p. 25. Despite active American interest in healthy diphtheria carriers and the problems of monitoring them, public health experts acknowledged the difficulties of implementing the German typhoid prevention system: see Charles E. A. Winslow, 'Some factors in the spread of typhoid fever', *American Journal of Public Hygiene*, 18(2) (1908): p. 32. For difficulties in managing diphtheria carriers see Charles V. Chapin, 'The methods of release of diphtheria patients in Providence', *American Journal of Public Hygiene*, 16(4) (1906): p. 30.

danger presented by convalescents or even the apparently healthy. In a lecture delivered in Berlin in November 1902, and subsequently summarized in the *British Medical Journal*, Koch expressed the view that the viability of the typhoid bacillus in water and soil was very limited, and that the detection of the organism in humans offered the key to controlling the disease. Investigations in Berlin had shown that many apparently healthy people who had been in contact with typhoid patients but had never themselves had the disease nonetheless excreted typhoid bacilli in their faeces. Case-to-case transmission, Koch declared, was the principal source of endemic typhoid.[30] The British reaction was cautious: Koch had done himself few favours with the announcement in 1901, similarly startling to accepted scientific opinion, that bovine tuberculosis was not transmissible to humans.[31] The *British Medical Journal*, for example, commented of his new statement on typhoid, 'It used to be said of Dupuytren that his motto in surgical practice was *Faire autrement. Professor Koch seems to have taken the same model for his own public deliverances*' (italics in original).[32] Returning to the issue, a later commentary held the sanitary line: intermediate channels infection could not be neglected, even if the primary source lay elsewhere.[33]

Koch's concern was primarily with endemic typhoid in rural areas where it was not always possible, in the circumstances of the early twentieth century, to put systems of good sanitation, pure water, and general cleanliness into place. In a novel field experiment, conducted in an area in the city of Trier where typhoid had 'got a firm hold', Koch and his assistants conducted bacteriological analyses of material from primary typhoid cases notified to local doctors, and then from their families. Although only eight cases had been notified, 72 people were shown bacteriologically to be suffering from typhoid, 52 of them children. As soon as cases were discovered, isolation and vigorous disinfection followed. Within three months the disease had been eradicated from the locality. The programme had, however, required special laboratory facilities and highly trained staff, and Koch admitted that it could not practically be applied on any large scale. In principle, however, the method could be used against any infectious disease for which laboratory diagnosis was possible, especially diphtheria and tuberculosis. The bacteriological diagnosis of cases, Koch argued, offered a new offensive tactic against infectious disease—a radical departure from the traditional defensive sanitary tactics—and should constitute the basis for future action.[34]

The suggestion met with little enthusiasm from the British medical community. The bacteriological facilities necessary for the offensive approach were non-existent, the bacteriological methods still difficult and uncertain, typhoid death rates already substantially reduced, and the extensive testing of British populations on the

[30] Koch, 'Crusade', pp. 503–4.

[31] See Waddington, *Bovine Scourge*, pp. 12–130.

[32] Editorial, 'Robert Koch and his campaign against typhoid fever', *BMJ* (1903), i: p. 97. Guillaume Dupuytren (1777–1835), surgeon, developed the curative operation for the contracture of the thumb named after him.

[33] Editorial, 'The suppression of typhoid fever', *BMJ* (1903), i: pp. 506–7.

[34] Koch, 'Crusade', p. 503.

German model considered intrusive and unacceptable.[35] The campaign against endemic typhoid which was launched in south-west Germany in 1903, using Koch's methods and with the financial backing of the Imperial government, attracted no direct comment in the British medical press, and there was no reportage of the campaign's progress as it ran through to a conclusion in 1906. Of the bacteriological and epidemiological studies from the campaign published in that year, only the findings on the culture media best suited to the typhoid bacillus were noted.[36] It was not, however, that the British medical community was unaware of the German typhoid offensive. In March 1906, it was noted of an investigation into typhoid at Lincoln that it followed 'our standard methods' of inquiry and as such was 'as complete and perfect as possible under the circumstances'. Sufficient use was not, however, made of the most advanced bacteriological methods for detecting the typhoid bacillus: the writer considered that the British public were unlikely to accept the 'inquisitorial and harassing methods' used in Germany. He concluded on an ambiguous and unhelpful note:[37]

> But it is obvious that methods of this kind must be adopted if we are to obtain full information with regard to the secondary infections, and with regard also to the general etiology of the disease, and especially the incubating and mild or abortive cases which contribute such a large proportion to extensive epidemics.

The introduction of new bacteriological techniques into sanitary science could be seen to complicate rather than simplify the tasks of the sanitarian.

The problem with Koch's method for typhoid eradication, as far as the British were concerned, lay in the detail. Finding the blood-based Widal test slow and unsatisfactory as a diagnostic tool, Koch opted for a method based on human excreta. In tackling an epidemic outbreak, the excreta of *all* persons resident in the locality was to be tested, regardless of whether they were sick or well. The complete isolation of affected individuals and the repeated testing of their excreta over a period of weeks were also required.[38] Further, the 'rigid and thorough disinfection of all excreta' had to be enforced.[39] For the British, such measures represented a sanitary step too far. There was no legal provision for such action and without it the public health authorities were powerless. Moreover, the collection of sample excreta raised issues of intimacy, revulsion, and individual liberty which public health officials would find difficult to negotiate. In a country which was then rejecting the principle of compulsory vaccination against smallpox (effectively abolished in England and Wales in 1907), the imposition of forcible sampling of excreta, let alone the compulsory complete and possibly lengthy isolation of individuals

[35] Discussion following William G. Savage, 'Recent work upon the bacteriology of typhoid fever in its relationship to preventive methods', *Public Health*, 20 (1907–8): pp. 20–4.

[36] Editorial, 'Recent investigation on typhoid fever', *BMJ* (1906), ii: pp. 938–9.

[37] Editorial, 'Explosive epidemics of typhoid', *BMJ*, 1907, i: p. 754; Richard Reece, 'Report on the epidemic of enteric fever in the city of Lincoln, 1904–5', MOAR LGB, BPP 1907, xxv, Appendix A no 8, pp. 61–145.

[38] Koch, 'Crusade', p. 504.

[39] Winslow, 'Some factors', p. 132. The Americans too found this measure troublesome to enforce.

who were perfectly well, must have seemed a recipe for further popular revolt. No radical programme for typhoid eradication was undertaken in England and Wales or in Scotland, and even when some provision was made for tackling the issue of carriers in the 1920s, suspects were not required by law (except for dairy workers in Scotland) to provide samples for bacteriological analysis. Compliance had in every case to be negotiated between suspect, health officer, and general practitioner. The problem of the healthy carrier remained, as it remains throughout the world today, 'a standing danger to the community'.[40]

HEALTHY HUMAN CARRIERS

The publication in April 1906 of the German study reporting, as an outcome of the eradication campaign, the discovery of chronic healthy carriers of typhoid seems to have passed the British medical establishment by, just as the findings of the American commission report had.[41] The information appears to have reached the public health community in July 1907 via the annual report of the sanitary commissioner with the Government of India, which was extracted and published in the medical officers' journal, *Public Health*.[42] In that month, the Medical Officer of Health for Colchester, William Savage—an experienced laboratory bacteriologist who had been employed by the Medical Department—addressed the provincial meeting of the Society of Medical Officers of Health on the subject. He clearly intended to open up the topic for debate; the paper was published in the October issue of *Public Health*. Remarking that his audience was 'doubtless familiar' with the recent advances in knowledge concerning the transmission of typhoid, Savage also noted the lack of public response among British public health experts. There had been no discussion of the new knowledge and its implications for typhoid in Britain, or of how far this knowledge should modify current investigative methods.[43] He proceeded to outline the recent findings—typhoid bacilli might be passed in urine; chronic carriers existed; bacilli might be recovered from healthy people who had apparently never suffered from typhoid; some apparent cases were due to infection with other organisms, the so-called paratyphoids.[44] Knowledge of these facts, he argued, had so far made no difference to British preventive methods; he recommended that the urine and faeces of all typhoid cases should be bacteriologically examined and shown to be free from bacilli before the patient was certified free from infection, and that blood tests should be conducted to determine which

[40] Browning et al., 'Chronic enteric carriers', p. 3.

[41] P. Klinger, 'Über Typhusbazillenträger', *Arbeiten aus dem kaiserlichen Gesundheitsamte*, 24 (1906): pp. 91–6.

[42] Annotation, '"Carrier cases" of enteric fever', *PH* 19 (1906–7): pp. 604–7. The previous month had seen the case of the carrier Typhoid Mary reported in the USA: George A. Soper, 'The work of a chronic carrier typhoid germ distributor', *Journal of the American Medical Association*, 48 (1907): pp. 2019–22.

[43] Savage, 'Recent work', pp. 12–24.

[44] Identified in the years around 1900, the paratyphoid fevers are caused by *Salmonella* other than *Salmonella typhi*, are generally milder, and are grouped with typhoid under the term 'enteric fever'.

cases were paratyphoid. He did not, however, think it necessary to establish 'anti-typhoid Institutes' on the German model, or to emulate the elaborate German case-detection system.[45]

The subject of the healthy chronic carrier finally broke open in Britain the following year—a time lag which suggests limitations to German influences on social reform in Britain at this period.[46] In January 1908, Alex Ledingham, Medical Officer for Health (MOH) for Banff County, and his brother, John Ledingham of the Lister Institute, published a paper in the *BMJ* which was designed to activate interest in the subject among British doctors.[47] Following this publication, the major medical journals began carrying reports of carrier outbreaks; there were discussions at the Sanitary Institute and the Royal Society of Medicine; and the Medical Department commissioned its inspector Theodore Thomson and John Ledingham of the Lister Institute to review existing knowledge of the subject.[48] Thomson and Ledingham concluded that the danger associated with known carriers might easily be exaggerated, and that the need for such measures as long-term isolation of patients was unproven. Instead, they argued, the danger of individual carriers was greatest where they were employed in particular occupations—such as in the food industries—and where they and their associates had unclean personal habits. In effect, they located the carrier within the existing framework of environmental approaches to the typhoid problem. Every convalescent typhoid patient should be told of the possibility of long-term infection, and of the need for 'scrupulous care in the hygiene of the toilet'.[49] This emphasis on personal hygiene fitted neatly with both political necessity and the existing environmental approach to typhoid, while legitimating the extension of preventive concern into the private sphere of personal habits.

Doubts remained, however, both in Britain and elsewhere, regarding the precise significance of chronic carriers in the etiology of typhoid. Between November 1909 and March 1910, for example, there were prolonged debates on the question in the French Academy of Medicine.[50] The resolution put to the assembled Academicians, that the chronic carrier played a part in maintaining endemic typhoid only exceptionally, was rejected, but by a mere three votes (18 to 15).[51] British debates, as at the Royal Society of Medicine in March 1908, reflected similar reservations.[52] Theodore Thomson, commenting on the French debates in his Presidential

[45] Savage, 'Recent work', pp. 18–19.

[46] The case for German influence has been discussed by E. P. Hennock in *The Origin of the Welfare States in Britain and Germany 1850–1914: Social Policies Compared* (2007).

[47] Alex Ledingham and John C. G. Ledingham, 'Typhoid carriers', *BMJ* (1908), i: pp. 15–17.

[48] Theodore Thomson and John C. G. Ledingham, 'Memorandum on the progress . . . ', MOAR LGB, BPP, 1909, xxix, Appendix B no 1, pp. 696–9; John C. G. Ledingham, 'Report on the enteric fever "carrier"', MOAR LGB, BPP, 1910, xxxix, Appendix B no 1, pp. 292–430.

[49] MOAR LGB, BPP, 1910, xxxix, p. 13.

[50] *Bulletin de l'Académie de Medicine*, 3rd series, 62 (1909): pp. 207–90, 305–17, 382–99, 409–26, 491–510, 544–98, 627–32; *Bulletin de l'Académie de Medicine*, 3rd series, 63 (1910): pp. 10–57, 75–101, 119–36, 155–83, 202–11, 239–44.

[51] *Bulletin de l'Académie de Medicine*, 3rd series, 63 (1910): p. 40.

[52] *PRSM*, 1 (February 1908), Section of Epidemiology and State Medicine: pp. 175–228.

Address to the Epidemiological Section of the Society in 1910, observed sapiently that the judgement likely to find favour with the majority was that voiced by the French pioneer of typhoid immunization, Hyacinthe Vincent; that new conceptions initially attracted both extreme partisans and impassioned detractors; and that the truth would be found to lie in-between.[53]

For many British public health men, the significance of the carrier was diminished by the recent history of typhoid, which supported the effectiveness of environmental measures. Death rates had declined pretty uniformly across England and Wales, but the geographical pattern of distribution remained unchanged. There were proportionately more deaths in the north-east, in Durham; in certain towns in Staffordshire, Lancashire, and the West Riding; and in parts of Wales. These were mostly areas where privy midden conservancy systems survived; towns such as Oldham, which exchanged dry conservancy for water carriage around 1900, experienced sharp drops in typhoid incidence.[54] As Thomson noted, the carrier had doubtless been around during the whole period of the decline in typhoid deaths, and the environmental measures taken in the misguided belief that the bacillus lived and throve outside the human body must nonetheless have greatly reduced the chances of infection by carrier.[55] General improvements such as scavenging and the paving of streets had also played a part: clean environments outside the home tended to encourage cleanliness within, and this promoted clean habits in the occupants, which were the chief safeguard against infection by carrier. It was an argument with distinct attractions, given the administrative difficulties presented by chronic carriers. How was the risk of each individual to be assessed? What measures were appropriate for different types of carrier? How could they be detected when individuals would not co-operate with bacteriological testing? The chronic carrier did not come under any of the regulatory clauses in the existing English public health acts.[56] In these circumstances, the temptation was to play down the role of the carrier.[57]

THE PERSISTENCE OF TYPHOID

Recognition of the healthy carrier did not, therefore, signal a resolution of the typhoid problem or any immediate transformation in public health policy toward the disease. Most immediately, it helped to reinforce the logic of the preventive measures being undertaken by the British Army in India, and those applied during

[53] Theodore Thomson, 'The enteric fever carrier', *PRSM*, 4(2) (1910–11): p. 24.

[54] MOAR LGB, BPP, 1910, xxxix, p. 11; A. M. N. Pringle, 'The relation of soil pollution to endemic conditions', *PH*, 15 (1902–03): p. 637.

[55] Thomson, 'Enteric fever carrier', p. 25.

[56] David S. Davies, '"Carriers" in disease with special reference to "typhoid carriers"', *Journal of the Sanitary Institute*, 32 (1911): pp. 6–16.

[57] Sheldon F. Dudley, 'The carrier problem', *PH*, 36 (1922): p. 62; John C. G. Ledingham, 'The carrier problem in relation to enteric fever and diphtheria', *Jnl State Med*, 34 (1926): p. 63; Harold Kerr, 'Disposal of refuse in relation to the enteric group of diseases', *PRSM*, 17 (1926): p. 41.

World War I. The control of typhoid among British and American troops fighting in the Great War was one of the most notable medical features of that campaign, achieved through a combination of scrupulous sanitary training, environmental hygiene, and immunization.[58] The military control of typhoid in wartime was not to be repeated in civilian life after the war, at least in part because mass immunization was neither a popular nor a practical possibility, as the Americans also found.[59] Typhoid continued to exist as a residual endemic disease, and in the 1920s the preventive focus remained on local incidents. The war years did, however, cover a change in pattern. Before 1914, the disease had been concentrated in the northern industrial centres; now it was tending to become diffused at a low level over the whole country.[60] In 1913, excess mortality was in the towns, excepting only London. Death rates stood at 5.1 per 100,000 per annum for the county boroughs, 4.2 in other urban areas, 3.3 in rural areas, and 2.3 in London. After the war the rate was much the same in both towns and countryside, at around 1 per 100,000. Although not by any means a universal European pattern, 'Scandinavia', Denmark, and Holland had similar experiences.[61]

Surveying the typhoid pattern across the years since 1870, the new Chief Medical Officer (CMO) to the new Ministry of Health, George Newman, ascribed important roles in the decline of the disease to improved water supplies, more efficient scavenging, the number of patients isolated in hospital since 1893 (over 50 per cent in London from 1902), higher standards of domestic hygiene, and a growing 'sanitary conscience' regarding clean food.[62] He cited the views of Colston Williams, the County Medical Officer for Glamorgan, a coalfield area where typhoid death rates had fallen from 22 to 3 per 100,000 between 1890 and 1920. Williams had also stressed 'the increasing awareness that life at a higher level of decency and self respect is possible'. He attributed that awareness first to education which stimulated social aspirations after better things, and second to the 'steady upward trend in real wages'. Illustrating the benefits of education, Williams instanced the sharp fall in infant mortality in Glamorgan, ascribing it to the 'beneficent influence' of health visitors and infant welfare centres.[63] Both health visitors and infant welfare centres probably also addressed wider issues of domestic management.[64] It was notable, for example, that typhoid death rates fell faster among women and children in both England and Wales and in Scotland

[58] For typhoid and the war see Hardy, '"Straight back to barbarism"', pp. 265–90.

[59] Charles R. Grandy and C. J. Andrews, 'Municipal control of typhoid fever', *American Journal of Public Health*, 3 (1913): pp. 746–9.

[60] Chief Medical Officer's Annual Report, Ministry of Health (CMOAR) (1923), p. 41. In America male typhoid deaths fell compared to female immediately after the war, apparently due to the military immunization programme. No similar fall was noted in England, but total typhoid death rates were much lower than in America, and women had for decades had lower typhoid death rates than men.

[61] CMOAR (1927), p. 31.

[62] CMOAR (1923), pp. 23–7.

[63] CMOAR (1923), p. 22.

[64] For the work of the infant welfare centres see Deborah Dwork, *War is Good for Babies and Other Young Children* (1987); Lara V. Marks, *Metropolitan Maternity: Maternal and Infant Welfare Services in Early Twentieth Century London* (1996).

throughout the period from 1870 to 1920 than they did among men.[65] Glasgow's MOH considered that this fact strengthened the argument for the significance of domestic hygiene: women and children lived more continuously in the domestic environment, and might be expected to be more strongly affected by its circumstances than men.[66]

Against this changed demographic pattern, the inter-war years saw a continuation of the longer established epidemiological pattern of endemic prevalence punctuated by outbreaks of greater or less note. On average, George Newman noted some four to six such episodes annually. In the investigation of these outbreaks, environmental considerations retained a high profile, partly because of the recognized importance of water and milk as vehicles for sudden explosive incidents, and partly because of frequent difficulty in tracing the source of the infection. At Barnes, for example, in the early summer of 1930, prolonged inquiries by both the local MOH and the Ministry of Health's investigator into both places and persons failed to uncover the source of a geographically dispersed and socially diverse outbreak.[67] Such difficulties were generally most acute in urban areas: in the country the detection of carrier infection, if not exactly easy, was potentially easier than in the complex urban ecology, although the transmission of infection from urban areas to rural ones had been recognized well before identification of the carrier.[68] Discussing in 1923 the 21 carriers identified in his county since 1908, James Watt, MOH for Aberdeenshire, suggested that endemic typhoid in rural areas was maintained by carriers.[69] Watt quoted the American pathologist Frederick Gay on the methodology of carrier detection: 'carriers usually become recognised by careful epidemiological surveys in connection with repeated cases . . . in a given locality in association with some particular individual over a period of time.'[70] Watt went on to specify the principal difficulty in establishing the identity of carriers: obtaining the necessary samples of stools and urine, especially as several samples were usually needed. These could only be obtained by favour.[71]

Bacteriology, therefore, did not play a leading part in the chain of epidemiological investigation between the wars. The formula remained essentially that described by the *BMJ* in 1903: tracing the intermediate channels of infection back 'step by step [until we arrive] at the primary source from which the

65 CMOAR (1923), p. 20; Archibald K Chalmers, 'The influence of sanitation on the decline of enteric fever in Scotland', *Jnl State Med*, 32 (1924): pp. 519–20.

66 Chalmers, 'Influence of sanitation', pp. 519–20.

67 CMOAR (1930), p. 55.

68 See for example Maclean Wilson, 'An outbreak of enteric fever at Chester-le-Street', MOAR LGB, 1894, xl, Appendix A no 7, pp. 527–31. Chester-le-Street, then a village, lay on the old post road between Durham and Newcastle.

69 James Watt, 'Typhoid carriers in Aberdeenshire', *Journal of Hygiene*, 22 (1923–24): pp. 417–37.

70 Frederick P. Gay, *Typhoid Fever Considered as a Problem of Scientific Medicine* (1918). I have been unable to pinpoint this specific quotation in Gay. On the contrary, Gay notes (p. 127) 'the failure of epidemiologists to trace epidemics, to say nothing of individual cases, back to the previous individual from which infecting dose was derived'.

71 Watt, 'Typhoid carriers', p. 417. On the problems of inter-war typhoid management see Anne Hardy, 'Scientific strategy and ad hoc response: The problem of typhoid in America and England, c. 1910–1950', *Journal of the History of Medicine and Allied Sciences,* 69 (2014): pp. 1–37.

contamination arose'.[72] The detection of carriers did not become the central focus of inquiry, even though repeated experience showed their significance as sources of infection, sometimes through personal habits, sometimes through the accident of sanitary defects. The first point of outbreak inquiry remained a medical and environmental survey and not a laboratory-based investigation: this method allowed identification of the channel of infection by which the source and possible originator of an outbreak might be discovered. Notification of cases and deaths was key to both the identification and the investigation of outbreaks, and the 'golden rule' was never to accept a notification at face value. Details had to be obtained from the general practitioner who had issued the certificate. His co-operation was considered essential: he diagnosed and treated the cases, and was familiar with their circumstances. 'You cannot work out the epidemiology of an outbreak of typhoid without the co-operation of the [general] practitioners', recorded the *Medical Officer* in 1934.[73]

A number of notable outbreaks during the 1930s demonstrated the varied nature of the continuing typhoid problem. The Dumfriesshire village of Ecclefechan experienced an explosive outbreak (61 cases) in September 1930, suggesting infection by milk or water. The pipes carrying the village drinking water supply from its upland spring were found to cross a field drain, at which point the clay bonding holding the joints of both sets of pipes had been washed away. A middle-aged man long employed on the farm where the spring was sited proved to be a faecal carrier; he was subsequently found employment in one of the county hospitals, where it was hoped he would be 'innocuous' in the future. Yet as the damaged pipes and the carrier had co-existed for years without causing a problem, the timing of the outbreak still required explanation.[74] Some 37 cases of 'true typhoid' were reported in West Hartlepool in 1929, which were traced back to dressed crab bought from a local fish shop. The woman who had prepared the crab was suffering from 'one of those obscure and long drawn out attacks which do not completely interfere with getting about and doing business': she was an ambulant case of typhoid. The outbreak had repercussions. One of the victims was reported to have become a carrier, and 'an exceedingly awkward one'.[75] Four years later Hartlepool was still much troubled by sporadic typhoid, with many minor outbreaks that were a constant worry to the MOH. Local suspicion was directed to shell-fish pollution and the condition of the foreshore near the outfall of the Seaton Carew sewer. However, as was pointed out, it was not sewage that infected people but people who infected sewage, and with 'almost unequivocal evidence' of typhoid carriers in the town it seemed likely that the disease would remain endemic.[76]

The Hartlepool and Ecclefechan episodes illustrate some of the problems associated with carrier cases in the years to 1932: the management of known carriers

[72] Editorial, 'The suppression of typhoid', *BMJ*, 1903, i: p. 507.
[73] Editorial, 'Enteric and drought', *MO*, 51 (1934): p. 91.
[74] John Ritchie and Edward Armstrong, 'A water-borne epidemic of typhoid fever', *Jnl Hyg*, 32 (1932): pp. 417–30.
[75] Editorial, 'Typhoid fever in West Hartlepool', *MO*, 44 (1930): pp. 53–4.
[76] Notes and Comments, 'Typhoid in West Hartlepool', *MO*, 47 (1932): pp. 62–3.

and the puzzles of circumstance where an unidentified carrier had existed harmlessly for years before causing an outbreak. The discovery of the Vi (Virulence) antigen of typhoid in that year (Chapter 5) made the identification of carriers and the connection of carriers and cases somewhat easier.[77] The outbreak at Malton in the North Riding of Yorkshire in 1932, also a carrier outbreak, had several resonances with earlier Victorian inquiries. First, the investigation was performed by William Vernon Shaw, a Ministry of Health inspector with a formidable epidemiological reputation,[78] whose hallmark was a Victorian thoroughness in inquiry. Second, the Medical Department had investigated typhoid in Malton before: the local Sanitary Authority was caught red-handed neglecting to provide safe water supplies. Well into the twentieth century, local narratives of sanitary progress could differ from the mainstream. The case clearly provoked a good deal of wry relish in George Newman, for the Medical Department had, 40 years previously, urged the authority to abandon the existing water supply, which injunction the authority had ignored.[79] 'The story is an old one', Newman recorded, 'and in this particular area has been repeated during successive generations of the Malton Sanitary Authority'.[80] One reader of Shaw's report found the story 'hardly credible in 20th century England'.[81] Bacteriology here played a pivotal role in confirming Shaw's deductions and identifying the source of the outbreak. Given the relevant biological specimens, and using the new antigenic technique, the Ministry of Health laboratory was able to isolate from Malton patients a strain of typhoid with identical cultural reactions to that recovered from the carrier. It was markedly different from the strain responsible for a simultaneous outbreak elsewhere.[82]

By the mid-1930s, bacteriology was beginning to perform—and be acknowledged to perform—signal services to epidemiology, as its techniques became more sophisticated. An extensive outbreak of milk-borne typhoid occurred in the South Coast towns of Bournemouth, Christchurch, and Poole in summer 1936.[83] More than 700 cases were recorded between July and September, and the infection was eventually traced to a carrier occasionally resident in a house in rural Dorset.[84]

[77] On the importance of this development see CMOAR (1932), p. 189. The Vi antigen persisted in the blood of chronic carriers once the illness was over, meaning they could be identified by a simple blood test.

[78] Notes and Comments, 'The Malton typhoid outbreak', *MO*, 49 (1933): p. 122; Editorial, 'The South Coast typhoid epidemic of 1936', *MO*, 57 (1937): p. 245; Anon, 'William Vernon Shaw', *BMJ*, 1937, i: p. 250.

[79] Robert Bruce Low, 'The outbreak of enteric in certain villages situated on the river Rye in North Yorkshire, and the water supply of Malton Urban Sanitary District', MOAR LGB, BPP, 1894, xl, Appendix A no 8, pp. 595–602.

[80] 'Introduction' to William Vernon Shaw, 'An outbreak of enteric fever in the Malton Urban District', *Reports on Public Health and Medical Subjects*, no 69 (1933): p. 2.

[81] Notes and Comments, 'Malton typhoid outbreak', p. 122.

[82] William Vernon Shaw, 'An outbreak of enteric fever in the Malton Urban District', *Reps on PH*, no 69 (1933): p. 13.

[83] More extended accounts of this outbreak are given in John Hassan, *The Seaside, Health and the Environment in England and Wales since 1800* (2003), pp. 130–3; Hardy, 'Scientific strategy', pp. 30–1.

[84] William Vernon Shaw, 'An outbreak of enteric fever in the county borough of Bournemouth and the boroughs of Poole and Christchurch', *Reps on PH*, no 81 (1937). Hassan, *The Seaside*, notes the

Shaw's investigation followed a painstaking process of elimination through the dairy's numerous suppliers, interrogating farmers and their families as to relevant illness and dairy hygiene practice, and examining local circumstances until a local source was identified. Shaw's report was described as 'the clearest cut piece of epidemiology on record',[85] but had it not been for the new technique of antigenic analysis, the linking of the carrier at the big house in rural Dorset to the epidemic in the coastal towns would have been impossible.[86]

Not all outbreaks proved amenable to bacteriological elucidation. The 1938 Croydon typhoid epidemic, which became something of a cause célèbre in the preventive community,[87] was thought to have occurred through pollution of the local water source by one of the workmen engaged in construction work on its plant, who happened to be a urinary carrier. Some 300 cases and 43 deaths resulted—'a disaster which ought to have been avoidable'.[88] The outbreak began slowly. The first case, notified on 16 October 1937, was thought to be due to the patient having eaten infected shell-fish during a recent holiday on the continent. There was another case on 25 October, and four on 29 October. By the time the Ministry of Health was informed, on 1 November, the tally was a total of seven cases, three of whom had only been diagnosed on admission to hospital with indefinite febrile symptoms. Because the number of cases was as yet relatively small, and the local water supplies were supposedly chlorinated, the idea that the infection was associated with water simply did not occur to the local officers.[89] It was only when the Ministry's Dr Conybeare arrived on 3 November, and a plotting of the distribution of cases on a map revealed a coincidence with the high-level supply from the Addington spring reservoir, that the connection was made. In this instance, traditional epidemiological mapping methods supplied what laboratory analysis could not.

Beyond these highly publicized epidemic outbreaks lay a persistent tally of household and sporadic cases linked to carriers or unrecognized cases. In Bradfield, Berkshire, a farming family was stricken in 1937, after a visitor suffered 'a suspicious illness' while staying in the house some weeks previously.[90] Household outbreaks were said to be very common, especially in villages, and were usually caused by infection carried by a visitor, whether carrier or unwitting patient. These

official secrecy in which details of this outbreak were shrouded (p. 132). This may have resulted from the identity of the carrier, Captain Angus Hambro (1883–1957), MP for South Dorset 1910–22, for North Dorset 1937–45, and High Sheriff of Dorset 1934–35, as revealed by Mary Graham, *The Typhoid Epidemic in Bournemouth, Poole and Christchurch 1936* (1997), pp. 7–8.

[85] Editorial, 'South Coast typhoid epidemic', *MO*, 58 (1937): p. 245.

[86] Shaw, 'An outbreak of enteric', p. 16.

[87] This was partly because of the intense newspaper interest in the outbreak, but particularly because Lord Dawson of Penn and Sir Kaye Le Fleming took it upon themselves in a letter to *The Times* (22 November 1937, p. 13) to offer hostile criticism of the preventive services and, by implication, of the Croydon MOH: see the various editorials and comments in *PH*, 51 (1937–38), pp. 61–2, 119–21; 137–55; 159–61; 179–82; 183, and *MO*, 58 (1937): pp. 222–3; *MO*, 59 (1938): pp. 54, 59, 74, 78–9; *MO*, 60 (1939): pp. 10, 275.

[88] Editorial, 'The report on the Croydon Inquiry', *PH*, 51 (1937–38): p. 159.

[89] Notes and Summaries, 'The Croydon typhoid inquiry', *PH*, 51 (1937–38): p. 137.

[90] Notes and Comments, 'Typhoid fever in West Berkshire', *MO*, 58 (1937): p. 153.

little episodes went unrecognized because the families were not familiar with the symptoms of typhoid, and because they happened in districts where no one was expecting typhoid to occur.[91] The persistence of typhoid in the inter-war period was the result not only of such accidental contaminations as occurred at Croydon, but also the fact that domestic and personal hygiene remained questionable. Throughout the inter-war period, water closet provision and hand-washing facilities remained inadequate in homes, schools, restaurants, kitchens of all types, and public places (Chapter 9). Mild, ambulant, and unrecognized cases, as well as carriers, served to perpetuate endemic typhoid infection and to precipitate occasional larger outbreaks.

CONTROL AND THE CARRIER

Recognition of the chronic carrier did not significantly change the practices of public health administrators and epidemiologists in Britain in the 1920s.[92] By the 1930s, however, the central role of the carrier in propagating typhoid, as demonstrated by repeated experience, had become accepted and was utilized by epidemiologists investigating outbreaks. Preventive concern focused on methods of limiting the epidemic potential represented by carriers, and to a large extent environmental safeguards were still seen to be essential.[93] The principal risks were contamination of water, milk, and food—the last a concern which featured increasingly through the 1930s. Water-borne typhoid was, nationally, of greatly decreased importance by this period, although the potential for damaging pollution was repeatedly demonstrated, as at Ecclefechan, Malton, Croydon, and elsewhere. It was, however, the duty of local authorities to ensure that recognized supplies of drinking water were safeguarded, as they could be by filtration and chlorination; legal powers existed to effect such protection. If individuals chose to drink from doubtful water sources, they did so at their own risk, and it was considered that the carrier could not be held responsible.[94] Milk, which had been known to act as a vehicle of infection since the 1870s, continued to pose a problem (Chapter 4). The application of protective techniques of heat treatment and pasteurization remained patchy, especially in rural areas. Medical pressure for pasteurization, especially with a view to preventing the transmission of bovine tuberculosis, had been growing, but even among the medical profession there were voices arguing against pasteurization. It was not before the 1950s that near-universal coverage was achieved.[95] Moreover,

[91] Notes, 'Typhoid fever'.

[92] Sheldon F. Dudley, 'The carrier problem', *PH*, 36 (1922): p. 62; Ledingham, 'The carrier problem', p. 63.

[93] Ledingham, 'The carrier problem', p. 63.

[94] John Ritchie, 'The problem of the carrier in enteric fever', *PH*, 46 (1933): p. 294.

[95] See Peter J. Atkins, 'The pasteurisation of England: The science, culture and health implications of milk processing, 1900–1950,' in *Food, Science, Policy and Regulation in the Twentieth Century*, edited by David Smith and Jim Phillips (2000), 37–51; Peter J. Atkins, *Liquid Materialities: A History of Milk, Science and the Law* (2010), pp. 223–77.

the new practice of bulking milk supplies offered novel opportunities for extensive infection, as was seen in Dorset in 1936. The social, economic, and technical developments that led to the emergence of a large-scale, bulk-supply food and drink industry brought the prospect of food-borne infections being channelled to larger numbers of people than ever before.[96]

The safety of both water and milk could, however, be effected by external technological controls. The hygienic behaviour of the human animal, of the individual carrier, was less amenable to external sanitary management. As the secondary, environmental sources of infection were brought within the domain of modern, scientific, sanitary practice, so the behaviour of the human animal, the ultimate primary source of typhoid infection, became of greater moment. The unknown carriers of West Hartlepool, for example, stood as a continual reminder to the preventive community of the dangers inherent in carrier status. Over the years various measures were proposed and discussed for identifying and managing chronic carriers, but none ever achieved general acceptance in the British public health community. Were typhoid patients to be kept in hospital until they were bacteriologically free of infection? Were typhoid convalescents to be registered and monitored? Should typhoid carriers be registered? Should they be subjected to compulsory treatment? Should they be quarantined and confined?[97]

Before 1914, the public health acts contained no provisions that could be used for dealing with chronic carriers. In England and Wales the only regulations on the supervision of carriers before World War II were given in the Public Health (Infectious Diseases) Regulations (England) 1927. These enabled an MOH to prevent persons judged to be enteric carriers from being employed or concerned in the preparation or handling of food and drink for human consumption for a specified period. However, the regulations did not enable the MOH to take action unless disease had already broken out. Not surprisingly, they were later described as 'a complicated process for obtaining powers to do nothing'.[98] In Scotland, the Scottish Carrier Regulations 1921, and later provision under Section 13 of the Public Health (Infectious diseases) Regulations (Scotland) 1932, permitted the certification of carriers for three months, imposing certain restrictions on behaviour during that time. At the end of that time further examination and re-certification had to take place. As John Ritchie pointed out, the procedure might be of some use with convalescent carriers, but it was hopelessly impracticable as a means of controlling chronic carriers.[99] The difficulty of managing and monitoring a chronic carrier over the course of a lifetime inevitably led to an emphasis on education, despite recognition that human waywardness meant this might not be enough. John Ledingham noted that 'persuasion and instruction will do more to reduce infection from declared carriers than any compulsory order rigidly applied'.

96 Ritchie, 'Problem', pp. 292–3. See also Chapter 4.

97 See, for example, David S. Davies, 'Carriers in disease with special reference to "typhoid carriers"', *Journal of the Sanitary Institute*, 32 (1911): pp. 6–16; Ledingham, 'The carrier problem', pp. 82–5.

98 Notes and Comments, 'Typhoid carriers', *MO*, 62 (1939): p. 252.

99 Ritchie, 'The problem of the carrier', p. 295.

Yet he argued that communities must, for their own security, have full powers to retain declared carriers on a permanent register, to insist on notification of all changes of address, to examine their discharges at any time, and to remove them to hospital for the purpose if necessary.[100]

By the 1930s, with increasing confidence in chlorinated water supplies and dairy hygiene, the risk of infection through food had come to be considered 'the real crux' of the carrier question.[101] While the domestic circumstances of the private home remained a problematic preventive target, the question of carriers working in the food trades or related occupations had been under consideration since Mary Mallon's case received extensive publicity around 1907.[102] Following the Mallon case, a number of American health authorities had adopted more or less rigorous monitoring of food handlers, but the record was not encouraging. Between 1920 and 1928 just one typhoid carrier was detected in 81,982 examinations made in Newark, New Jersey.[103] It was noted with interest that in New York City most carriers were still discovered through the occurrence of actual cases of typhoid, despite the programme for the detection and control of carriers, and it was noted in 1940 that New York State had become convinced that food-handler examinations were unwarranted, being so time-consuming and expensive as to be quite impractical.[104] The American example and the food-handler issue were frequently discussed among British MOHs. Much of the discussion turned, however, on the desirability of improving general standards of personal hygiene: if a reasonable standard of ordinary cleanliness, such as washing hands before touching food, could be enforced, much gastric illness would be prevented.[105] Concern over typhoid carriers lingered well into the 1950s, although Britain experienced no significant upsurge in typhoid infections during World War II, and unlike many European countries did not see a greatly increased prevalence persisting into the post-war years.[106] In 1945, the Emergency Public Health Laboratory Service—reiterating the desirability of detecting, whenever practicable, patients likely to become chronic typhoid carriers—set out in detail the methods by which this was to be achieved.[107] Two years later the CMO, Wilson Jameson, resumed the discussion.[108] This was the view from the laboratory and from Whitehall. The view on the ground remained sceptical: 'The detection of carriers is not difficult but exceedingly troublesome, so it is not feasible except in suspects.'[109]

[100] Ledingham, 'The carrier problem', pp. 84–5.

[101] Ritchie, 'The problem of the carrier', p. 294; Ledingham, 'The carrier problem', p. 85; Browning et al., 'Chronic enteric carriers', p. 21.

[102] For the Mallon case see Soper, 'A chronic carrier'; Leavitt, *Typhoid Mary;* Judith Walzer Leavitt, '"Typhoid Mary fights back". Bacteriological theory and practice in early twentieth century public health', *Isis*, 83 (1992): pp. 608–29.

[103] Charles V. Craster, 'The medical examination of food handlers', *PH*, 43 (1930): pp. 102–5.

[104] Editorial, 'Routine examination of food handlers', *PH*, 53 (1940): p. 167.

[105] Annotation, 'Medical examination of food handlers', *MO*, 43 (1930): p. 17.

[106] CMOAR (1948), p. 8.

[107] Ministry of Health, 'The detection of typhoid cases', *MBMH*, 4 (1945): p. 224.

[108] CMOAR (1947), pp. 49–50.

[109] Notes and Comments, 'Epidemic typhoid', *MO*, 76 (1946): p. 158.

The effectiveness of modern methods of carrier detection and control, where they could be rigorously implemented within a manageable geographical compass, were vividly demonstrated in Southern Ireland, where a highly successful campaign was waged between 1920 and 1950.[110] From 1922–32 clean water supplies were provided, sewage schemes implemented, ashpits abolished, and house refuse collections initiated in towns and villages throughout the country. Typhoid incidence fell from several thousand cases per year to an average of 400 between 1930 and 1945. The health authorities then moved to tackle the residual carrier problem, and in eight years had reduced annual incidence to fewer than 50 cases. Significantly, the number of carriers found in the towns and villages was very small. Over 95 per cent were found in rural areas, where incidence of the disease had not decreased, and over 60 per cent were from households with a previous history of typhoid.[111] Two factors were said to be critical to the success of the very detailed Irish programme: first, the co-operation of family doctors, which was essential in obtaining the necessary samples of blood, faeces, and urine; second, the establishment of a central typhoid typing laboratory (1947), which mapped the distribution and occurrence of the different phage types and facilitated the identification and management of problem carriers (for the introduction and importance of phage-typing see Chapter 5).[112] The two-stage Irish control programme for typhoid mirrored, in a much tighter time-frame, the loose pattern of the English and Scottish operations against the disease which had effectively spanned a century. In all three countries the development of the new technique of phage-typing, supplemented by adequate public health laboratory provision, provided the key to solving the riddle of endemic typhoid.

The methods of observational epidemiology, as pioneered in England by William Budd and John Snow, set the example for outbreak investigation as it was developed under John Simon and his successors at the Medical Department after 1860. The pathways of infection discovered by these methods, and increasingly taken into account in public health practice, contributed toward the reduction in typhoid prevalence in England and Wales, and in Scotland, in the later decades of the nineteenth century. Yet low-level endemic typhoid persisted, and it was only with the microbiological discoveries of the 1930s that Britain emerged in the post-World War II era as a virtually typhoid-free country. Since the 1950s, typhoid has become a rare disease in the west, yet it remains endemic in large parts of the world, and eternal vigilance remains the price of safety in countries where it is successfully controlled. Imported infections and potential carrier status among travellers and migrants present a continuing public health threat.[113] The methods so painfully developed for the control of typhoid between 1870 and 1945 are not applicable to

[110] A similar campaign was successfully waged in Norway. See Morten Hammerborg, 'The campaign to eradicate typhoid fever in Western Norway', in *Healthcare Systems and Medical Institutions*, edited by Astri Andresen et al. (2009), pp. 170–85.

[111] John D. MacCormack, 'Typhoid fever control', *PH*, 67 (1953–4): p. 130.

[112] MacCormack, 'Typhoid fever control', pp. 130–1.

[113] See S. J. Olsen et al., 'Outbreaks of typhoid fever in the United States, 1960–99', *Epidemiology and Infection*, 130 (2003), pp. 13–21; F. J. Cooke et al., 'Cases of typhoid fever imported into

the lesser *Salmonella*. Carrier status among non-typhoid *Salmonella* and other gastro-intestinal infections remains highly problematic, and gastro-enteric illness an enormous and expensive burden. Human and animal carriers of gastro-intestinal infections, poor food-handling practices, and deficient personal hygiene lie at the core of this problem.[114]

England, Scotland and Wales (2000–2003)', *Transactions of the Royal Society for Tropical Medicine and Hygiene*, 101 (2007): pp. 398–404.

114 Kathryn Senior, 'Estimating the global burden of foodborne disease', *The Lancet Infectious Diseases*, 9(2) (2013): pp. 80–1.

2

The Hygiene of the Sea

For many centuries the seas around Britain were regarded as a natural good, as providers of food and livelihood, as an obstacle to invasion, and, from the eighteenth century increasingly, as a source of inspiration, recreation, and entertainment. Traditionally too, sea waters were regarded as pure and purifying, as were moving waters generally. The late eighteenth century even saw a fashion for drinking sea water as a medicinal tonic, akin to the waters of the inland mineral spas at Bath, Malvern, Harrogate, and elsewhere.[1] For as long as urban development remained limited and the disposal of human wastes achieved by dry conservancy systems, the innocence of the sea was maintained. Indeed, the idea persisted well after massive urban growth and the introduction of water carriage systems for human wastes resulted in polluted shorelines and coastal waters. The advent of bacteriology did not initially dent the purifying reputation of the sea: in 1895 the Norwich physician Sir Peter Eade noted that 'the accepted view has been that current water, and especially sea water, was an immediate and complete destroyer of these living germs'.[2] Yet from the 1860s onwards, increasing levels of sewage pollution in British rivers had raised the question, What becomes of pollution?[3] What happened when sewage entered moving water? Was it indeed purified and rendered innocuous?

By the 1880s, the public health community had generally accepted that cholera and typhoid could be transmitted in drinking water contaminated with the specific infection of these diseases. Partly because of the tradition of the purifying sea, partly because epidemiological evidence was lacking, and partly because it was assumed that the gastric action of the sea creatures concerned would destroy any pathogenic organisms,[4] it was not until the 1890s that the question of disease transmission from specifically polluted water through fish and shell-fish taken from contaminated

[1] Alain Corbin, *The Lure of the Sea: The Discovery of the Seaside 1750–1840* (1995), pp. 57–78; John Walton, *The English Seaside Resort: A Social History, 1750–1914* (1983); Alan Durie, 'Medicine, health and economic development: Promoting spa and seaside resorts in Scotland c. 1750–1830', *Medical History*, 47 (2003): pp. 195–216; John Hassan, *The Seaside, Health and the Environment in England since 1800* (2003).

[2] Sir Peter Eade, 'Typhoid fevers and oysters and other molluscs', letter, *British Medical Journal* (*BMJ*) (1895), i: pp. 121–2.

[3] Christopher Hamlin, *What Becomes of Pollution: Adversary Science and the Controversy on the Self-Pollution of Rivers in Britain 1750–1914* (1987). Hamlin also notes (p. 270) that bacteriology had 'remarkably little' effect on water analysis. See also John Hassan, *A History of Water in Modern England and Wales* (1998), chapter 2.

[4] Eade, 'Typhoid fevers', pp. 121–2.

estuarine, coastal, and deep sea waters began to attract attention. With the introduction of water-borne sewage disposal systems, coastal towns and cities from the 1870s began discharging their untreated sewage wastes directly into the sea, while London developed a system of transporting sewage sludge out to sea beyond the Thames estuary. As noted by John Hassan, 'the pumping of raw sewage a short way into the sea was virtually universal before 1914'.[5] Before the 1890s, cases of gastric illness associated with fish and shell-fish were attributed to ptomaine poisoning, to the toxins of decay rather than specific infection. Stale fish were often popularly blamed for stomach troubles, as were a wide range of other foodstuffs depending on season.[6] Moreover, although tradition held that shell-fish should not be eaten in months whose name did not contain an 'r'—the early summer months when native shell-fish were breeding—they were a cheap popular luxury, enjoyed by all social classes. Indeed the oyster had a special reputation, not just as an aphrodisiac, but as a restorative and medicinal food, widely recommended to invalids and convalescents.[7] It was only in the 1890s that epidemiology and bacteriology began to cut through this haze of positive cultural assumptions and link the consumption of specifically polluted fish and shell-fish to typhoid and gastro-enteritis.

The connection between sewage contamination of oysters and gastric illness among consumers remains important to twenty-first-century outbreak investigation.[8] Despite established systems of sanitary safeguard and surveillance, layings may still be accidentally polluted, or molluscs contaminated in culinary handling, as several recent, highly publicized instances have made clear. The possibility of such contamination is taken seriously in modern public health inquiries, but when the idea was first introduced it was bitterly contested by the shell-fish trade, and scientific experts were involved on both sides of the argument. The identification of oysters as purveyors of typhoid infection provides a classic example of expert disagreement, with the fish trades invoking the expertise of their chosen bacteriologists against the findings of the public health investigators at the Local Government Board. The controversy over oyster-borne typhoid was just one facet of a wider concern with the faecal pollution of coastal waters, but it provided enough scientific evidence to undermine the tradition of the purifying sea.

Unease over the condition of the fish trades surfaced in London around 1890. The city possessed two fish markets, the ancient riverside mecca at Billingsgate and the newer Farringdon Retail Market, opened by the City Corporation in November 1888. Billingsgate remained of central importance, however, as the major national entrepot of the trade in fish, and more especially in shell-fish. In 1890, Billingsgate was reported to receive 136,000 tons of land- and water-borne (rail and steamer) fish a year, together with 125 million oysters, one million lobsters,

[5] Hassan, *Seaside*, pp. 43–6, 49–51.

[6] Owen H. Peters, *Observations on the Natural History of Epidemic Diarrhoea* (1911), pp. 83–5.

[7] For the culture of oyster eating see Anne Hardy, 'Exorcising Molly Malone: Typhoid and shellfish consumption in urban Britain 1850–1950', *History Workshop Journal*, 55 (2003): pp. 73–90.

[8] See E. Alfano-Sobsey et al., 'Norovirus outbreak associated with undercooked oysters and secondary household transmission', *Epidemiology and Infection*, 140 (2012): pp. 276–82.

500,000 crabs, 300 million shrimp, three million whelks, 30 million mussels, 40 million cockles, and 100 million winkles ('littorinas of the pin').[9] By 1905, the amount of wet fish coming in to London was estimated at well over 200,000 tons, coming both by sea and by rail.[10] It was through Billingsgate that the Worshipful Company of Fishmongers exercised careful control over the English fish trades generally, with a view to regulating standards and maintaining consumer confidence in this fragile product.[11] Initial concerns over the impact of sewage pollution on the quality and hygiene of fish supplies were reinforced in the mid-1890s by evidence that both cholera and—more alarmingly, since it was an indigenous disease—typhoid were transmitted by contaminated shell-fish. As powerful medical voices began to endorse and publicize the dangers of shell-fish, a severe public reaction followed.

Before the 1890s, public health concerns over food supply quality had related to decayed or diseased foods and to adulteration, in which area England and Wales passed pioneering legislation in 1872–5.[12] Concern with the bacterial contamination of foods by faecally polluted water came later. Over a period of some ten years from 1895 serious damage was done to the British shell-fish trades while scientific experts clashed over the likelihood of typhoid transmission by shell-fish. If the pronouncements of different authorities and their relationships to the interests represented offer a classic example of adversary science, the shell-fish story is also an example of problem-solving by technical fix. The problem presented by coastal and deep-sea waters polluted by human effluent to human food supplies and health was overcome without engaging with its fundamental environmental causes. The wider issue of the hygiene of the sea was shelved before World War I, but remained as a source of anxiety to later public health practitioners.[13] The food scares which erupted meanwhile around faecally contaminated shell-fish may be the first documented food scares, reflecting a shift in public perceptions of disease agents from smell to filth contamination, as well as a first popular expression of the disgust for bodily secretions, especially faeces and animal products, which appears to be common to human societies.[14]

[9] 'London's fish supply', *Fish Trades Gazette* 24 January 1891, p. 10.

[10] Medical Officer's Annual Report, London County Council (1905), Appendix III, p. 1.

[11] John W. H. Eyre, 'The oyster and the public health', *Public Health,* 38 (1924): pp. 20–1.

[12] For the history of food adulteration law see John Burnett, *Plenty and Want: A Social History of Food in England since 1815,* 3rd edn (1989), chapter 10; Michael French and Jim Phillips, *Cheated Not Poisoned? Food Regulation in the United Kingdom, 1875–1938* (2000).

[13] Hassan, *Seaside,* 136–59; Robert Neild, *The English, the French and the Oyster* (1995), pp. 116–17.

[14] Valerie Curtis and Adam Biran, 'Dirt, disgust, and disease. Is hygiene in our genes?', *Perspectives in Biology and Medicine,* 44 (2001): pp. 17–31. See also David S. Barnes, 'Confronting sensory crisis in the Great Stinks of London and Paris', in *Filth. Dirt, Disgust and Modern Life,* edited by William A. Cohen and Ryan Johnson (2005), pp. 103–29; David S. Barnes, *The Great Stink of Paris and the Nineteenth-century Struggle against Filth and Germs* (2006), pp. 3–11.

SHELL-FISH

The first definite medical concern about shell-fish and typhoid surfaced in 1880, when Sir Charles Cameron, Medical Officer of Health (MOH) for the city of Dublin, expressed the view that endemic typhoid in his city was maintained through the consumption of sewage polluted shell-fish.[15] By 1890 the condition of many fishing grounds, notably of the estuaries and coastal waters where shell-fish were laid prior to marketing, were beginning to worry health officers. In 1888, a Board of Trade Fisheries Inspector, Charles Fryer, found oyster beds in the Thames Estuary badly affected by untreated London sewage, the creatures filthy, with blackened shells, and none of the fine green weed 'that betokens health'.[16] By 1890, the Fishmongers Company was anxious about the discharge of sewage effluent and refuse into the estuaries of the country's large rivers, especially of the Thames, while the industry journal, the *Fish Trades Gazette* (*FTG*), reported widespread problems of sewage dumping in major fishing grounds from the Mersey to Bridport in Somerset.[17] Mortalities of up to 50 per cent were being recorded among oysters laid on flats in the lower Thames reaches. Although the owner of the layings carefully explained that these molluscs were for 'culinary purposes' only, a Local Government Board inspector present ventured the opinion that he should not care to eat those particular oysters.[18] Billingsgate itself was coming in for criticism: one contemporary declared it to be 'as unsuited for a fish market as a sewer would be for a larder', its porous unglazed brickwork acting as a 'sponge' for bacteria.[19] Reaction from the fish trades was jovial, however, with much banter on the subject of smells, rather than on harmful bacteria.[20]

Late in 1891, trade anxieties sharpened, when Prince George (later King George V, 1910–36) fell ill with typhoid, reportedly from eating sewage-contaminated oysters while visiting Dublin. 'The position of Dublin today may be the position of the Thames Estuary tomorrow', warned the *Fish Trades Gazette*, urging action before worse followed.[21] While no scare materialized on this occasion (after all, the oysters in question had been taken from the Liffey, not an English river), the Prince's illness was significant for the English shell-fish trade. He was attended both by his regular physician and by William Broadbent, a well-known authority on infectious diseases. Broadbent was a popular society physician who had already been suggested several times for 'the medical knighthood'. His successful management of the Prince's illness was duly crowned by appointment as the Prince's Physician in Ordinary in 1892, and by a baronetcy in 1893.[22] Broadbent's standing

15 Charles A. Cameron, 'Oysters and typhoid', *BMJ* (1880), ii: p.71.

16 'Prince George and the poisonous oysters', *FTG*, 28 November 1891, p. 8.

17 'The annual reports', *FTG*, 13 June 1891, p. 8.

18 'Our note book', *FTG*, 3 October 1891, p. 10.

19 J. Hamilton-Lawrence, *Report upon the Fish Markets, Fish Trade Abuses, Fish Frauds and Adulterations and Fish Supply of the Metropolis*, 2nd edn (1890), p. 2.

20 *FTG*, 8 March 1890, p. 10; *FTG*, 1 November 1890, p. 9.

21 'Prince George', *FTG*, p. 8.

22 Anon, 'Sir William Broadbent', *Munk's Roll of the Royal College of Physicians*, vol 4, p. 169.

as a physician of high repute was thus confirmed. Two years later, his pronouncement that there was indeed a connection between oyster-eating and typhoid infection proved a weighty contribution to an escalating, and critical, oyster scare.

Suspicions of a connection between oysters and typhoid were, therefore, already current in the early 1890s, if not influential with the general public. A turning point came in early 1895. Cholera had again visited England briefly and all but innocuously in 1893, resulting in a scatter of cases across the Midlands and north-east, for which no immediately obvious cause, as in a contaminated water supply, could be determined. As cholera was an important epidemic disease, the Medical Department of the Local Government Board naturally investigated the reasons for its importation and spread. The Department's inquiry into the distribution of cholera cases in 1893 was published early in 1895, although its conclusions were known to the medical community several weeks before the official publication. On the local evidence, CMO Richard Thorne Thorne suggested that these anomalous English cholera cases were caused by consumption of sewage-polluted shell-fish taken from estuarial waters at Cleethorpes and Grimsby.[23] As cholera, like typhoid, was by now well known to be communicable by the faecal–oral route, pathways of infection that worked for cholera could be assumed also to work for typhoid. In the circumstances of January 1895, the connection was quickly made by Britain's medical community.

Already in December 1894, an unusual prevalence of typhoid among the wealthier sections of London society had been attributed to oysters, which were a standard seasonal celebratory fare.[24] On 12 January 1895, Sir William Broadbent published a 'Note on the transmission of the infection of typhoid fever by oysters' in the *British Medical Journal* (*BMJ*). He had, he recorded, occasionally seen cases of typhoid apparently attributable to oysters, but it was only during the previous autumn that he became convinced of the connection. 'The contamination of oysters by typhoid can only be accidental', he noted, 'and is therefore probably preventable'. He then described the 'six separate incidents' that had convinced him. First, a young man convalescent from influenza, who developed bronchial catarrh and was confined to his room for three weeks: he consumed oysters freely during that time, and was the only member of a large household with 'faultless' sanitary arrangements to be stricken. Second, two young men living in the same house, who had enjoyed an oyster supper after visiting the theatre together ten days previously; third, a clergyman and his 12-year-old daughter at Daventry, the only members of the household to have eaten oysters sent down from London; and finally, several cases among City gentlemen who had eaten oysters at lunch, and were similarly the only members of their households to suffer.[25] Broadbent's cases represent a wonderful window on the oyster-eating habits of the English middle class, but,

[23] Correspondence, 'Typhoid fever and oysters', *BMJ* (1895), i: p. 217 (26 January); 'Reports and Papers on Cholera in England in 1893, with an Introduction by the Medical Officer of the Local Government Board', BPP, 1894, xl, p. xxix.

[24] Annotation, 'Typhoid and oysters', *BMJ* (1894), i: p. 41.

[25] Sir William Broadbent, 'A note on the transmission of the infection of typhoid fever by oysters', *BMJ* (1895), i: p. 61.

given his popular profile, and standing as Physician-in-Ordinary to the Prince of Wales, they were also highly damaging to public confidence in the safety of English oysters.

Barely had Broadbent pronounced when news of a typhoid outbreak at Wesleyan University, Connecticut, USA, in October/November 1894 was published in the medical press.[26] There had been 25 cases, 13 very severe, with four deaths. None of the 50 women students at the college had suffered: the damage had been done at a series of fraternity suppers held during freshman initiations on 12 October. This was the first major outbreak of oyster-borne typhoid recorded. In the words of Wesleyan's biology professor Herbert W. Conn, who investigated the outbreak for the State Board of Health, it was 'especially interesting . . . a more typical example of an outbreak of typhoid due to a single source of infection has hardly been found in the history of medicine, and the example furnishes a demonstration of a new source of danger for this disease'.[27] Conn's conclusion was stark: 'One thing is sure. The public health is placed in jeopardy when oyster dealers, for the sake of producing plumpness, place oysters in the mouths of freshwater creeks in close proximity to sewers.'[28] Never mind the current English worries over sewage-polluted oyster layings: in Britain as in America, it was a common belief among oyster cognoscenti not only that sewage was rendered harmless by sea water, but also that it was beneficial in fattening and enhancing the flavour of shell-fish destined for the table.[29]

The accumulated effect of these revelations, all published in the *British Medical Journal* during January 1895, was an immediate and thorough-going food scare—an early example of the effectiveness of a media and medical generated food scare in changing popular patterns of consumption both temporarily and in the longer term.[30] Such scares seem largely to be associated with widely available foods which are not subject to technical controls (as water and milk became) such as, at various times, shell-fish, eggs, and beef. Victorian oysters were subject to no regulation, and as late as March 1896, in a month when business was normally buoyant, the oyster trade was reported to be 'almost at a standstill'.[31] Already on 12 January the *FTG* had lamented of the medical journals,

> Will they ever have done with scaring the public? . . . The *British Medical Journal* . . . will make our grey hair go down in sorrow to the grave. And all on account of oysters . . . Are the public to forego oysters at the bidding of medical alarmists at the end of the nineteenth century? Why the very idea is absurd.[32]

26 Annotation, 'Typhoid fever and oyster eating', *BMJ* (1895), i: pp. 92–3 (12 January).

27 'Copy of a report on an outbreak of typhoid fever at Wesleyan University by Professor H. W. Conn', BPP, 1896, xxxvii, Appendix 3, p. 274.

28 'Copy of a report', p. 285. For Conn, see Henry J. Conn, 'Professor Herbert William Conn and the founding of the Society', *Journal of Bacteriology*, 12 (1948): pp. 275–96.

29 James G. Bertram, *The Harvest of the Sea, a Contribution to the Natural and Economic History of the British Food Fishes* (1865), p. 374.

30 See T. Baird, 'Some notes on the purification of oysters', *Medical Officer*, 88 (1952): p. 203.

31 'The English oyster scare', *FTG*, 16 March 1895, p. 13.

32 'Oh, those medical papers', *FTG*, 12 January 1895, p. 8.

By mid-February, however, the tone was less ebullient. The oyster, it was reported, was ill in bed and unlikely to get up for some time. Time was, the writer declared, when the medical profession 'gave us a lift'. Now it had laid down a law that 'every bi-valve is a bacillus in ambush, consequently the public won't buy the bi-valve any more'.[33] The impact of the scare was later confirmed by the Medical Department's investigator. The English oyster trade had been temporarily paralyzed, with such severe financial loss to the oyster merchants and their staff that representations had been made to the Board of Trade. Not only public health was at stake as a result of the oyster merchants' practices and the recent medical revelations, but also the future of that large national industry.[34]

The Medical Department's response to this crisis, although stated to be the result of the 1893 cholera inquiry, was to undertake an inquiry into conditions in the English coastal oyster industry, supplemented by a bacteriological investigation of the various known pathogenic 'sewage' organisms in relation to oysters. This was notably more comprehensive than the Department's contemporary response to reports of meat-poisoning and contaminated milk: it involved both the traditional epidemiological survey—the coastal inquiry—and utilization of bacteriology in exploring the economy of potential pathogenic organisms in nature. It seems likely that the human dimension of the problem facilitated this broader investigative approach: here was a direct connection to existing problems of sewage management and disposal. It had, indeed, already been noted in this connection that 'man had only himself to blame . . . the mollusc was only the unwilling vehicle of infection'.[35] Whereas the possible environmental sources of *Salmonella* infections in animals potentially led medical epidemiologists into the uncertainties of veterinary epidemiology (a subject then virtually non-existent), and of professional entanglement with veterinarians and the powerful agricultural industry, in addressing problems created by human excreta they were on home ground.

The Medical Department's inquiry into oyster layings was undertaken by another of its star investigators, Herbert Timbrell Bulstrode, who had joined the Department in 1890, not long after qualifying as an MD. Published in November 1896, the inquiry offered a thorough survey of the English oyster industry, as well as a detailed account of the local conditions existing in oyster beds around the coasts of England and Wales.[36] Bulstrode investigated 54 sites with exemplary thoroughness, but his conclusions were not entirely satisfactory: it was difficult to demonstrate any substantial risk of sewage pollution in most of the layings examined, but only a few of them could be held to be free of the possibility of chance infection. In

[33] 'The oyster's lament', *FTG*, 16 February 1895, p. 14.

[34] MOAR, LGB, BPP, 1896, xxxvii, 'Supplement to the Medical Officer's twenty-fourth annual report, on oyster culture in relation to disease', p. 30 (hereafter 'Oyster culture').

[35] H. J. Lewis-Johnston, 'The possible conveyance of certain water borne diseases, especially typhoid fever, by oysters and other molluscs', *BMJ*, 1895, i: p. 559.

[36] Herbert Timbrell Bulstrode, 'Report on an inquiry into the conditions under which oysters . . . are cultivated and stored along the coast of England and Wales', BPP, 1896, xxxvii, Appendix no 1, pp. 29–198. For Bulstrode see Anon, 'Herbert Timbrell Bulstrode', *Lancet*, 1911, ii: pp. 332–4.

the event, Bulstrode condemned 14 layings and approved 8, finding 22 to be associated with various degrees of risk. Although commended for its 'unbiased character' by both the *Lancet* and the *BMJ*, in the hope that it would serve to draw public and official attention to the issue, the latter was concerned lest, by apparently minimising the risks of direct sewage contamination, the whole question should be 'put back'.[37] Bulstrode's report was a miracle of scrupulous, almost loving, attention to the detail of the coastal environment and the condition of shell-fish in the layings investigated, but the responses from the fish trades would confirm his findings to be a mixed blessing.

Bulstrode's report was accompanied by Edward Emmanuel Klein's inquiry into the bacteriology of oyster-borne disease.[38] Although Klein was a controversial figure, who often got things wrong, his bacteriological work 'as applied to sanitary science' was recognized to have permanent value.[39] Unlike Bulstrode's pioneering investigation, Klein's was not a new area of inquiry. The first experiments on the survival of cholera and typhoid bacilli in sea water had been published in 1889. Both had survived three to four weeks in sterilized sea water, but rapidly disappeared in the natural medium—a result attributed to an unsuccessful evolutionary struggle with other water organisms, apparently endorsing the tradition of the purifying sea. By the mid-1890s, further confirmatory and contradictory studies had been published, and the problematic nature of available bacteriological techniques in securing dependable results recognized.[40] Yet the question of the viability of these organisms in sea water remained, and was recognized to be important because, as the *BMJ*'s investigator phrased it, 'those interested in denying the possibility of infection through oysters have made use of these results in support of their statements'.[41] It was in this context that Klein's investigation was of special significance. Although Klein was able to add judicious weight to existing research indicating that shell-fish could carry the infections of typhoid, cholera, and gastroenteritis, he was only able to detect the typhoid bacillus itself once in a number of oysters placed in contaminated water. It was a result which Thorne Thorne confessed to finding disappointing. The bacteriologist, Thorne Thorne concluded, 'can . . . tell us of impurity and hazard—often indeed, of the precise nature of specific hazard—but not of purity and safety'. For these desiderata, in his view, observational epidemiology was the answer: 'We must go, with the aid of what the bacteriologist has been able to teach us, in search of the conditions surrounding and affecting the culture and storage of oysters along our coasts.'[42] For the expert assessors in the Medical Department, bacteriology offered indicative not confirmatory knowledge.

37 Editorial, 'Oysters and disease', *BMJ*, 1896, ii: p. 1663.

38 'Report by Dr Klein on his bacteriological researches', MOAR, LGB, BPP, 1896, xxxvii, Appendix no 2, pp. 109–51.

39 The most informative of his obituaries is that by William Bulloch, 'Emmanuel Klein, 1884–1925', *Journal of Pathology and Bacteriology*, 28 (1925): pp. 684–97.

40 See G. E. Cartwright Wood, 'Special report to the British Medical Journal on the circumstances under which infectious diseases may be conveyed by shellfish with special reference to oysters', *BMJ* (1896), ii: p. 759.

41 Wood, 'Special report', p. 759.

42 Thorne Thorne, 'Introduction' to 'Oyster culture', p. 26.

THE FISH TRADES AND THE EXPERTS: BACTERIOLOGY IN THE COMMUNITY

The immediate impact of the medical pronouncements of January 1895 suggests the extent to which the public was already sensitized to the idea of oyster-borne illness, as well as the degree of popular anxiety about typhoid. The *BMJ* published its report on typhoid in London on 5 January: by 12 January reports in the *FTG* testified to widespread dismay in the trade, and to the active interest of the press at large.[43] Cartwright Wood's observation of 1896, that interested parties had made full use of conflicting bacteriological evidence, was well substantiated by the *Gazette*'s reportage between January 1895 and the eventual denouement of debate in 1902–3. As the Medical Department was well aware, the shell-fish trades were an important industry, estimated to be worth £2,500,000 a year.[44] As an unregulated industry, the trades were combative and enterprising in their own defence. Among the layings condemned by Bulstrode was that at Southend-on-Sea, an important supplier to the London market, but also a popular holiday destination for East-Enders, for whom shell-fish were traditional celebratory fare. A newspaper attempt in December 1896 to discover whether Southend oysters had been withdrawn from the market as a result of Bulstrode's 'damaging document' ascertained that 4,000 Southend oysters were dispatched to London every day, but their final destination remained a mystery: 'they seemed to disappear somehow en route'. Shopkeepers, it might be inferred, concealed their place of origin.[45] At London Bridge, one dealer was found advertising his stock as 'non-typhoidal oysters', while another in Little Queen Street submitted his to the public analyst and received a certificate of 'absolute purity', which he displayed in his window.[46] The *FTG*, meanwhile, was much dismayed by Bulstrode's condemnations: his reputation was such that his negative opinion was likely to be very damaging to the trade. By way of counter-blast, it suggested that the whole question be referred to scientists at the Marine Biological Laboratory, Plymouth, or to the Scottish Fisheries Board, or indeed to 'The Right Honourable Thomas Huxley' who, during a previous scare, had pronounced there to be no connection between cholera and the consumption of mackerel.[47]

Beleaguered as they were by the collapse of their market, the shell-fish trades were perfectly ready to exploit scientific uncertainties, and to wield denigration as a weapon against the medical profession. The *BMJ*'s fears that Klein's bacteriological report would 'put back' the issue of sewage pollution, for example, were amply justified by subsequent events. Of Thorne Thorne's disappointment at Klein's inconclusive results, the *FTG* noted, 'What would the man have? Would evidence

[43] 'Oh, those medical papers', *FTG*, 12 January 1895, p. 8; 'Typhoid and oysters', *FTG*, 19 January 1895, pp. 6–7.

[44] J. M. Tabor, 'The position of the oyster industry in Great Britain', *FTG*, 9 September 1899, p. 57; Wood, 'Special report', p. 759.

[45] Annotation, 'Oysters and typhoid fever', *BMJ* (1896), ii: p. 1736.

[46] 'Our trawl net', *FTG*, 12 January 1895, pp. 10–11.

[47] 'Our trawl net', *FTG*, pp. 10–11.

that might have ruined an industry been more pleasing to him?' It was more kindly to Klein—'on the whole, Dr Klein has played the part of Balaam, and his report may be used as a counterblast to Dr Bulstrode's alarming indictment': Bulstrode's remarks did not carry the weight they would have done had Klein's research backed them up.[48] And finally and specifically, the *FTG* noted the *BMJ*'s interpretation of the Medical Department report—it suggested that germs were so diluted by sea water that there was little chance of them being absorbed by the oyster: 'We thank thee . . . for teaching us these words.'[49]

The Medical Department's oyster investigations made an immediate issue of polluted shell-fish and how they were to be judged. Medical journals were ranged against the trade, and scientists disputed bacteriological standards of purity and impurity. The *Lancet* promptly suggested the registration of all oyster layings, fattening beds, and storage ponds.[50] The *BMJ* called for the Local Government Board to be empowered to close dangerous oyster beds.[51] The *FTG* expressed a preference for regulation by the Board of Trade, 'which according to the *Lancet* has no expert sanitary advice at its disposal'.[52] The battle lines were clearly drawn between the sanitarians on the one hand, and the fish trades on the other. Bacteriology, however, lay in-between—its uncertainty of expertise laid it open to competitive exploitation by both sides.

Despite a low opinion of doctors and scientists, and of MOHs in particular, the *FTG* was perfectly willing to use science to fight its corner, exploiting the uncertainties of bacteriology, and divisions and disagreements among its practitioners. During the 1890s, the journal repeatedly drew attention to the issues surrounding bacteriological analysis, the methods by which shell-fish (especially oysters) were judged to be safe or hazardous, and techniques for ensuring their purity. Indeed, the bacteriology of shell-fish can here be viewed as an example of boundary territory, in which different forms of expert knowledge competed for responsibility.[53] A favourite fish trade authority was William Abbott Herdman, professor of natural history at Liverpool University, marine biologist and oceanographer, an energetic advocate of co-operation between scientific research and the fishing industry. Herdman had founded the Liverpool Marine Biological Committee in 1885, which in 1887 opened its own research laboratory, initially at Puffin Island, Anglesey, and later at Port Erin, Isle of Man. In 1891, Herdman was brought into yet closer connection with the fishing industry, when he was invited by the newly established Lancashire Sea Fisheries Committee to organize their marine research laboratory at Liverpool, and became their chief scientific adviser.[54] Following the

[48] 'The oyster report II: Dr Klein as Balaam', *FTG,* 19 December 1896, pp. 8–9.

[49] 'The oyster report', pp. 8–9.

[50] Annotation, *Lancet,* 1896, ii: p. 1695.

[51] Editorial, 'Oysters and typhoid fever', *BMJ* (1896), ii: p. 1736.

[52] 'The oyster report III', *FTG,* 26 December 1896, pp. 8–9.

[53] On boundary science see Robert E. Kohler, *Landscapes and Labscapes: Exploring the Lab-Field Border in Biology* (2002); Olga Amsterdamska, 'Demarcating epidemiology', *Science, Technology and Human Values,* 30 (2005): pp. 17–51.

[54] 'Sir William Abbott Herdman (1858–1924)', *Oxford Dictionary of National Biography,* vol vi, pp. 761–2; Anon, 'Sir William Abbott Herdman FRS', *Nature,* 114 (1924): pp. 165–6.

oyster scare of January 1895, Herdman joined with Rubert Boyce, professor of pathology at Liverpool, to research into the effects of pollution on oysters.[55] Their initial results were published in the Lancashire Sea Fisheries Committee's annual report, and emphasised that oysters could be cleaned by natural methods: their occasional transmission of disease germs to humans was not sufficient reason for the public to avoid 'an important and highly-esteemed food matter'.[56] According to Herdman and Boyce, the typhoid bacillus could not flourish in clean sea water, and their experiments 'seemed to show' that it decreased in numbers in its passage along the oyster's alimentary canal. Their preferred cleaning method was the French 'dégorgeoir': tanks of clean water in which oysters were placed for a short while before dispatch to the consumer.[57] In 1897, as befitted a friend of the industry, Herdman again urged 'the exercise of common-sense by the public and of moderation by some sanitary reformers . . . do not insist on conditions which will make it impossible to rear any oysters at all'.[58]

Herdman was clearly identified with fish-trade interests, and from 1898 was working with the newly formed British Oyster Industries Association to ensure improved conditions within the trade. Nonetheless, he sought to maintain the authority of science. 'The oyster, like the woman, is better not to have had a damaged past', he declared in 1898, and that 'more or less damaged character' necessitated that it 'come into court—the scientific laboratories—and request the fullest possible investigation'.[59] In the wider food industries too, Herdman's position was seen as a rational counterbalance to sanitary over-enthusiasm. The journal *Food and Sanitation*, for example, accepted the Herdman/Boyce claim never to have found naturally occurring typhoid bacilli in any oyster, whether obtained from markets or the sea: 'they give the whole case against oysters away'.[60]

The questions of the authority of laboratory findings and of sanitary 'over-enthusiasm' were especially pertinent at the end of the 1890s in regard to the imminent introduction of legislation to regulate the oyster industry. In May 1899, the Local Government Board formulated its Oyster Bill, which provided for the inspection of layings, a ban on removing oysters from unsanitary grounds, and the regulation of oyster imports from abroad, measures which were to be the responsibility of the county and borough sanitary authorities.[61] These authorities were already responsible for sewage disposal: as the fish trades pointed out, they were unlikely to require themselves to undertake the expensive removal or relocation of sewer outfalls. The Bill appeared to take it for granted that the oysters must give

[55] Anon, 'Sir Rubert Boyce MB Lond, FRS', *BMJ* (1911), ii: pp. 53–4.

[56] 'Oysters and "orrors"', *FTG*, 4 April 1896, p. 8.

[57] William A. Herdman and Rubert Boyce, *Oysters and Disease*, Lancashire Sea Fisheries Memoir no 1 (1899), p. 38.

[58] 'Oysters for ever', *FTG*, 13 February 1897, p. 8.

[59] 'The oyster question', *FTG*, 10 September 1898, p. 14.

[60] 'A word to Medical Officers', *FTG*, 6 January 1900, p. 8. According to the British Library Catalogue, *Food and Sanitation* was discontinued in 1893.

[61] Since the bill was not taken forward, it was not printed. For details of this story, see Neild, *The Oyster*, pp. 105–6; Anne Hardy, 'Lord Gifford's oysters: state, trade and the courts in England, 1895–1905', in *Citizens, Courtrooms, and Crossings*, edited by Astri Andresen et al. (2008), pp. 87–94.

way before the sewers, and that the outfalls must not be interfered with; there was no suggestion of any possible compromise or of compensation to oyster growers for loss of business.[62] And who was to decide whether the risk of pollution was serious, or not worth troubling about? The local fish trades clearly did not trust local MOHs to act impartially.[63] Both the British Oyster Fisheries Association and the National Sea Fisheries Protection Association objected.[64] In July the Bill was referred to a Select Committee, and in August withdrawn: in a pattern common in food regulation, the Committee had substituted an interested organization, the local Sea Fisheries Committees, for the LGB as supervisory authority—a solution which the Board of Trade found impractical.[65]

The central issue of the Oyster Bill lay in the interests represented by the potential supervisory authorities. The Local Government Board and its delegates were seen to act in the interests of human health; the Sea Fisheries Committees in the interest of the fish. Proponents of the former were angry,[66] but a stalemate had been reached, and this was recognized in the abandonment of the Bill. Moreover, the newly established (1888) County Councils were beginning to take steps to combat river pollution, and there were signs that the oyster industry too was beginning to take remedial action: in Kent and Essex, the Sea Fisheries Committees were standardly opposing new sewerage schemes that were likely to contaminate oyster beds, and a number of independent oyster bedders also took action; even the British Oyster Trades Association was reported to have begun to flex muscle.[67] Launching an offensive, the *FTG* declared in February 1901 that nearly all oyster beds in England had been purified.[68] By September 1901, the trade was beginning to feel more secure. First, it had been established that the Sea Fisheries Committees had the power to forbid the deposit of crude sewage in areas under their jurisdiction; second, the court case of Lord Gifford versus the City of Chichester had determined that sanitary authorities could be deemed responsible for damaging sewer discharge and made to pay compensation; and third, the Board of Trade had declared that all new sewage schemes were liable to be disapproved unless they satisfied the requirements of the Board and of the Fisheries Committees as to the purity of the effluent.[69]

The trades also responded to the scientific threat. Early in 1901, the *FTG* began to instruct its readers in the language of bacteriology: 'a subject but little

62 'The Government's Oyster Bill', *FTG*, 20 May 1899, p. 12.

63 'The Oyster Bill', *FTG*, 27 May 1899, p. 14; 'The Oysters Bill—objections from Essex', *FTG*, 17 June 1899, p. 18.

64 'Our trawl net', *FTG*, 24 June 1899, p. 13.

65 'Fish trades in parliament', *FTG*, 5 August 1899, p. 9. See also Nield, *The Oyster*, pp. 105–6. For similar results in milk regulation see Keir Waddington, *The Bovine Scourge: Meat, Tuberculosis and Public Health, 1850–1914* (2006), pp. 171–3.

66 See Annotation, 'The Government Oysters Bill', *Lancet*, 1899, ii: pp. 295–6; Annotation, 'Mr Chaplin's Oyster Bill', *Lancet*, 1899, ii: pp. 351–2; Annotation, 'Amendments to the Oysters Bill', *BMJ*, 1899, ii: p. 294; Annotation, 'The abandoned Oysters Bill', *BMJ*, 1899, ii: pp. 421–2.

67 'The oyster trade', *FTG*, 15 December 1900, p. 23; *FTG*, 29 December 1900, p. 17. For action against river pollution see Hassan, *History of Water*, pp. 35–9.

68 'The oyster trade', *FTG*, 9 February 1901, p. 27.

69 'The oyster trade', *FTG*, 7 September 1901, p. 15.

known to oyster dealers, but one which, in their business, is continually cropping up.'[70] The frequent conjunction of oysters and microbes in press reports, the journal noted, made it important for the trade to be familiar with the action of bacteria, and of typhoid bacteria in particular. A series of five 'discussions' followed, dealing with bacteria generally, typhoid bacilli, the work of scientists demonstrating that 'typhoid bacilli do not flourish in sea water' and the virtual absence of bacteria in general in fresh oysters, the distribution of typhoid bacteria in nature, and the action of septic tanks in rendering sewage harmless. How effective this educational effort proved remains uncertain, but in 1904, in the midst of yet another oyster crisis, one of the *FTG*'s correspondents noted how the enforced idleness of the oyster merchants had encouraged them to inform themselves on bacteriological subjects: 'The readiness with which the crack-jawed names of different bacteria are bandied about . . . and the depth of knowledge and the subtlety of argument displayed, raise an apprehension as to whether oyster merchants will not all take to bacteriology as a profession.'[71] For the oyster trade at least, joining the bacteriologists had become an alternative to beating them.

THE FISH TRADES AND PUBLIC OPINION

The importance of learning the language of bacteriology was underscored by the oyster traders' experience through the 1890s, which amply demonstrated that both press and public were highly sensitive to the risk of typhoid, and that the influential public health lobby listened to the pronouncements of bacteriologists. Initially, the *Fish Trades Gazette* took a robust attitude towards critics of the shell-fish trades, which it kept up for much of the 1890s. It was, for example, adept at picking up and republishing the opinions of other contemporary newspapers and journals.[72] Thus it quoted the sensationalist London paper *The Star*, which, it claimed, had summed up the Medical Department Report 'in one Anglo-Saxon word—Rot!' In the *Star*'s opinion, 'We are not a bit awed at the learned twaddle of these well-meaning bacteriologists, who would find microbes in heaven, and would have issued a report condemning manna if they had been employed by Moses to report upon its collection and storage.'[73] The *Star* clearly had a low opinion of bacteriologists (as well as a respect for Moses), for months later it was poking fun at 'medical oysteria', declaring that 'if Dr Klein had been a contemporary of Moses he would have found bacilli in the water that gushed from the rock'.[74] On accumulated evidence, including the reported opinions of its contemporaries, the *FTG*

70 'The oyster trade', *FTG*, 1 April 1901, p. 27.

71 'Our trawl net—Oyster merchants in a new profession', *FTG*, 9 January 1904, p. 18. There are parallels here with the uses made of bacteriology by anthrax-affected workers and typhoid-affected civilians: see Rosemary Wall, *Bacteria in Britain, 1880–1939* (2013), chapters 3 and 6.

72 Or even of inventing them: see n. 60.

73 'Our trawl net', *FTG*, 19 December 1896, p. 9.

74 'Our trawl net', *FTG*, 18 September 1897, p. 9.

had decided, by December 1896, that the Medical Department was 'ignorant and short-sighted'.[75]

Beyond the bacteriologists and the Medical Department, the *FTG*'s writers took a particularly dim view of MOHs, perhaps considering them an inferior variety of medical practitioner and playing on differences in expertise.[76] Dr Laing of Cowpen, Northumberland, was 'an irresponsible person' for attributing typhoid to mussels from the river Blyth.[77] In December 1896, MOHs were accused of trying to foster the oyster scare: 'Who on earth is Dr A. Wynter Blyth, Medical Officer of Health for Marylebone, that we should accept him as an authority?'[78] The paper became increasingly truculent about 'medical alarmists'—a view that stayed with it for many years. In 1900, for example, it reprimanded the MOH for Folkstone for blaming typhoid on oysters from Whitstable: although a bacillus 'common to sewage' had been found, the typhoid bacillus had not—'there is no reliable evidence whatsoever that the disease was so caused'. This was in line with the contemporary debates and uncertainties on the precise relations between sewage contamination, specific disease organisms, and proof of dangerous contamination of food and water, and the *FTG* made it the vehicle for a more generalized attack on the public health administration, and on the medical profession as a whole, flagging, it seems, medicine's lack of specific scientific expertise against its favoured experts, the bacteriologists:[79]

> This was another illustration of the haphazard way in which many medical officers accept unhesitatingly, and repeat, statements which, to a critical mind, would not be accepted for a moment without verification. The cause of this ready belief is probably because medicine is not a science. Medicine is based on empiricism and not on rationalism, and men trained to believe what they are told by authority, without reasons being adduced to support statements they are asked to believe, are liable to carry this uncritical and unsceptical mental receptivity with them in all the questions with which they are called upon to deal.

In picking up on weaknesses in medical logic, the *FTG* was, like other opponents of public health expertise such as the anti-vaccinationists, seeking to exploit and undermine medical authority to its own advantage.[80]

The trade line on the general public and the influence of the press on popular opinion was no more flattering than its opinion of the medical profession. Columnist P. Quant declared that it 'takes very little to frighten the public. A couple of

[75] 'Oyster report III', *FTG*, 26 December 1896, pp. 8–9.

[76] For MOHs' variable expertise see Jeanne Brand, *Doctors and the State. The British Medical Profession and Government Action in Public Health* (1965), pp. 109–11.

[77] 'Our trawl net', *FTG*, 2 May 1896, p. 9.

[78] 'Our trawl net', *FTG*, 26 December 1896, p. 10. Alexander Wynter Blyth was an eminent MOH and public analyst, holding the combined post for Marylebone from 1882 to 1912, and Analyst to 1921: Anon, 'Alexander Wynter Blyth', *Journal of the Chemical Society, Transactions*, 119 (1921): pp. 546–7.

[79] 'The oyster trade', *FTG*, 17 November 1900, p. 86.

[80] See for example Nadja Durbach, *Bodily Matters: The Anti-vaccination Movement in England, 1853–1907* (2005), pp. 150–69.

paragraphs in the medical papers extensively copied into other journals throughout the country are quite sufficient to ruin a good industry'. The medical press, he admitted, had to live: 'it can only live by working up sensations of some kind or another'. If the medical press were self-interested promoters of damaging allegations, the public was sadly gullible: 'People nowadays do not think for themselves—they allow the newspapers to do all their thinking for them. We are a nervously over-excitable people.'[81] Publicity in the lay press, whether in newspapers or other journals, was clearly thought important in shaping popular opinion and the fortunes of trade. In 1900, for example, the *FTG* welcomed an item in the *Daily Express* headed 'Oysters Acquitted', which summarized the report of the British Oyster Industries Association and indicated that conditions of oyster culture had significantly improved: 'More of this kind of publicity is required.' As the *FTG* specifically noted, 'Now that the trade is practically, if not absolutely purified, the public certainly ought to be informed, both for their own benefit and for the benefit of the trade.'[82]

The Oyster Industries Association, founded like so many food and farming organizations to safeguard the interests of the trade,[83] came in for repeated criticism for not doing enough to publicize improvements. In particular, the *FTG* felt that action should be taken at the beginning of the oyster season in August—which happened to coincide with the British Medical Association's annual meeting. Inevitably, papers on typhoid were read at the latter, 'in all of which reference is made to oysters', which the daily press then seized on, resulting in the annual renewal of the oyster scare.[84] As the trade remained depressed through 1901 and 1902, the calls became more urgent:[85]

> Improving the trade depends upon *publicity*. It was by the public condemnation of oysters that the trade was reduced . . . if public condemnation took five or six years to reduce the trade to its present level it will take forty years to restore it to its previous level if the fact that oysters are clean remains unpublished.

There were signs of recovery at the beginning of the 1902 season, and a degree of equilibrium appeared to have been reached.[86] The *FTG* responded sharply to the publication of Klein's latest researches into typhoid in cockles and mussels, demonstrating its grasp of contemporary bacteriological understanding: Klein's research was conducted in the laboratory, it noted, 'which in no way imitates the conditions found in nature', where sunlight and harmless bacteria combined to destroy potential pathogens. Given this fact, the great majority of mussel beds must be

[81] P. Quant, 'Fish snacks', *FTG*, 6 November 1897, p. 10.

[82] 'The oyster trade', *FTG*, 15 December 1900, p. 23.

[83] Thus the National Federation of Butchers and Meat Traders Associations was founded in 1888 to defend butchers against prosecutions for the sale of tuberculous meat: see Waddington, *Bovine Scourge*, p. 90. The Federation's other interests are chronicled in Richard Perren, 'Filth and profit, disease and health: Public and private impediments to slaughterhouse reform in Victorian Britain', in *Meat, Modernity and the Rise of the Slaughterhouse*, edited by Paula Young Lee (2008), pp. 127–50.

[84] 'The oyster trade', *FTG*, 10 August 1901, p. 35.

[85] 'Shell-fish trade at Billingsgate', *FTG*, 8 February 1902, p. 28–9.

[86] 'Shell-fish trade at Billingsgate', *FTG*, 23 August 1902, p. 29; *FTG*, 18 October 1902, p. 29.

free from pollution.[87] Yet despite the vigorous claims of the *FTG*, and stirrings to action among oyster bedders and the Oyster Industries Association, 'practically, if not absolutely purified' proved not to be good enough. A seminal crisis broke over the English oyster industry in December 1902.

CRISIS, 1902

Mayoral banquets were an integral part of the annual tradition of local government in provincial England, and they commonly took place in the late autumn, in the last week of November. Within weeks of the banquets held at Southampton and Winchester in November 1902, typhoid had broken out among the guests who had assembled at the different feasts. At Winchester 63 people fell ill and four died, and at Southampton 55 fell ill. At Portsmouth at the same time, 22 persons fell ill after eating oysters from the same source as those supplied to the banquets, although guests at the town's mayoral feast went unscathed: their oysters had come from Whitstable, and not from Emsworth near Chichester.[88] By mid-December, the *Daily Mail* was said to be 'working up' a campaign against Emsworth oysters, and oyster sales had again plummeted. In keeping with the generally short duration of food scares, however, it was later admitted that damage to the Christmas trade had not been as great as expected.[89]

In light of this fresh disaster, the Fishmongers' Company finally took decisive action. The Company's inspectors were instructed to stop the sale of shell-fish coming from any known contaminated source. In late December, therefore, cockles which had been deposited in Lea Creek prior to boiling were banned: bacteriological examination had shown them to be dangerously infected and unfit for human consumption.[90] Although this prohibition applied only to the London markets, it was important to the shell-fish industry generally, as a great many provincial centres were supplied through Billingsgate. The Company was nothing if not thorough. In the months that followed, it instituted a programme of sampling and testing oysters from beds supplying the London market, having them analysed, and closing those reported as likely to endanger public health.[91] By September 1903, even the *FTG* had come round to the idea that all polluted oyster beds must be closed.[92] And finally, the Company appointed Edward Klein as its official bacteriologist, responsible for the testing and monitoring of layings, for devising

[87] 'Shell-fish trade at Billingsgate', *FTG*, 23 August 1902, p. 29.

[88] Herbert Timbrell Bulstrode, 'Report upon alleged oyster-borne enteric fever and other illness following on the mayoral banquets at Winchester and Southampton', BPP, 1904, xxvi, Appendix A no 9, pp. 129–89. For an account of this outbreak from a more economic and administrative perspective see Neild, *The Oyster*, pp. 106–16.

[89] 'Our trawl net', *FTG*, 20 December 1902, p. 19; 'The oyster trade', *FTG*, 27 December 1902, p. 16; 'Oysters for London', *FTG*, 3 January 1903, p. 23.

[90] 'Oysters for London', *FTG*, 3 January 1903, p. 23.

[91] 'Our trawl net: Opening of the oyster season', *FTG*, 8 August 1903, pp. 16–17.

[92] 'Our trawl net—Cleethorpes again', *FTG*, 26 September 1903, p. 19.

bacteriological tests of purity for shell-fish, and for developing methods to ensure that they reached market in a safe and saleable condition.

The bacteriological wrangles were not yet over, however, for the question of just what constituted the measure of safety remained. Over Christmas 1903, the well-established oyster merchants Messrs Gann were prosecuted for selling polluted 'Princess' oysters unfit for human consumption. The case of 'Gann's Princesses' became something of a *cause célèbre* in the trade: it turned on Klein's judgement that the 'B. coli communis' found in considerable numbers in eight of twelve oysters sampled made them 'decidedly sewage polluted, and . . . not fit for human consumption'. On a previous occasion, however, Klein had allowed that the presence of 'small quantities' of the bacteria did not mean the oysters were not 'pure': where was the dividing line? Was it an arbitrary one drawn by Klein himself? If Klein was an eminent bacteriologist, noted the *FTG*, again exploiting the uncertainties and disagreements of bacteriology, so was Alfredo Kanthack, who in 1896 had declared to the British Association that bacillus coli existed everywhere in nature and that it was 'absurd to assume' that its presence in the digestive tract signalled direct faecal contamination.[93] In his recently published report on the mayoral banquet fiasco, moreover, none other than Timbrell Bulstrode had noted,[94]

> Negative bacteriological evidence may be highly misleading, and as regards positive evidence, it is desirable that there should be some agreement among bacteriologists as to the precise significance, both as regards presence and number, of B.Coli Communis and B. Enteritidis Sporogenes before a bacterial standard can be applied either with safety to the consumer or justice to the oyster industry.

A week later, the *FTG* saw its stand on Klein's 'extraordinary ruling' triumphantly justified, when the interim report of the Royal Commission on Sewage Disposal declared itself 'dead against the bacteriological test, seeing no grounds for condemning oysters for the mere presence of b. coli or the like'.[95] Kanthack's opinions were again invoked in direct contradiction to Klein, and his status as a scientist proclaimed: he had been Klein's predecessor at St Bartholomew's Hospital, but also Professor of Pathology at Cambridge. Twisting the truth a fraction, the *FTG* continued: 'When he died, in 1897, he was described in *Nature*, which is the leading scientific journal, as the ablest and most brilliant exponent of bacteriology we possessed.'[96] There was no suggestion that bacteriological understanding might have moved on in the intervening five years—indeed, the evidence did not suggest that it had. A further cynical note on bacteriologists was added by 'a correspondent':[97]

93 'Gann's princesses', *FTG*, 2 January 1904, p. 20. Kanthack, appointed Professor of Pathology at Cambridge University in 1896, was considered one of the 'ablest and most indefatigable' exponents of pathology. See Anon, 'Professor Alfredo Autunes Kathack', *Nature*, 59 (1899): pp. 252–3.

94 Bulstrode, 'Report upon alleged oyster-borne enteric fever', p. 152.

95 'Our trawl net—Royal Commission on Sewage Report', *FTG*, 9 January 1904, p. 18.

96 'Our trawl net—Dr A. A. Kanthack and B.Coli Communis', *FTG*, 9 January 1904, pp. 145–6. For *Nature*'s actual description see n. 93.

97 'Our trawl net–Oyster merchants and a new profession', *FTG*, 9 January 1904, p. 18.

> The competition in the profession does not appear to be keen, for illogical reports seem to pass unchallenged, and the fees appear to be remunerative. Moreover, a little tact and a few contradictory reports enable a bacteriologist employed in any branch of the investigation to keep the ball rolling indefinitely.

When further reading of the Royal Commission report threw up a divergence of opinion between Klein and Alexander Houston, the Commission's chosen bacteriological expert, the *FTG* reported with glee. Klein had told the Commission that his standard was based on the view that the normal oyster did not contain b. coli communis; Houston, however, had examined over one thousand oysters, and found that nearly every one contained that which 'Dr Klein said the normal oyster did not harbour—b. coli communis and allied bacteria'.[98]

The Royal Commission on Sewage Disposal had been appointed in 1898 to inquire into the methods of treating and disposing of sewage. Its fourth report, however, diverged into the issue of the impact of sewage pollution on shell-fish. Its members included a number of eminent scientists and public health experts: Sir Michael Foster MP, founder of the Cambridge School of Physiology, William H. Power, then Chief Medical Officer, Sir William Ramsay (Nobel Prize winner in chemistry, 1904), and Dr James Burn Russell, MOH for Glasgow City (1872–98), and latterly a member of the Scottish Local Government Board. That a Commission with such a membership should come out against Klein's bacteriological standard for oysters, and assent to the proposition that b. coli communis was not significant in public health terms was little short of astonishing. But Alexander Houston's investigations on behalf of the Commission into the ecology of b. coli had demonstrated that the organism was widely distributed in nature, and in areas far removed from sources of human faecal pollution. Although in general oysters stored in pure water contained very many fewer b. coli than those stored in polluted waters, it did happen that the occasional mollusc from these pure waters contained as many as if it had been stored in sewage. The 'mere presence' of b. coli and related bacteria, the Commissioners concluded, was no justification for the wholesale condemnation of shell-fish. And, they warned further, 'It is clear . . . that a single examination of chance samples of oysters might be most misleading as to the bacterial flora of the whole oyster contents of a laying or pond.'[99] This was unwelcome news to the medical community. The *Lancet* reflected the general dismay when observing that the report was remarkable from the purely scientific standpoint: for the first time in the history of bacteriology, 'a check has been administered to that young and vigorous pursuit'. The journal prophesied that the result would be improvements in bacteriological technique, and more careful interpretations in the discipline's 'unfolding of nature's story'.[100]

[98] 'Sewage and shell-fish', *FTG*, 16 January 1904, p. 19. On Sir Alexander Houston FRS, bacteriologist and drinking water expert, see M.H.G., 'Sir Alexander Cruickshank Houston 1865–1933', *Obituary Notices of Fellows of the Royal Society*, vol 1, pp. 334–44; Emma M. Jones, *Parched City. A History of London's Public and Private Drinking Water* (2013), pp. 105–21.

[99] Royal Commission on Sewage Disposal, Fourth Report, BPP; 1904, xxxvii, pp. 32–3.

[100] 'Our trawl net', *FTG*, 23 January 1904, p. 21.

TOWARDS A RESOLUTION

Yet if the Royal Commission report was seen as a set back for bacteriology, there was little evidence on the ground, in the ongoing polluted shell-fish drama, that this was so. The Fishmonger's Company showed no sign of having their faith in Klein undermined, and continued to retain his services. The trades themselves soon had cause to be grateful to Klein's research. In 1905, at the Company's instigation, Klein published the results of experiments undertaken to assess the vitality of typhoid bacilli in oysters, cockles, and mussels.[101] He was able to demonstrate that the numbers of typhoid bacilli in oysters were greatly reduced after four days in water changed every day, and disappeared after six days. Similar experiments on cockles and mussels were, however, much less satisfactory. As regards oysters, the trade found this result 'welcome and reassuring', but it was still not enthusiastic about bacteriologists: 'What we really want is that bacteriologists should be tried by a jury of their peers.' Klein's research indicated, however, that there was no reason to restrict the sale of oysters from any area, however polluted, provided that they had first been placed in clean sea water, changed frequently, 'for a given period to be decided on'.[102] On balance, the *FTG* concluded, the trade 'cannot fail to be grateful to the Fishmongers' Company'.[103]

Klein's name remained closely associated with the bacteriology of shell-fish for several decades. The Fishmongers' Company was anxious to develop bacteriological controls for shell-fish that would both protect the consumer and be flexible enough to meet the needs of the trade in assessing the hygienic quality both of layings and of supplies for the retail market. Two different tests were adopted, which remained in use into the 1930s.[104] The first was Klein's 'Short Method', suitable for the assessment of shell-fish in the market, because results could be obtained within 24 hours or so. Using b. coli as the index of cleanliness (despite all previous reservations), the proportion of contaminated oysters in a sample of ten provided the guideline for cleanliness. Any sample containing 30 per cent or fewer clean fish was rejected; those at 40–50 per cent clean were subjected to further analysis, and then if required a review of the topography of the layings from which they came; samples rating 60 per cent and above clean were 'safe' for market. For the evaluation of conditions in shell-fish layings, Alexander Houston's 'Long Method' was favoured. Far more complex than Klein's in technique, results were only obtained after a period varying between seven to ten or 14 days.[105] If the conclusions of the Royal Commission revealed divisions between bacteriologists and sharpened the search for bacteriological standards for evaluating sewage pollution in shell-fish, it was less successful in moving the administrative authorities towards reforming techniques of sewage disposal, or in developing an administrative

[101] Edward Klein, *Report of Experiments and Observations on the Vitality of the Bacillus of Typhoid and of Sewage Microbes in Oysters and Other Fish* (1905).

[102] 'Dr Klein's report', *FTG*, 29 July 1905, p. 16.

[103] 'B. coli communis', *FTG*, 5 August 1905, p. 16.

[104] John H. Eyre, *Bacteriological Techniques*, 3rd edn (1930), pp. 560–1.

[105] Eyre, *Bacteriological Techniques*, p. 559.

framework for the environmental protection of shell-fish layings. The Commission proposed the establishment of separate Rivers Boards under a central administrative and executive authority to administer and enforce the Rivers Pollution Prevention Act 1876, and to police the condition of shell-fish layings.[106] This proposal remained 'in the air'.[107] Various minor attempts to deal with the situation were made by the legislature. The Public Health (Regulations as to Food) Act 1907 enabled the local authorities to make regulations, but it was not until 1915 that the Local Government Board produced the Public Health (Shellfish) Regulations which forbade the sale of shell-fish likely to endanger public health. These offered no guidance to medical officers of health on how to decide whether shell-fish in the market were clean or sewage polluted, and to a large extent remained a dead letter. The safeguarding of British shell-fish supplies against sewage pollution and contamination with pathogenic bacteria remained, essentially, in the hands of the trade itself, and of the Fishmongers' Company.[108]

By the 1920s, the furore over sewage-polluted shell-fish had all but died away, and even two further oyster outbreaks after mayoral banquets at Portsmouth and Wallasey in 1924 seem not to have provoked significant reaction, perhaps because bacteriological evidence was lacking in one case, and the oysters locally sourced in the other.[109] The actions of the Fishmongers' Company, the development of bacteriological tests, and of new commercial techniques for the purification of shell-fish all contributed to a reduction in levels of public anxiety. The events of the years 1895–1905 had not been without their effect, however. Public tastes had begun to change, and to veer away from the consumption of shell-fish as a cheap and easy luxury.[110] New generations of consumers were influenced by the scares, by the warnings of MOHs, even by cooking manuals, to view shell-fish with suspicion and to avoid them, while declining stocks, sharply raised prices, and economic depression in the inter-war period also contributed to reduced consumption.[111] The enormous trade in imported American oysters disappeared and, except in bastions like the East End of London, indulgence in shell-fish as a holiday treat waned. Whereas shell-fish had been an integral part of the holiday culture of Southend and Blackpool in the early years of the century, cockles and oysters had by the inter-war period been replaced as holiday fare by fish and chips.[112] Although the traditional oyster feasts that marked the opening of the oyster season in August continued to be reported, and were reported in *The Times* until just after World War II, the shell-fish trades were in difficulty, partly due also to declining yields

[106] Royal Commission on Sewage Disposal, Fourth Report, pp. 22–8.

[107] John H. Eyre, 'The control and marketing of shell-fish', *Journal of the Royal Sanitary Institute,* 49 (1928–29): pp. 275–82.

[108] Eyre, 'Control and marketing', p. 282.

[109] CMOAR (1924), p. 185; Anon, 'Oysters and paratyphoid', *MO,* 33 (1925): pp. 224–5.

[110] See for instance 'The foods we grew to hate', *The Times,* 15 July 2002, p. 5. 'Deliquescent texture' was cited as a quality which many of these foods, including oysters, have in common; clearly texture is also an element in exciting disgust.

[111] Hardy, 'Molly Malone', pp. 82–6; Neild, *The Oyster,* pp. 146–51.

[112] Notes and Comments, 'Fried fish', *MO,* 50 (1933): pp. 149–50.

from the native oyster layings.[113] The association between typhoid and shell-fish had, however, been deeply implanted in the national psyche. The outbreak of typhoid at Croydon in 1937, which was due to contaminated drinking water, was followed by a serious slump in shell-fish consumption: typhoid was still greatly feared, and any foodstuff popularly associated with its transmission suffered repercussions when the public became alarmed.[114]

The solution to the problem of sewage-contaminated shell-fish was brought about not by central government intervention, or by local authority action, but rather by the efforts of the fish trades themselves, through the Fishmongers' Company, and utilization of the disputed, but nonetheless valued, techniques of bacteriology. Once the problem of disease transmission by contaminated shell-fish had been identified, and as the circumstantial evidence accumulated and public anxiety escalated, so it became imperative for the industry to establish a basis for the retrieval of public confidence. Yet despite the disappearance in the twentieth century of cholera and typhoid as scourges of developed societies, shell-fish continue to generate outbreaks of gastro-enteritis. The immediate causes of infection may lie in the environmental circumstances of layings or in the hygiene of the kitchen where the creatures are prepared. Raw or undercooked shell-fish present a continuing hazard to diners at festive occasions and in restaurants. In recent years, norovirus has more commonly been reported as the infecting agent than typhoid or *Salmonella*, and some outbreaks have attracted much publicity. In January and February 2009, for example, at least 240 diners at a world-class English restaurant were infected with norovirus in what has been described as the world's largest restaurant outbreak. Epidemiological investigation confirmed transmission by oysters contaminated during preparation by infected kitchen staff—agents also blamed oysters for an outbreak of norovirus affecting 63 diners at the restaurant then known as the world's best in Copenhagen, Denmark, in February 2013.[115] By contrast, an outbreak involving over 200 individuals and associated with steamed oysters consumed at a North Carolina restaurant in December 2009 was shown to have been caused by molluscs taken from sewage-polluted layings.[116] While purification methods for raw shell-fish have greatly improved since 1900, sewage pollution and poor kitchen hygiene continue to render them a hazard in the kitchens of the developed world, and the consumption of molluscs gathered from beaches and estuaries remains a risky business also.

113 Neild, *The Oyster*, pp. 139–51.

114 R. W. Dodgson, 'Shellfish and the public health', *Proceedings of the Royal Society of Medicine*, 31.1 (1937–38): p. 925; Editorial, 'Shellfish and the public health', *MO*, 56 (1936): p. 62.

115 Neild, *The Oyster*, p. 117; Richard Milne, '"World's best restaurant" forced to eat humble pie', *Financial Times*, Weekend Section, 9 March 2013, p. 1. For the English outbreak, see A. J. Smith et al., 'A large food-borne outbreak of norovirus in diners at a restaurant in England between January and February 2009', *Epidemiology and Infection*, 140 (2012): pp. 1695–1701. A restaurant run by the same English chef was again in trouble in 2014: <http://www.theguardian.com/lifeandstyle/2014/feb/02/heston-blumenthal-dinner-restaurant-closed-norovirus>, accessed 21 April 2014.

116 Alfano-Sonsey et al., 'Norovirus outbreak', p. 280.

3

Things with Wings

As public health consciousness of the pathways of potential infection that existed in nature for disease transfer to humans expanded from the 1890s, it came to encompass not only fish and shell-fish but also insects, wild fowl, and domestic poultry. The piecemeal process of discovery that proceeded from the observational approach to epidemiology added two further creature-related pathways for *Salmonella* infections in the first three decades of the twentieth century: flies and duck eggs. As with seafood, this creature-related transmission of enteric infection was partly due to human habits and practices. Faecal contamination of natural and built environments by human activity caused otherwise innocent creatures (which might nonetheless themselves have some unpleasant habits) to play a critical part in cycles of infection between human animals. In Victorian cities a horse-dependent transport system and still imperfect disposal systems for human and equine excreta ensured that flies were well supplied with food and breeding grounds. In rural areas, the answering of 'the call of nature' by humans could and did infect local soils, water sources, and water fowl. In both cases human activity created and perpetuated cycles of infection, as is still the case in many areas of the developing world.[1] The public health responses to these two phenomena of infection were very different, and illustrate the ways in which human perceptions of risk may be changed. Flies were linked to the pressing public health issue of infant mortality around 1900 and were the subject of a vigorous public health awareness campaign in the early twentieth century, which focused on the creation of disgust for their habits and built effectively on their fondness for faeces, human and animal. By contrast, duck egg infections attracted little public attention in Britain before much-publicized hospital outbreaks in 1949 and 1950. Since hen eggs were then newly cheap and accessible, a food scare turned into a food trend.

When flies began to be associated with the transmission of typhoid and infant diarrhoea in the years around 1900, the environmental conditions which generated the fly problem fell within the remit of local authority public health departments. As had been the case with shell-fish, once the public health association had been made, efforts were put in train to confirm the pathway in the laboratory. Whatever the strength or weakness of the bacteriological case against flies, the insects' unpleasant habits, and the fact that they were a public and domestic nuisance,

[1] For modern conditions and prevention, see <http://www.who.int/water_sanitation_health/resources/vectorcontrol/en/>; <http://www.who.int/sanitation_health_resources/en/>, accessed 3 June 2014.

enabled the local authorities to take action. By contrast, transmission by duck eggs never became a serious public health issue in Britain. Unlike the fly nuisance, it was not associated with any significant human problem, it could not firmly be associated with disgust, and bacteriological confirmation of the validity of the epidemiological deduction did not produce any determined preventive response.

FLIES, FOOD, AND DIARRHOEA

The existence of transmission links between insects and animals, and insects and humans, was demonstrated first by Patrick Manson's elucidation of the causes of filariasis (1878), second by the discovery of the tick-borne nature of Texas cattle fever by Theobald Smith (1893), and then by Ronald Ross's painstaking discovery of the role of the mosquito in transmitting malaria (1898). While these discoveries belonged essentially to the fields of tropical disease, veterinary medicine, and agricultural entomology, they had their resonances with public health and preventive medicine more generally. As the English pathologist George Nuttall noted in 1899, these 'brilliant researches . . . have at last aroused more general attention to the part which insects play in the propagation of disease'.[2] At this date, however, relatively little work had been done on insects as the carriers of disease. Nuttall himself made a signal contribution by gathering together all the references he could trace into one mighty publication, which became a standard reference point for those interested in the subject thereafter.[3] Also in the years around 1900, the circumstances of war in both Britain and America drew attention to the possibilities of the housefly, *musca domestica*, as a vehicle of infection for enteric diseases.[4] Observations by Walter Reed and his team of investigators during the Spanish–American war (1898) suggested that typhoid was spread among the troops through the agency of flies, although no experimental proof was provided to support the observation.[5] The Cuban campaign of the following year strengthened the suspicion,[6] while British military authorities were making the same connection almost

[2] George H. F. Nuttall, 'The part played by insects, arachnids and myriapods in the propagation of infective diseases of men and animals', *British Medical Journal* (1899), ii: p. 642. Nuttall, later the first Quick Professor of Pathology at Cambridge University, had a lifelong interest in the part played by insects in the spread of disease: George Stuart Graham-Smith, 'George Henry Falkiner Nuttall (1862–1937)', *Journal of Hygiene*, 38 (1938): pp. 129–39.

[3] George H. F. Nuttall, 'On the role of insects, arachnids and myriapods as carriers in the spread of bacterial and parasitic diseases of man and animals', *Johns Hopkins Hospital Reports*, 8 (1900): pp. 1–154. For the importance of this work, see Leland O. Howard, 'A fifty year sketch history of medical entomology', *Smithsonian Report for 1921*, pp. 565–86; Leland O. Howard, 'A history of applied entomology', *Smithsonian Miscellaneous Collections*, 84 (1930): whole issue.

[4] See also John F. M. Clark, *Bugs and the Victorians* (2009), pp. 220–1.

[5] On the American experience see Naomi Rogers, 'Germs with legs: flies, disease and the new public health', *Bulletin of the History of Medicine*, 63 (1989): p. 605.

[6] M. A. Veeder, 'House flies as spreaders of disease in camps', *New York Medical Record*, 54 (1898): pp. 429–30.

simultaneously, first in Ceylon in 1900, and then in South Africa during the Boer War.[7]

A number of scientists and medical men in both England and America had earlier raised concerns about the transmission of disease by houseflies.[8] The discoveries that granular ophthalmia was transmitted by flies, and that the creatures could harbour tuberculosis bacilli in their guts, sharpened medical alertness to the possibility of fly-borne transmission of other infections.[9] In the early 1890s, in the context of resurgent pandemic cholera, the role played by flies in the dissemination of that disease became widely discussed.[10] With meat, shell-fish, and foods such as watercress and ice cream becoming suspect as vehicles of enteric infection in the 1890s, it was perhaps not surprising that British civilian doctors too, perhaps coincidentally, began linking the incidence of typhoid and infant diarrhoea to the seasonality of the common housefly. The Medical Officer of Health (MOH) for Gorton, Manchester, for example, first made this observation in 1898, and by 1903 his colleague at Manchester, James Niven, had begun a series of investigations and inquiries into the matter.[11] Interest among London MOHs was reflected in the LCC MO's annual report by 1907, when Shirley Murphy remarked that although more evidence was needed to confirm the fly transmission of diarrhoea and enteric infection, the sheer physical discomfort caused to human beings justified further effort being made to control the fly nuisance.[12] In 1903 Arthur Newsholme, then MOH for Brighton, whose information was garnered through his department's programme of household inspections and concern for domestic hygiene, graphically described how food in the homes of the poor could hardly escape faecal contamination:[13]

> The sugar used in sweetening the milk is often black with flies which have come from a neighbouring dust-bin or manure-heap or from the liquid stools of a diarrhoeal patient in a neighbouring house. Flies have to be picked out of the half-empty can of condensed milk before its remaining contents can be used for the next meal . . .

[7] Edward L. Munson, *The Theory and Practice of Military Hygiene* (1901), p. 685; Ernest E. Austen, 'The house fly and certain allied species as disseminators of enteric fever among troops in the field', *Journal of the Royal Army Medical Corps*, 2 (1904): pp. 653–65.

[8] Sir John Lubbock, 'The fly in its sanitary aspect', *Lancet* (1871), ii: p. 270; Note, 'The pestiferous fly', *Lancet* (1873), i: p. 156; G. E. Nicholas, 'The fly in its sanitary aspect', letter, *Lancet* (1873), ii: p. 724.

[9] Annotation, 'Flies as carriers of contagion', *Lancet* (1889), ii: pp. 232–3.

[10] M. Simmonds, 'Fliegen und choleraubertragnung', *Deutsche Medicinische Wochenschrift*, 17 (1892): p. 951; C. F. Francis, 'Cholera caused by a fly?', *BMJ* (1893), ii: p. 65; W. Moore, 'Diseases probably caused by flies', *BMJ* (1893), ii: p. 1154; R. Macrae, 'Flies and cholera diffusion', *Indian Medical Gazette*, 29 (1894): pp. 407–12; E. H. Sibthorpe, 'Cholera and flies', *BMJ* (1896), ii: p. 700; W. T. Buchanan, 'Cholera diffusion and flies', *Indian Medical Gazette* (1897): pp. 86–97.

[11] See Nigel Morgan, 'Infant mortality, flies, and horses in later-nineteenth-century towns: a case study of Preston', *Continuity and Change*, 17 (2002): pp. 99–100; MOAR, Manchester (1903), pp. 123, 164–70.

[12] Medical Officer's Annual Report, London County Council (1907), p. 63; Appendix II: 'Report by the Medical Officer presenting a report by Dr Hamer on the extent to which the fly nuisance is produced in London by accumulations of offensive matter'.

[13] MOAR, Brighton (1903), p. 21. For Newsholme's work at Brighton, see John M. Eyler, *Sir Arthur Newsholme and State Medicine, 1885–1935* (1997), chapter 2.

The belief that flies might carry enteric infection rested essentially on traditional epidemiological observation, and on an assumed analogy to cholera. Nuttall, for example, who recorded both bacteriological and observational reports in proof of fly-borne cholera transmission, found them 'absolutely convincing'. Although he admitted that the evidence for fly-borne typhoid transmission had not been worked out as for cholera, he nonetheless felt it 'safe to assume that the experience garnered in connection with cholera also applies to typhoid fever'.[14] Following the traditional, observational method, the reporting that now began on the possible links between flies and enteric infections included such evidence as the greater prevalence of typhoid among mounted troops in India (where the difficulties of sanitary latrine management were notorious) over infantry; the low rates of typhoid fever in Hull, where privy middens were cleaned once a week, compared to high rates in York where they were cleaned once a month; and the coincident seasonal patterns of flies, summer diarrhoea, and typhoid.[15] The MOH for Coventry, investigating in August 1907 the 'inordinate' number of infant deaths in the north-east quarter of his city, where refuse was tipped, was repelled by what he found: 'I have never seen anything like it before . . . they literally swarmed; it was quite impossible for the householders to pick up any food which had not immediately before been covered with flies'.[16] No other cause for the unequal distribution of deaths from diarrhoea in the city was either apparent or needed to be sought, he decided.[17]

Although research into the conveyance of bacteria by flies was being pursued at University College London as early as 1885, bacteriological interest in fly transmission surged once the subject had been raised by public health observers.[18] The bacteriologists got to work, initially in the laboratory, later in the field. Members of the Royal Army Medical Corps were notably assiduous in pursuing this lead, in view of the continuing problems with endemic typhoid in India. In 1902, Major R. H. Firth and Major W. H. Horrocks published the results of their laboratory experiments with flies, as well as with soil and fabric, in transmitting typhoid. In respect of the fly, bacteriological findings confirmed suspicion. The authors concluded,[19]

> ordinary house flies (musca domestica) can convey enteric infecting matter from specific excreta or other polluted material to objects on which they may walk, rest or feed. That such infective matter appears to be attached not only to their heads (mandible probably) but also to their legs, wings, and bodies. It has not yet been proved that the enteric bacillus passes through the digestive tract of the fly.

[14] Nuttall, 'On the role of insects', pp. 30–1.

[15] Major A. R. Aldridge, 'The spread of the infection of enteric fever by flies' *JRAMC*, 3 (1904): pp. 649–51; Major N. Faichnie, 'Fly-borne enteric fever: the source of infection', *JRAMC*, 13 (1909): pp. 580–4; J. E. Sandilands, 'Epidemic diarrhoea and the bacterial content of food', *Journal of Hygiene*, 6 (1906): p. 90.

[16] E. H. Snell, 'Insanitation and infantile mortality', *Journal of the Royal Institute of Public Health*, 16 (1908): p. 16.

[17] Snell, 'Insanitation', p. 17.

[18] W. H. Symons, 'Flies and refuse heaps', *Journal of the Sanitary Institute*, 37 (1916): p. 128.

[19] Major R. H. Firth and Major W. H. Horrocks, 'An inquiry into the influence of soil, fabrics and flies in the dissemination of enteric fever', *BMJ* (1902), ii: p. 941.

At this date, however, very little was known of the habits and natural history of the housefly.[20] As Canadian Dominion entomologist Charles Gordon Hewitt later recalled, when asked, around 1904, for information about the housefly, he was surprised to find that existing knowledge on the insect was 'extremely meagre'.[21] That inquiry started Hewitt on an investigative track that culminated in 1912 in the publication of his popular and widely influential study of the habits of *musca domestica* and its role in spreading disease.[22]

Hewitt was not the only investigator to develop an interest in the housefly in these years. In 1906, Liverpool Corporation commissioned a special inquiry into the life cycle of the fly, and the nature and extent of its breeding grounds, from Robert Newstead, lecturer in medical entomology at the Liverpool School of Hygiene and Tropical Medicine, and from 1912 Professor of Entomology at Liverpool University.[23] Ernest Austen, who had joined the Natural History Museum's Zoological Department as an entomologist in 1889, also went on to explore the natural history of the fly,[24] and in 1908 the Local Government Board authorized a series of investigations into flies, employing a range of experts in various fields, including Austen; Hewitt; Nuttall; Jephson, of the Quick Laboratory in Cambridge; George Stuart Graham-Smith, later lecturer in bacteriology at Cambridge University; and their own Dr Monckton Copeman.[25] The publications resulting from this enterprise covered several pertinent topics, from the identification of flies found in houses to flies as carriers of infection; the examination of flies for the presence of colon bacilli; their range of flight; their hibernation patterns; and their part in the dispersal of the eggs of parasitic worms.[26] At much the same time, American entomologists such as Leland O. Howard of the US Department of Agriculture also began exploring the natural history of the fly and its role in disease transmission, and launched vigorous anti-fly campaigns in their own country.[27] Military and civilian concern with the role of the housefly in transmitting disease

[20] For the role of entomologists in the 'fly danger campaigns' of the early twentieth century, see Clark, *Bugs*, pp. 216–36.

[21] Charles G. Hewitt, *House Flies and How They Spread Disease* (1912), p. vii. For Hewitt see P. W. Riegert, 'Charles Gordon Hewitt', *Canadian Dictionary of Biography Online*, accessed 17 May 2013.

[22] Hewitt, *House Flies*.

[23] Robert Newstead, *Preliminary Report on the Habits, Life-cycle and Breeding Places of the Common House Fly (Musca domestic Linn) as Observed in the City of Liverpool, with Suggestions as to the Best Means of Checking its Increase* (1907); Robert Newstead, *Second Interim Report on the House-fly, as Observed in the City of Liverpool* (1909). See J. W. Munro, 'Robert Newstead', *Obituary Notices of Fellows of the Royal Society*, 22 (1953): pp. 548–53.

[24] Edward E. Austen, *The House Fly as a Danger to Health and How to Deal with It* (1913).

[25] See MOAR, Local Government Board (LGB) (1909–10), *British Parliamentary Papers* (BPP) 1910, xxxix, p. 31; MOAR, LGB (1910–11), BPP, 1911, xxxii, pp. 68–73; MOAR LGB (1912–13) BPP, 1912, xxxvi, Report by Dr Graham-Smith, Appendix B no 4, pp. 590–615; Report by Dr Graham-Smith, Appendix B no 5, pp. 616–21.

[26] For a brief account of these publications see J. Spottiswode Cameron, 'House flies', *Jnl San Inst*, 35 (1914): pp. 172–3.

[27] Rogers, 'Germs with legs', pp. 605–15. Leland Ossian Howard (1857–1950), Director of the Entomology Division of the US Department of Agriculture, 1894–1927: see *Encyclopaedia Britannica* online; Arnold Mallis, *American Entomologists* (1971), pp. 79–86.

was, within the space of a decade, translated into a new scientific subdiscipline—domestic medical entomology—which adopted, as did medical entomology generally, the relatively new scientific perspective of bionomics: the study of the life of organisms in their natural habitat, and their adaptation to their surroundings.[28]

FLIES AND THE URBAN ECOLOGY

In preventive and epidemiological terms, biological interest in the fly centred on its breeding and feeding habits. Considered in terms of natural history, shell-fish became harmful through human carelessness, whereas flies became so through their own habits. *Musca domestica* breeds in the warmth of stored manure or fermenting refuse. The whole cycle from egg-laying to fly emergence takes between ten days and two months depending on warm or cold weather, and it is an omnivorous feeder, with a preference for animal and human excreta, carrion, and any accessible foodstuffs. 'Born in a dunghill', wrote the director of the Lister Institute graphically in 1913, 'it spends its days flitting between the sugar basin, milk pan, and any faecal matter available'.[29] In partially modernized Victorian cities, in a horse-centred economy, domestic flies found generous provision both for breeding and feeding, as they also did on battlefields and in military encampments, especially in the tropics. In the first decade of the twentieth century, the disposal of human and animal excreta, as of urban wastes, remained an imperfect practice. Horse manure and stable litter not only accumulated at a frightening rate, but were economically valuable: to a man keeping just one horse, Nigel Morgan has noted, a midden stack could be worth 30 shillings a year.[30] Local authorities across the country kept depots for the storage of town refuse before sorting and disposal, and these were often notorious as noisome breeding grounds for countless swarms of flies.[31]

Nor were horses the only problem. In towns where the water carriage of human wastes had not yet been achieved, privies, ashpits, and middens provided ample fly access to human excreta, especially where accumulations were not removed more often than once every few months. In Morgan's case study, for example, Preston ashpits were emptied once in three, six, or twelve months, and it was not until 1905 that they were emptied once a week.[32] Where the training of urban man remained defective, yards, pavements, and floors were also used for excretory purposes. This was especially true for young children. The MOH for Mansfield found that even

[28] On the history of medical entomology see Howard, 'History', p. 465 *et seq.*; see also John F. M. Clark, 'Sowing the seeds of economic entomology: houseflies and the emergence of medical entomology in Britain', in 'Insects and illnesses: contributions to the history of medical entomology', edited by Mario Coluzzi et al., *Parassitologia*, 50 (2008): pp. 321–8. 'Bionomics' is a now rarely used term for ecology.

[29] Charles J. Martin, 'Insect porters of bacterial infections', *BMJ* (1913), i: p. 2.

[30] Morgan, 'Infant mortality', p. 101.

[31] Symons, 'Flies and refuse heaps', pp. 128–35.

[32] Morgan, 'Infant mortality', p. 110.

where water closets were provided, children in some families used floors or pavement.[33] And finally, urban slaughterhouses and knackers' yards were also noted as sites of prolific fly density. Flies caught by Liverpool health department staff in the slaughtering room of a knacker's yard—the most unsavoury site investigated—carried the theoretically impossible load of a million million bacteria in their guts, while those caught in eating houses close to slaughterhouses also carried enormous loads.[34]

There was no disputing either that domestic flies had ample access to foods intended for human consumption, although this was more especially the case in poor districts, where the fly populations were much denser, as was found in Coventry, Brighton, and Liverpool.[35] Indeed, investigation showed that town-bred flies rarely travelled far from the localities where they hatched, because that was where food was plentiful.[36] In poorly furnished houses, in the age before domestic refrigeration, foodstuffs were often kept uncovered on tables or other surfaces, sometimes outside the back door, and were open to attention from flies, as was food exposed in shops and on stalls.[37] By 1912, scrupulous bacteriological investigation had shown that, while flies did carry bacteria on their heads, bodies, and legs, they also defecated very frequently, at least ten times an hour, and regularly regurgitated the contents of their crops (vomit drops).[38] The last two characteristics were considered probably to be the most important pathways of infection, as externally carried bacteria would soon die from exposure to light and air. Modern research has shown the vomit drop to be the more significant medium of infection, and also that the fly gut is not in fact a favourable environment for *Salmonella* organisms.[39] In all, as Charles Martin noted, 'the fly's 'hairy, probably sticky feet and the habit of regurgitating and defecating at frequent intervals suggests it to be an excellent inoculating agent for any bacteria it may pick up in the satisfaction of its unsavoury tastes'.[40]

Nonetheless, the evidence incriminating flies as major transmitters of infant diarrhoea and enteric diseases remained circumstantial.[41] Although laboratory experiments repeatedly demonstrated that houseflies were capable of carrying pathogenic bacteria on their bodies and in their guts, these studies were problematic since they were conducted using artificially infected flies. 'Wild flies', however, carried so many 'allied, almost indistinguishable types' of bacteria in their guts that

33 Owen H. Peters, *Observations on the Natural History of Epidemic Diarrhoea* (1911), pp. 60–2; G. Lissant Cox et al., 'The number and varieties of bacteria carried by the common house-fly in sanitary and insanitary city areas', *Jnl Hyg*, 12 (1912): p. 302.

34 Cox et al., 'Numbers and varieties', p. 302.

35 Sandilands, 'Epidemic diarrhoea', p. 90.

36 Cox et al., 'Numbers and varieties', p. 303; Charles G. Hewitt, 'Observations on the range of flight of flies', *Reports on Public Health and Medical Matters*, New series no 66 (1912).

37 Notes and Comments, 'Dirt in food', *Medical Officer*, 5 (1911): p. 264.

38 George S. Graham-Smith, 'Observations on the ways etc flies carry and distribute pathogenic bacteria', *Reps on PH*, no 53 (1910); Martin, 'Insect porters', p. 2.

39 Martin, 'Insect porters', p. 2; D S Kettle, *Medical and Veterinary Entomology*, 2nd edn (1995), p. 256.

40 Martin, 'Insect porters', p. 2.

41 Notes and Comments, 'Flies and accumulations of manure', *MO*, 5 (1911): p. 201.

isolation and identification were extremely difficult, and required the application of 'all known tests'.[42] By 1912 few experiments had been made with naturally infected wild flies, and still fewer researchers had attempted to count the numbers of bacteria which any one fly might carry.[43] In Liverpool, a concerted effort by local pathologists and bacteriologists to assess the habits and infecting capacities of wild flies in the city brought no conclusive result. It was clear that flies captured in the suburbs, where infant diarrhoea was rare, carried fewer bacteria than those captured in the city, where diarrhoea was common, but the team found it impossible to correlate exactly the numbers and varieties of bacteria carried by inner-city flies with the numbers of cases and deaths from diarrhoea in individual streets.[44] One of the principal difficulties remained, of course, infant diarrhoea's unidentified causal organism. As O. H. Peters noted in his exhaustive study of diarrhoea in Mansfield, direct evidence of fly causation was necessary before the theory warranted practical adoption.[45] In the absence of such evidence, however, medical officers and bacteriologists still sought to establish a connection, as did James Niven in his studies in Manchester. For Niven, flies were the only factor that fitted the essential epidemiological requirement for a transmitting agent whose rise and fall coincided with the rise and fall in the incidence of diarrhoea.[46]

THE DECLINE OF SUMMER DIARRHOEA

The search for the specific bacterial agent of infant diarrhoea had begun early, but proved an exceptionally complex and contentious bacteriological exploration.[47] In the years around 1900, however, death rates from infant diarrhoea became an increasingly sharp preventive concern—partly because they seemed to be holding up the infant mortality rate, which unlike other age-specific death rates stubbornly refused to fall, and partly because political concerns over high levels of infant death were raised by debates over physical degeneration and the prospects of a major European war.[48] Because typhoid death rates had fallen markedly since 1870, and because the disease was known to be spread mainly by contaminated food and water, the possible fly transmission of typhoid attracted little attention from the preventive community.[49] By the outbreak of World War I, infant mortality and infant diarrhoea deaths had alike also developed a steady downward curve, but between 1900 and 1915 their pattern was unsteady enough to keep medical interest focused on the problem. Although summer diarrhoea was a worldwide phenomenon,

42 George S. Graham-Smith, *Flies in Relation to Disease. Non-blood Sucking Flies* (1913), p. 6.

43 Cox et al., 'Number and varieties', pp. 290–1.

44 Cox et al., 'Number and varieties', p. 310.

45 Peters, *Observations*, pp. 143 *et seq.*; 167.

46 James Niven, 'Summer diarrhoea and enteric fever', *Proceedings of the Royal Society of Medicine*, 3 (2) (1909–10): p. 140. John Robertson of Birmingham was also of this opinion: Notes and Comments, 'Flies and diarrhoea', *MO*, 4 (1910): p. 111.

47 See Martin, 'Bacterial porters', p. 4.

48 Deborah Dwork, *War is Good for Babies and Other Young Children* (1987).

49 J. Beatty, 'Summer diarrhoea and infection', *Jnl Roy Inst PH*, 15 (1907): pp. 14–15.

its clinical features were not always identical. In America, by the first decade of the twentieth century, a large proportion of cases had been demonstrated to be due to various dysentery bacilli (*Shigella*), but in London the dysenteries were absent, and expert opinion favoured a causal organism among the *Salmonella*.[50]

English experts admitted that summer diarrhoea might be 'an illness conditioned by several allied bacilli', but were generally united in the view that it was 'a clinical entity pursuing a very definite course', and as such a legitimate study.[51] The 'somewhat definite' group of symptoms characterizing British summer diarrhoea were vomiting, sickness, copious diarrhoea, rice-watery and green stools, and finally convulsions.[52] Moreover, it was not simply an affliction of infants. Many observers emphasized its familial nature.[53] The exact bacterial cause of early twentieth-century British summer diarrhoea remains in doubt, however, and it is possible, even likely, that the causal organism changed over time.[54] In 1938, for example, it was noted that the symptoms now observed in infant diarrhoea were very different from those of the old, fatal *cholera nostras* dominant in the age of fatal summer diarrhoea, although the latter was still occasionally to be found.[55]

The dubious ground that lay between the epidemiologically observed correlation in incidence of summer diarrhoea and fly prevalence, and the failure of the bacteriologists firmly to establish the precise modes and circumstances in which flies delivered a fatal dose of bacteria, was never satisfactorily cleared. The most the bacteriologists could do was to point to the very large numbers of bacteria coming from houseflies struggling in liquid, and the bacterial multiplication that resulted from keeping milk and other foodstuffs at room temperature for prolonged periods after initial infection by flies had taken place.[56] In 1917 it was noted that although bacillary enteritis was often found in flies under natural conditions, in no case had *musca domestica* been demonstrated to be the exclusive vector of any disease.[57] Both the principal authorities writing on house flies after World War II expressed similar doubts. Luther West of Northern Michigan University remarked on 'the terrible hazards to health wherever flies have unrestricted access both to human faeces and human food', but cautioned nonetheless,[58]

[50] John C. G. Ledingham, 'The bacteriology of summer diarrhoea', *Jnl San Inst*, 30 (1909): p. 350; Niven, 'Summer diarrhoea', p. 133.

[51] Niven, 'Summer diarrhoea', p. 133; see also Sandilands, 'Epidemic diarrhoea', p. 91; Peters, *Observations*, pp. 19–23.

[52] Niven, 'Summer diarrhoea', p. 132.

[53] William Johnston, 'The etiology of summer diarrhoea', *Transactions of the Epidemiological Society*, 4 (1876–81): p. 204; Edward Ballard, 'The causation of the annual mortality from "diarrhoea"', MOAR, LGB (Supplement, 1887), BPP, 1889, xxxv, pp. 29–35; William Russell, 'Summer diarrhoea—its cause and prevention', *Journal of State Medicine*, 9 (1901): pp. 141–6, 141; Peters, *Observations*, pp. 11–16.

[54] Maternity and Child Welfare Group, 'Gastro-enteritis in childhood', *Public Health*, 67 (1953–4): p. 88.

[55] Notes and Comments, 'Sonne dysentery', *MO*, 60 (1938): p. 174. See also Notes and Comments, 'Infantile diarrhoea', *MO*, 67 (1942): p. 154.

[56] Cox et al., 'Numbers and varieties', p. 308; Martin, 'Insect porters', p. 6.

[57] William Nicholl, 'Flies and bacillary enteritis', *BMJ* (1917), i: p. 870.

[58] Luther S. West, *The Housefly* (1951), pp. 265, 272.

> A moderate viewpoint on the medical importance of filth-feeding *Diptera* should always be maintained. Flies are rarely the *sole* transmitting agency in any epidemic and in most cases their role, however important, must logically be considered subordinate.

Bernard Greenberg of the University of Illinois similarly emphasized that while flies had, by 1965, been found to harbour 100 different species of pathogenic organisms, and had been accused of transmitting 65 different diseases, including dysentery, salmonellosis, and cholera, the evidence was still only circumstantial.[59] This position has not changed.[60] Critically, as Greenberg pointed out, the human body requires the introduction of at least a million or more bacteria to give a high likelihood of salmonellosis; flies of themselves cannot deliver such a formidable bacterial load by direct contact. Small deposits of infection, probably through vomit drops, in media such as milk and other foodstuffs, can, however, multiply so rapidly in warm weather when foods are not refrigerated that the threshold of infection might quickly be reached.[61]

Despite the lack of binding threads, it has been argued that public health campaigners in America found the concept of fly-borne enteric infection useful as a means of bridging the gap that existed in the public consciousness between Victorian sanitary theory and twentieth-century bacteriology. In making this argument, Naomi Rogers suggests that in nineteenth-century America flies were widely regarded as useful scavengers and friendly domestic insects, and that popular attitudes towards them were transformed as a result of the anti-fly campaigns launched after 1911.[62] In Britain, however, the evidence for such a scenario is more mixed. Evidence for favourable attitudes towards the fly in Britain certainly exists: in 1871 the eminent naturalist Sir John Lubbock reviled an elementary school textbook that declared that 'the fly keeps the warm air pure and wholesome by its swift and zigzag flight', while as late as 1896 Major-General Sibthorpe of the Indian Army considered them useful scavengers that destroyed rather than conveyed cholera infection.[63] There is, however, also evidence for revulsion and exasperation: town refuse depots and the fly populations they generated were the subject of popular complaint by the 1890s, and MOHs reported such observations as 'a perfect plague of flies', 'spent eightpence a week on fly papers, had three over the bed', 'something shocking, couldn't get our food'.[64] The evidence of language also suggests that flies had long been popularly viewed with distaste. The term 'fly-blown', meaning full of flies' eggs, tainted, putrid, impure, dates back to the

[59] Bernard Greenberg, 'Flies and diseases', *Scientific American*, 213(1) (1965), p. 92. Greenberg was a specialist in forensic entomology: see Anthony DeBartolo, 'Fly expert lands amid murder', *Chicago Tribune*, 12 July 1988: <http://www.hydeparkmedia.com/greenberg.html>. For infectious doses of *Salmonella* see American Public Health Association/World Health Organization, *Control of Communicable Diseases Manual*, 19th edn (2008).

[60] Kettle, *Entomology*, pp. 254–5.

[61] Greenberg, 'Flies', p. 96.

[62] Rogers, 'Germs with legs', p. 599.

[63] Annotation, 'The fly in its sanitary aspect', *Lancet*, 1871, ii: p. 270; Notes, 'Cholera and flies', *BMJ* (1896), ii: p. 700.

[64] Cox et al., 'Numbers and varieties', p. 302.

sixteenth century, and the word 'fly-trap' entered the English language in 1855.[65] Charles Dickens provides evidence for the existence of fly traps ('a paper fly-cage') in 1838, and Henry Mayhew was informed that fly papers 'came, generally, into street traffic' in London in the summer of 1848.[66] The very fact that fly papers were commonly available in the streets and grocers' shops of Victorian cities suggests that numerous citizens regarded the fly as more of a nuisance than a sanitary benefit. In 1898, the London County Council introduced new regulations on the storage of stable manure that were designed to reduce the fly nuisance, following which the number of complaints about stables declined.[67] Municipal authorities throughout Britain were engaged in anti-fly campaigns on grounds of the nuisance flies constituted well before the epidemiologists and bacteriologists began gathering ammunition against the fly as a transmitter of disease.

The literary campaign to popularize the evils of the housefly took off in Britain slightly later than in America, in 1912–13 as against 1911, the year which saw the publication of Leland Howard's *The House Fly: Disease Carrier* in the United States. The book was published in England the following year, which also saw the appearance of Charles Hewitt's *House Flies and How They Spread Disease* in the Cambridge Manuals of Science Popular Series. Edward H. Ross's *The Reduction of Domestic Flies* and Edward Austen's *The House Fly as a Danger to Health*, a British Museum publication, appeared in 1913, as did Graham-Smith's more scientific *Flies in Relation to Disease*, again published by Cambridge University Press. Both the Natural History Museum and the journal *Medical Officer*, with a readership among local government staff, designed and marketed anti-fly posters aimed at raising disgust for distribution to health departments, maternal and child centres, and schools. MOHs mounted public campaigns of advice and instruction on anti-fly measures, but continued to take action against accumulating domestic refuse and stable manure. The MOH for York, for example, expressed the view that such measures were much more effective than the 'swat that fly' campaign urged by 'a certain brand of leaflets'.[68] As elsewhere, the York health department's own anti-fly publicity campaign predated the upsurge of interest reflected by the anti-fly publications of 1912–13.

The impact of both the popular anti-fly campaign and the new knowledge of the fly's supposed ability to spread infection are therefore difficult to assess in the British context. The evidence suggests that flies were popularly disliked and regarded as a nuisance well before they became scientifically associated with germs and the transmission of disease. Moreover, the evidence also indicates that rising popular standards of environmental comfort and cleanliness—or reactions against the newly intolerable nuisance that soaring urban horse populations created—had already instigated municipal action against urban fly populations in

[65] *Oxford English Dictionary.*

[66] Charles Dickens, *Oliver Twist* (Penguin edn, 2003), p. 294; Henry Mayhew, *London Labour and the London Poor* (1968), vol 1, p. 435.

[67] MOAR, Kensington (1898), p. 141.

[68] Spottiswode Cameron, 'House flies', pp. 179–81.

the 1890s by regulating the methods and frequency of disposal of stable manure, and improving the efficiency of scavenging and removal of refuse from municipal dumps. Surveying the London scene in 1907, Shirley Murphy reported that the stable manure nuisance was less frequently mentioned by his colleagues than in some previous years. A year later he noted that the removal of stable manure was now being done to the required frequency: three times a week at not less than 24-hour intervals.[69]

Whether such campaigns were sufficiently widespread to have begun to affect fly prevalence by 1900 is a moot point, but one that may perhaps have some bearing on the vexed issue of summer diarrhoea and the decline in infant mortality that set in from around 1901. Horses, stable manure, and flies were inextricably linked, and Britain's urban horse population expanded rapidly in the late nineteenth century thanks to the continued growth of the railway network, which generated a significant demand for onward road transport services for both goods and passengers. F. M. L. Thompson pinpointed 1902 as the year in which Britain's horse population peaked, and Nigel Morgan has linked the rise in Britain's horse population to the sharp rise in deaths from summer diarrhoea that occurred in the 1890s.[70] By 1902, however, horsepower was encountering a serious competitor. Morgan cites Dr Pilkington, MOH for Preston, lamenting in 1907 the difficulty of avoiding urban stable middens as long as there were urban stables, 'until the services of the horse are entirely superseded by the motor engine'.[71] In the first decade of the twentieth century, cars were already having an impact on urban environments. In 1909, Murphy recorded a 'constant decrease' in the amount of stable manure produced in London, as horses were replaced by motor traction.[72] It was a transition hastened during World War I by the army's insatiable demand for horses, and soaring costs of horse fodder at home.[73]

While many factors were probably involved in triggering the beginning of the decline in infant mortality, and by no means all contemporaries accepted the paramount role some suggested for the fly in the causation of summer diarrhoea,[74] the twentieth-century histories of horse, motor car, fly, and diarrhoea do present some intriguing parallels. George Stuart Graham-Smith produced two reports in the inter-war period detailing the coincidental declines of horses, flies, and summer diarrhoea.[75] Using the records of licences issued for horse-drawn vehicles (there are no statistics for the numbers of urban horses), Graham-Smith charted a persuasive

69 MOAR, LCC (1907), p. 83; MOAR, LCC (1908), p. 63.

70 Francis M. L. Thompson, *Victorian England: The Horse-drawn Society* (1970), p. 10; Morgan, 'Infant mortality', p. 127.

71 Morgan, 'Infant mortality', p. 101.

72 MOAR, LCC (1909), p. 75.

73 James Munson, ed, *Echoes of the Great War. The Diary of the Reverend Andrew Clark, 1914–1919* (1985), p. 166.

74 Beatty, 'Summer diarrhoea', p. 16; Arthur Newsholme, 'Domestic infection in relation to epidemic diarrhoea', *Jnl Hyg*, 6 (1906): pp. 139–48; Peters, *Observations*, pp. 87–8.

75 George Stuart Graham-Smith (1875–1950), FRS 1919, was an early protégé of Nuttall with a lifelong interest in flies as vectors of disease: E. T. C. Spooner, 'George Stuart Graham Smith', *Jnl Hyg*, 49 (1951): pp. 13–21.

picture. In 1906–16, the number of horse-drawn vehicle licences fell by one third; between 1916 and 1921 the numbers were almost stable; from 1921 to 1927 they decreased almost uniformly. By 1927, the total stood at less than a quarter the number for 1906. By contrast, the number of motor vehicle licences had increased from 67,000 to nearly 2 million over the same period. The diarrhoea death rate, meanwhile, fell steadily from 1913.[76] Ten years later, Graham-Smith recorded not only a continuing fall in deaths from summer diarrhoea, but also a decrease in horse-drawn vehicles, from 237,342 in 1922 to 14,195 in 1936. By 1936, the number of licensed motor vehicles had reached 2,706,555.[77] By 1925, he suggested, the number of breeding places for urban flies had fallen to such a low level that even in the very hot summers of 1932–5, flies no longer exercised any serious influence on the dissemination of disease.[78]

The decline in infant deaths due to diarrhoea has also been associated with the introduction of safer methods of artificial feeding from the early years of the twentieth century,[79] and with improving maternal and infant care.[80] Historically, the evaluation of the factors driving the decline in infant mortality is complex.[81] While contemporaries admitted complexity, however, it was noted that the fall in diarrhoea mortality was 'dramatic and sudden, far too much so to be accounted to gradual improvement in hygiene and infant care', and that it could be correlated 'with great nicety' to the replacement of the horse by the motor car from 1918.[82] The downward trend of infant mortality in other European countries also showed a close, inverse relationship with car registrations, and British cities where horse transport lingered into the 1930s, such as Liverpool and Glasgow, were still experiencing 'the true epidemic diarrhoea of infants' in that decade.[83] If the bacteriologists had failed in their endeavour to pin down the fly as the principal transmitter of infantile diarrhoea, the statistics of rising car registrations and falling numbers of horses continued to suggest the validity of that particular epidemiological deduction.

The enormous fly populations which afflicted Victorian cities during the summer and autumn months and the nuisance they demonstrably caused to residents were probably at least as important as any bacteriological demonstration of their infecting capacity in stimulating public health action against them. The observed feeding and breeding habits of these creatures were sufficiently productive of

[76] George S. Graham-Smith, 'The relation of the decline in the number of horse-drawn vehicles, and consequently of the urban breeding grounds of flies, to the fall in the summer diarrhoea death rate', *Jnl Hyg*, 29 (1929–30): pp. 122–38.

[77] George S. Graham-Smith, 'Further observations on the relation of the decline in the number of horse-drawn vehicles to the fall in the summer diarrhoea death rate', *Jnl Hyg*, 39 (1939): pp. 558–62.

[78] Graham-Smith, 'Further observations', p. 561.

[79] Notes of the Week, 'Dried milk and reduced mortality', *MO*, 29 (1923): p. 45.

[80] See Dwork, *War is Good*; Lara V. Marks, *Metropolitan Maternity: Maternal and Infant Welfare Services in Early Twentieth Century London* (1996).

[81] See for example, Naomi Williams and Chris Galley, 'Urban–rural differentials in infant mortality in Victorian England', *Population Studies*, 49 (1995): pp. 401–20.

[82] Notes and Comments, 'Infantile diarrhoea', *MO*, 67 (1942): p. 154.

[83] Notes and Comments, 'The trend of infant mortality', *MO*, 54 (1935): p. 149.

revulsion to assist materially in support for anti-fly campaigns. Nonetheless, these campaigns, when set against the factor of rapidly diminishing urban horse populations, were not universally effective. Although flies occupied relatively little space in inter-war issues of *Medical Officer,* a report on Manchester's energetic annual anti-fly campaign described numerous shortcomings, and concluded that 'the fly, on the whole, has proved too many for us, aided by human allies in all sorts of places'. Urban allotment holders clung to horse manure for mulching; railway workers failed to clean up spillages of horse manure and fly larvae that fell among the tracks during loading, and iron foundries used stable manure in the making of cores for hollow castings.[84] Stable manure had values that ensured its continued use in many quarters until World War II.

AVIAN HABITS

Flies were not the only winged creatures whose feeding habits attracted the attention of epidemiologists and bacteriologists. Gulls were an early subject of investigation as a potential nuisance, their delight in urban refuse heaps making the bacteriological content of their excreta a matter of concern.[85] In the first half of the twentieth century, however, the chief concerns about salmonellosis and feathered creatures centred rather on the domestic duck. The pathway of *Salmonella* infection through eggs, which became of acute public interest in the 1980s, emerged as a preventive issue only gradually and comparatively late. Until World War II, eggs were of little concern to epidemiologists or to the public health organization as a whole. There was some interest among bacteriologists, curious about the inevitable question: how did the bacteria get into the egg? Early investigations into the distribution of *Escherichia coli* in nature had provided 'abundant evidence' of the presence of this supposed indicator of contamination with human excrement in the intestines of a number of different bird species, from ducks, pigeons, and sparrows to sea gulls and birds of prey.[86] Although this finding suggested that bird droppings might transmit infectious bacteria, it did not immediately translate into suspicion of other avian products, whether eggs or the flesh of the birds themselves. Indeed eggs, sealed in their natural protective coating, had long been regarded as one of the safest forms of food.[87] They were widely regarded as a valuable source of concentrated nutrients and a perfect invalid food, readily digestible when raw or lightly cooked (overcooked eggs were considered indigestible, and rigorously excluded from the diets of the sick).[88] Even in 1928, Herman Senn, a food writer alert to medical findings on food-borne disease, offered no warning against eggs in his

[84] Anon, 'Prevention of fly breeding', *MO,* 29 (1923): pp. 77–8.
[85] John W. H. Eyre, 'On the distribution of bacillus coli in nature', *Lancet* (1904), i: pp. 648–9.
[86] Eyre, 'Bacillus coli in nature', pp. 648–9.
[87] William M. Scott, 'Food poisoning due to eggs', *BMJ* (1930), ii: p. 56.
[88] Isabella Beeton, *Family Cooking,* new edn (1907), pp. 157, 176; Charles H. Senn, *Cookery for Invalids,* 6th edn (1915), p. 46.

Cookery for Invalids, although he did warn against the dangers of milk—a warning not included in the 1915 edition of the book.[89]

The earliest indications in Britain that eggs were involved in food poisoning came in 1913, when the Medical Department investigator, Spencer Low, found duck eggs implicated in an outbreak of salmonellosis caused by cream cakes at Yeadon in the West Riding. Low was intrigued enough by this possibility to do some research on his own account, discovering that a series of such outbreaks had already been reported in France, usually associated with wedding breakfasts or other festivities where whipped cream and/or cream cakes containing eggs were served.[90] These examples alerted the Medical Department, but despite careful attention to detail in reported outbreaks it was not until 1926 that its successor the Ministry of Health picked up on an apparent egg poisoning in Stepney, where a fatal case of *Salmonella typhimurium* was attributed to a fried duck egg.[91] A larger outbreak in Swansea the following year, due to egg sandwiches, and another at Darlington, where a cream for trifle had been lifted with the whipped whites of duck eggs—together with a family episode of violent gastro-enteritis at Portslade, from custard made with duck eggs—drove the message home: the Ministry's laboratory began inquiring into the conditions under which *Salmonella typhimurium* succeeded in entering duck eggs.[92]

The research was undertaken by Ministry of Health bacteriologist W. H. Scott, who published his findings in the *British Medical Journal* in 1930.[93] As Scott then noted, food poisoning from eggs had hitherto apparently been so rare in Britain as hardly to have been noticed: despite his own considerable experience as a bacteriologist, he admitted that he had been 'totally ignorant' of the considerable literature on food poisoning from eggs until he began investigations in 1927. Scott was especially impressed by a French thesis on poisoning by whipped cream, published by André Le Coq in 1906.[94] Le Coq demonstrated that the poisonous properties of creams prepared by mixing cream, gelatine, and the whipped white of egg had long been known. (Whipped whites lend lightness to the mixture.[95]) Such poisonings occurred most commonly in summer, and Le Coq was able to show that they were due to bacterial infection of the egg albumen. As to how the infection reached the egg, he suggested that it was introduced into the oviduct during copulation, the albumen being infected as it was deposited around the yolk. The greater frequency of infection in duck eggs might be explained by the fact that ducks 'practice their amours' in ponds and ditches where specific contamination of the water might easily be present, and they were also careless layers, freely dropping eggs into these unsatisfactory surroundings.[96]

Scott offered two further suggestions as to how duck eggs might become infected. The first came from Spencer Low, who in 1913 had concluded that the

[89] Charles H. Senn, *Cookery for Invalids*, 8th edn (1928), p. 38.

[90] CMOAR (1925), p. 173; Scott, 'Food poisoning', p. 57.

[91] CMOAR (1925), p. 173.

[92] CMOAR (1926), pp. 205–6; CMOAR (1927), p. 174.

[93] Scott, 'Food poisoning', p. 57.

[94] André Le Coq, 'Contribution à l'étude des empoisonnements par les gateaux à la crème'... [These]', (1906). I have been unable to trace a copy of this work.

[95] See Beeton, *Family Cookery*, p. 157.

[96] Scott, 'Food poisoning', p. 57.

infectious agent must have been present in one or more of a batch of 'cooking eggs', the whites of which were used to make whipped cream. Low suggested that infection of the ovary, oviduct, and egg with *Salmonella* could occur as part of a general infection of the bird.[97] Scott's attempt to test this hypothesis experimentally was, however, defeated by his ducks, which refused to lay eggs in the available animal house.[98] He remained hopeful that other experimenters with better facilities would succeed where he had failed; indeed, the confirmatory experimental evidence had been obtained by 1932.[99] Another possible route was more easily demonstrated experimentally. Both duck and hen eggs dipped in cultures of *Salmonella typhimurium* became infected within a few days if the shells remained moist. Infection did not take place if the culture was allowed to dry. Once infected, however, the bacteria multiplied rapidly as the egg aged, although not all eggs were susceptible: one in a batch of fifteen remained uncontaminated. After a fortnight at room temperature, however, infected eggs 'may then come to represent an enormous dose—a loopful of albumen or yolk . . . yielding countless colonies (of *Salmonella typhimurium*)'.[100] Such eggs, Scott noted, might smell no more than slightly stale and seem to the 'less discriminating cook' to be perfectly useable. Nor did he doubt that eggs were contaminated in ordinary farming practice. Ducks fed with cultures of *Salmonella typhimurium* or *Salmonella enteritidis* discharged the bacteria in enormous numbers in their droppings for at least a week; and where their bedding was allowed to remain moist for this period, any eggs left there were readily infected. The casual laying habits of ducks, dropping eggs into the ponds and ditches where they fed, meant eggs could be gathered and marketed after specific infection had occurred. By contrast, Scott observed, hens' eggs were much less likely to become infected, either through the oviduct or a general infection.

The interest in egg infection displayed by the Ministry in the later 1920s and 1930s also sprang from a realization that the pattern of human *Salmonella* infection was more complex than suggested by the reported larger outbreaks of food poisoning. Epidemiological observation now began to suggest that single cases of food poisoning were far from uncommon.[101] As George Newman noted, 'there is one form of food which is naturally distributed in isolated portions, namely *eggs*'.[102] Scott too pointed to the egg as an obvious source for such isolated cases: 'an egg is one of the commonest and most conspicuously unshared . . . dishes in ordinary life, and in spite of its notorious innocence should not escape suspicion'.[103] From 1926 onwards, Newman regularly drew attention to the strong circumstantial evidence incriminating lightly cooked egg as a cause of severe and fatal food poisoning. It was

[97] Scott, 'Food poisoning', p. 57.

[98] For the deficiencies of the Ministry of Health's laboratory facilities, see Chapter 5.

[99] William M. Scott, 'Consequences of s. typhimurium infection of eggs', *Journal of Pathology and Bacteriology*, 35 (1932): p. 655; T. Dalling and G. K. Warrack, 'Ducks and salmonella infections', *Jnl Path and Bact*, 35 (1932): p. 23.

[100] Scott, 'Food poisoning', p. 57.

[101] CMOAR (1928), pp. 211–12; J. Smith, 'Sporadic infections in Aberdeen due to food-poisoning organisms of the salmonella group', *Jnl Hyg*, 33 (1933): p. 232.

[102] CMOAR (1928), p. 212.

[103] Scott, 'Food poisoning', p. 58.

not until 1937, however, following German legislation requiring the indelible stamping of all duck eggs offered for sale with the instruction to boil for eight minutes or thoroughly bake, that Newman issued a more specific warning:[104]

> Fried, lightly boiled, in creams, custard or mayonnaise, and most of all in the raw form of egg flips etc, ducks eggs are capable at all seasons of the year of producing severe gastro-enteritis and fatal septicaemia . . . thorough cooking of the eggs remains the only safeguard.

Although Scott had noted the risk of *Salmonella* infection from duck eggs to be comparatively remote, given the many thousands that were consumed daily across the country, reports of outbreaks and cases related to duck eggs continued to come in to the Ministry: in 1947, for example, fourteen outbreaks of *Salmonella*, amounting to 110 cases in total, were ascribed to duck eggs.[105]

A potentially more significant public health concern than sporadic cases and limited outbreaks due to duck eggs surfaced in the early 1930s. The inter-war period saw the further rapid development of two commercial trends already established before 1914: the globalization of trade, and the expansion of the British catering and prepared foods industries. Bulked, frozen liquid egg from China was reaching the British catering industry in quantity—an estimated 700 million eggs in liquid form were imported annually by 1935.[106] Public concern over possible health risks from imported liquid egg was being articulated in Parliament by 1932, and a bacteriological investigation conducted for the Scientific Poultry Breeders Association uncovered 'a disturbing degree of bacterial contamination'.[107] Analysis showed that frozen egg was sound if used frozen, but once thawed and at room temperature, marked bacterial multiplication took place. As the Deputy MOH for Chester noted, most bakeries at this period had few facilities for cold storage, and it seemed inevitable that eggs with a high bacterial content would be used in the preparation of made-up foods. The degree of excremental contamination was relatively high and the danger of imported gastro-intestinal infections might be real. His own experiments with samples taken from 14 lb tins of frozen liquid egg suggested that the danger might be 'neutralized' by cooking, but he remained sceptical.[108]

PRODUCERS AND CONSUMERS

The two strands of concern over duck eggs and imported liquid egg survived the war years and reappeared afresh in the later 1940s and 1950s.The experience of World War II meanwhile added another temporary dimension to the egg question, when consignments of spray-dried egg were found to be instrumental not just in producing human disease, but also in the introduction and dissemination of new *Salmonella* strains into Britain (Chapter 7). These concerns echoed those aroused

104 CMOAR (1937), pp. 112, 143–4.
105 CMOAR (1947), p. 54.
106 A. T. G. Thomas, 'The purity of imported eggs', *PH*, 48 (1935): p. 321.
107 Thomas, 'Purity', p. 321.
108 Thomas, 'Purity', p. 321.

by imported American meat at the time of the *Jungle* scandal earlier in the century, when conditions in the Chicago meat-packing plants were revealed, and indeed by the cattle plague epidemic of the 1860s.[109] By 1940, Britain's reliance on imported egg for the catering industry had become significant. With the outbreak of war, European sources of supply disappeared, and shipping losses meant both a reduction in the number of shell eggs imported and a drastic reduction in the amount of animal feeding stuffs coming into the country.[110] As a result of the latter, the native British poultry population was nearly halved for the duration of the war.[111] The Ministry of Food therefore resorted to American spray-dried egg (see Chapter 7). Routine bacteriological sampling undertaken between August 1942 and August 1945 and sampling for *Salmonella* between February 1943 and August 1945 showed an infection rate of 10 per cent.[112] By contrast, the small amount of dried egg imported from Australia went through a highly mechanized production process, and appeared to be free of infection.[113]

The Ministry of Food's bacteriological monitoring was not due to any application of current food hygiene standards, but was prompted by events on the ground: a sudden rise in reported episodes of human salmonellosis which became evident from late 1942. In 1943 and 1944, an unprecedented 454 outbreaks were recorded. This rise coincided with the release onto the open market in July 1942 of American spray-dried egg. The inference that a new source of *Salmonella* infection had been introduced into the country in the latter half of 1942 was, the subsequent Medical Research Council inquiry noted, 'very strong'.[114] At the same time Ministry of Health investigations into the specific causes of these outbreaks showed most to be caused by *Salmonella* types new to Britain, whose appearance closely paralleled the release of dried egg for retail distribution.[115] Although direct evidence incriminating the spray-dried egg was inevitably difficult to obtain, there was very little doubt the new foodstuff and the new pattern of *Salmonella* infection were linked.[116] Expert advice from the Medical Research Council suggested that if the egg was effectively cooked immediately after reconstitution, the risk of infection was minimized. Danger threatened only if the reconstituted egg was left standing for any length of time, allowing bacterial multiplication to occur.

109 Keir Waddington, *The Bovine Scourge: Meat, Tuberculosis and Public Health 1850–1914* (2006), pp. 145–7.

110 Graham S. Wilson et al., 'The bacteriology of spray-dried egg, with particular reference to food poisoning', Medical Research Council, *Special Report Series*, 260 (1947): 'Appendix by the Ministry of Food on practical problems presented by the bacteriology of spray-dried egg', p. 65 (hereafter MRC, *Report*).

111 R. F. Gordon, 'The poultry industry and the veterinary profession', *Veterinary Record*, 61 (1949): p. 724.

112 MRC, *Report*, pp. 2–5.

113 P. S. Waters and S. Mander, 'An investigation into the incidence of salmonellae in South Australian eggs and egg pulp', *MBMH*, 12(1953): pp. 127–9.

114 MRC, *Report*, p.10.

115 MRC, *Report*, p. 10; T. V. Cooper, 'Case of fever due to infection with *Bact. Oranienburg*', *MBMH*, 3 (1944): pp. 40–3.

116 MRC *Report*, p. 63.

Wartime conditions precluded any publicity, however: dried egg was too valuable a food source amid wartime scarcity to permit any danger of a food scare. As the reporter of the appearance of numerous cases of food poisoning due to *Salmonella* hitherto unknown or uncommon in Britain noted, 'It is hoped, when conditions are more favourable, to be able to present a report on these cases and to discuss the probable source of infection.'[117] The Ministry of Health was well aware of the connection between dried egg and *Salmonella* infections by the end of 1945, although reference was made to it only in connection with outbreaks of staphylococcal food poisoning by ice cream in three separate American barracks.[118] Local MOHs knew of an 'usual incidence of those states of ill-health characterised by belly-ache' during the war but, if aware of the dried-egg connection, kept their silence.[119] Instead, the Ministry began a campaign of public health education, issuing leaflets and instructions to civilians and Forces caterers, and ensuring that packets for domestic consumption carried advice on safe preparation and cooking. Recipe leaflets and the promotion of 'Food Facts' in the national and local press also followed.[120] Noting the 'very great tonnage' of dried egg imported in these years, and the *Salmonella* contamination rate of 10 per cent, the Ministry of Food robustly declared the number of related food poisoning cases ascertained to be very small, indicating the effectiveness of measures taken to minimize the bacteriological risk.[121] The new public health strategy of bacteriological sampling, facilitated by the recently established Emergency Public Health Laboratory Service, may have been a critical factor in this apparent success (for the Public Health Laboratory Service, see Chapter 5).

Despite the Ministry of Food's claims, the public education campaign seemingly had a limited impact on consumers. The 1947 Medical Research Council investigation noted specifically that very few doctors were aware of the *Salmonella* risk present in dried egg.[122] Nor were the dangers of duck eggs and imported liquid egg generally appreciated. Preventive awareness of these persisted after World War II: the researchers associated with the Public Health Laboratory Service (PHLS) were particularly interested in these pathways of *Salmonella* infection.[123] In 1949–50, however, widespread public mistrust of duck eggs was generated by two spectacular hospital outbreaks of *Salmonella typhimurium.* At both hospitals, the mischief lay in puddings made with duck eggs, which, being cheaper than hen eggs, were often used by canteens and institutions feeding large numbers of people.[124] At St Bartholomew's Hospital, London, in July 1949, a Queen of Puddings made

[117] Cooper, '*Bact. Oranienburg*', p. 41.

[118] G. C. Williams et al., 'Three outbreaks of staphylococcal food-poisoning due to ice-cream', *MBMH*, 5 (January 1946): pp. 17–25.

[119] Editorial, 'Food-spread disease', *MO*, 74 (1945): p. 49.

[120] MRC, *Report*, Appendix, pp. 65–6.

[121] MRC, *Report*, Appendix, p. 66. [122] MRC, *Report*, p. 63.

[123] Numerous reports are to be found in the *Monthly Bulletin of the Ministry of Health*, beginning with R. F. Gordon and A. Buxton, 'A case of food poisoning in man probably caused by the consumption of a duck egg', *MBMH*, 4 (1945): pp. 46–50.

[124] Salmonella Sub-Committee, 'Salmonella in duck eggs', *MBMH*, 13 (1954): p. 42.

with 200 duck eggs and sufficient for 700 portions caused illness in 136 staff and 60 patients. (Most of the latter had preferred the alternative rice pudding.)[125] Nine months later, in April 1950, a similar outbreak occurred among nursing and auxiliary staff serving a group of teaching hospitals in Belfast. The culprit on this occasion was lemon meringue pie.[126] Widespread publicity in the medical and lay press surrounded both these outbreaks, and seems to have engendered a deep and lingering suspicion of duck eggs across a broad section of the British public.[127] Further investigation by a special PHLS Salmonella Sub-Committee in 1950–2 re-emphasized the risks presented by duck eggs.[128]

Public suspicion was facilitated by market developments, which provided an easy alternative to duck eggs. The new methods of intensive farming introduced after the war were better suited to the production of hen eggs, now widely available and increasingly inexpensive. As laying ducks remained a small-time 'farmer's wife' activity, patterns of consumption and popular tastes shifted away from duck eggs. For city children born in the 1950s, duck eggs were an unknown experience. Well into the 1960s, hen eggs were considered decidedly safer than duck eggs, with human infections from shell hen eggs in Britain thought to be extremely rare.[129] It was, however, not unknown that *Salmonella* infection among chickens was very common in America at this date.[130]

During the 1950s, the PHLS established itself as a major contributor to public health activity and research in England and Wales. In that decade, preventive concerns over liquid egg re-emerged, with the PHLS acting as both organizer and initiator of relevant investigations. In 1954 an inquiry into the production of liquid egg in Northern Ireland found that 2.1 per cent of hen egg batches were infected with *Salmonella* (against 48.3 per cent of duck egg). Given the frequent use of bulked egg (liquid tinned or frozen eggs packaged by lb weight), any infection of either hen or duck eggs was a potential health hazard, as the author of the report, C. R. Murdoch of the Belfast hospitals' central laboratory, warned,[131]

> Any product of shell egg, hen or duck, liquid or frozen, should therefore be subjected to adequate sterilization before being used for human consumption, as it would appear that there is considerable risk of these products containing salmonellae.

Murdoch's investigation of Northern Irish egg sources spanned the years 1951–3. A similar study, involving 38 laboratories, was undertaken by the PHLS in England

[125] L. P. Garrod and M. B. McIlroy, 'Hospital outbreak of enteritis due to duck eggs', *BMJ* (1949), ii: pp. 1259–61.

[126] R. A. Neely and M. G. Wilson, 'Salmonella food poisoning due to duck eggs with a trial of chloramphenicol in a carrier state', *MBMH*, 10 (1951): pp. 96–100.

[127] B. N. Eedy, 'Salmonella food poisoning conveyed by a duck egg and associated with infection in a drake', *MBMH*, 9 (1950): pp. 213–14; Richard Hardy, personal communication, 16 April 1998.

[128] Salmonella Sub-Committee, 'Duck eggs', pp. 42–3.

[129] A. Bernstein, 'Salmonella infection of hen eggs', *MBMH*, 11 (1952): pp. 64–7; C. L. Broomhead and P. G. Mann, 'A family outbreak of Salmonella Thompson infection', *MBMH*, 18 (1959): pp. 124–7.

[130] C. R. Murdoch, 'The occurrence of salmonella in liquid egg', *MBMH*, 13 (1954): pp. 43–4.

[131] Murdoch, 'Occurrence', p. 45.

and Wales between 1 April 1953 and 31 March 1954. These results were more reassuring: the major contaminator, *Salmonella typhimurium*, was detected in 0.3 per cent of English hen eggs sampled and in 3.1 per cent of English duck eggs.[132]

In August 1954, however, there was a widespread outbreak of an unusual strain of Paratyphoid B in north-west London, apparently associated with the use of frozen imported Chinese egg by local bakeries in the preparation of cream cakes. As usual, the evidence was circumstantial, the only common factor being the use of a particular brand of frozen Chinese egg in every bakery implicated. On-site investigations showed there to be a considerable risk of *Salmonella* contamination of uncooked products such as cream when any contaminated ingredients were used in a cake mix.[133] A further investigation by PHLS scientists revealed a variety of *Salmonella* present in 27 per cent of cans of Chinese frozen egg sampled. *Salmonella* were also isolated from bakery products ready for retail distribution.[134] By 1960, it had been ascertained that an average of 10 per cent of imported liquid whole egg was contaminated with *Salmonella*, and guidelines for pasteurization were being drawn up—an instance in which the technological fix seemed easier and more effective than educating egg producers and packagers. As with milk, pasteurization seemed the only way of achieving a bacteriologically safe product.[135] The findings of the PHLS investigation, combined with publicity surrounding more than half a dozen outbreaks of food poisoning originating in contaminated bakery products between 1954 and 1963 brought public concern and parliamentary agitation.[136] In January 1964, the Liquid Egg (Pasteurization) Regulations 1963 came into force, designed to ensure that bulked liquid egg was effectively sterilized before being used for human consumption. Driven by a perceived public health need, the Regulations were made possible only by intensive research under the aegis of the PHLS to establish methods of pasteurization that resulted in a product which satisfied both the bakery and confectionery trade and public health requirements.[137]

Between 1926 and the early 1960s, therefore, English concerns over *Salmonella* infection in eggs focused almost entirely on duck eggs and imported liquid frozen egg. Laboratory research had determined the pathways of infection in duck eggs by the mid-1930s, and also helped to establish the risks associated with industrially bulked egg for commercial use. Conditions in the egg industries were changing, however. In the years after World War I, the national poultry industry had quadrupled, from 15 million birds in 1918 to 85 million by 1938. After 1945, expansion resumed. Whereas the national poultry sector had been worth £30

[132] PHLS, 'Salmonella in liquid egg, including frozen liquid egg', *MBMH*, 14 (1955): pp. 65–9.

[133] Kenneth W. Newell, 'paratyphoid B fever possibly associated with Chinese frozen egg', *MBMH*, 14 (1955): pp. 146–54.

[134] M. E. Smith and Betty C. Hobbs, 'Salmonellae in Chinese frozen egg', *MBMH*, 14 (1955): pp. 154–60.

[135] C. R. Murdoch et al., 'The pasteurisation of liquid whole egg', *MBMH*, 19 (1960): pp. 134–52.

[136] Parliament and Public Health, 'Paratyphoid', *MO*, 109 (1963): p. 321.

[137] Annotation, 'Pasteurization of liquid egg', *MO*, 110 (1965): p. 185. See also Murdoch et al., 'Pasteurisation', pp. 149–50.

million in 1938, the gross annual value by 1948 was estimated at more than £100 million.[138] National average egg consumption rose steadily, from an average of 145 a year in 1938 to 215 in the early 1960s.[139] By the 1960s, the great bulk of eggs consumed in Britain were hen eggs, but there was as yet no suggestion of any significant egg-related human *Salmonella* problem, despite veterinary anxieties over poor husbandry practices and a rising toll of disease among poultry.[140] The example of America, where several *Salmonella* were regularly present in poultry flocks, was regarded with foreboding. In 1956, William Savage noted birds as apparently the commonest reservoir of *Salmonella*, and suggested that they might constitute the primary source of *Salmonella* thompson and *Salmonella* newport, since the former at least was a common cause of disease in British poultry flocks and was not uncommon in imported eggs.[141]

The debates over *Salmonella* in eggs were, however, conducted mainly among bacteriologists, in the context of laboratory research, and increasingly among the veterinary profession after 1945. Despite repeated admonitions, the general public and the catering trades remained largely unconscious of the hazards presented by duck eggs until the 1950s. The investigators of the St Bartholomew's Hospital outbreak suggested that the risk of eating duck eggs unless thoroughly cooked was fairly well known in medical circles, but perhaps less so among caterers.[142] This observation, made in the middle of a concerted campaign for wider education of caterers and the public in food hygiene (Chapter 9), sounds a telling note. The translation of medical understanding into public knowledge proved harder than reformers in the immediate post-war years had envisaged. The duck egg scare, however, occurred at a time when a satisfactory alternative was readily available, resulting in a long-term shift in consumption patterns. If the public health problems posed by flies remained a concern in large parts of the world long after knowledge of their habits had generated an enduring disgust in Western populations, the issue of bacteriologically clean egg production resurged spectacularly in the 1980s when the health hazards presented by hen eggs became public knowledge. In the twenty-first century, duck eggs returned to the frame, in the context of the adventurous new gastronomy which was engulfing Britain and which led to a significant increase in duck egg consumption. The year 2010 saw the first duck egg-related outbreak of salmonellosis in Britain for 60 years, leading the industry to plan the implementation of an industry assurance scheme similar to that in place for hen eggs since the late 1990s.[143] It is still possible for the public health problems of the past to resurface in the present.

[138] R. F. Gordon, 'The poultry industry and the veterinary profession', *Vet Rec*, 61 (1949): p. 724.

[139] J. D. Blaxland, 'Poultry and public health', *Vet Rec*, 73 (1961): p. 507.

[140] Gordon, 'Poultry industry', pp. 724–6; Blaxland, 'Poultry', pp. 507–9.

[141] William S. Savage, 'Problems of salmonella food poisoning', *BMJ* (1956), ii: pp. 318, 320.

[142] Garrod and McIlroy, 'Hospital outbreak', p. 1260.

[143] D. J. Noble et al., 'Revival of an old problem: an increase in *Salmonella enterica* serovar Typhimurium definitive phage type 8 infections in 2010 in England and Northern Ireland linked to duck eggs', *Epidemiology and Infection*, 140(1) (2012): pp. 146–9. For hen eggs see C. L. Little et al., 'Public health investigations of *Salmonella* Enteritidis in catering raw shell eggs, 2002–2004', *Letters in Applied Microbiology*, 44(6) (2007): p. 596.

4

Other Animals

The nineteenth-century emphasis on the environmental causes and contexts of endemic typhoid highlighted the activities of humans as both source of infection and unthinking desecrators of natural surroundings. In this respect, the environment was regarded largely as playing an accidental role in the generation of disease: man was the perpetrator; air, water, and soil—and contaminated foodstuffs derived therefrom—merely the innocent vehicles of his self-destructive habits: the oysters that dealt death and discomfort to Victorian shell-fish eaters were not intrinsically dangerous. Danger had been imposed upon them by human carelessness. In the last decades of the century, however, nature began to assume a less benign aspect. The emergence of bacteriology and of a more sharply interrogative epidemiological style contributed to a creeping erosion of belief in nature's innocence, the opening up of a seam of doubt which, nevertheless, was a long time in achieving anything like popular or general scientific influence. The source of this seam of doubt lay in the animal kingdom, and in the dawning recognition that animals used as food by humans could of themselves transmit diseases not of human origin to their consumers.

Diseases passed from animals to humans through the food chain—through infected meat or milk—are of two types. One the one hand, there are those which transmit clinically identifiable diseases such as tuberculosis, which can be identified and eradicated by culling as a means to resolving the human public health problem. Infections with *Salmonella* or *E. coli*, on the other hand, are generally not clinically identifiable, since they inhabit healthy animal carriers which exhibit no recognizable symptoms. While a newly emergent disease, as BSE was in the 1980s, may take time to be established as a public health problem, preventive action can be taken once it has been identified as a danger to humans. Carrier infections, however, present an ongoing public health problem. Being invisible, and transmissible also by the faecal–oral route, they are generally not subject to control measures, except through scrupulous personal and food hygiene, emergency limitation measures where outbreaks occur, and latterly, in the case of *Salmonella enteritidis* in poultry, by vaccination.[1] As with sewage-contaminated shell-fish, meat and milk contaminated with pathogenic enteric organisms remain a continuing public health hazard.

While the adulteration and the deliberate poisoning of foods had long been recognized, the realization that animal foodstuffs could cause illness in humans seems to have come relatively late. Putrid meat was a long-standing concern, the

[1] See Hugh Pennington, *When Food Kills. BSE, E. coli and Disaster Science* (2003), chapter 2.

condition of the meat being assumed to cause illness. By the early nineteenth century, chemical poisons generated during decomposition were thought to blame; later the cause came to be thought to be putrefactive alkaloids, or ptomaines.[2] Ptomaine poisoning was the commonly used term for food poisoning until well into the twentieth century, much to the annoyance of those who considered the term a barrier to the proper understanding of the nature and risks of food poisoning.[3] From the middle years of the nineteenth century, however, growing scientific evidence that tuberculosis was transmissible from cattle to humans either in milk or in meat raised awareness of potential dangers in animal foodstuffs.[4] The first connections between specific disease in food animals and food poisoning in humans were made in Germany in the late 1870s;[5] in Britain the subject caught the attention of the Medical Department of the Local Government Board in the summer of 1880. The transmission of disease to humans by infected meat was to remain a public health issue in Britain for more than a century, until the high drama of the emergence of BSE in the 1980s finally forced acceptance of more rigorous veterinary surveillance and regulation of meat producers at the end of the twentieth century. Food poisoning via domestic food animals remains a hazard in modern public health systems, and regulation of the noxious trade of slaughtering continues to cause concern.

THE ENGLISH DISCOVERY OF MEAT-BORNE FOOD POISONING

In June 1880 the Medical Department's attention was drawn to a significant outbreak of food poisoning in Nottinghamshire, associated with a four-day sale of timber and machinery organized on the Duke of Portland's Welbeck Abbey estate.[6] The sale was attended by over 2,000 people from six counties, attracted both by the sale and by Welbeck's reputation as a remarkable place. Refreshments were provided on site from a popular hotel in Mansfield, and consisted of cold ham and roast beef, cold beefsteak pie, mustard and salt, bread and cheese, pickles, and 'Chutnee sauce', with bottled and draught beer, spirits, ginger beer, lemonade, and

[2] Elliott B. Dewberry, *Food Poisoning. Foodborne Infection and Intoxication*, 4th edn (1959), p. 6.

[3] William G. Savage, *Food Poisoning and Food Infections* (1920), pp. vii, 6–7; Allan Wotherspoon, 'Food poisoning', *Journal of the Sanitary Institute*, 58 (1937–8): p. 573.

[4] Anne Hardy, 'Animals, disease and man: Making connections', *Perspectives in Biology and Medicine*, 46 (2002): pp. 200–15; Keir Waddington, '"Unfit for human consumption": Tuberculosis and the problem of infected meat in late Victorian Britain', *Bulletin of the History of Medicine*, 77 (2003): pp. 636–61; Keir Waddington, *The Bovine Scourge. Meat, Tuberculosis and Public Health, 1850–1914* (2006), chapters 1, 4, 8, 9.

[5] See Dewberry, *Food Poisoning*, p. 9. For details of this research, see Robert von Ostertag, *Handbook of Meat Inspection*, translated Earley V. Wilson (1904), pp. 712–18.

[6] This account of the Welbeck incident is reprinted from Anne Hardy, 'Food, hygiene and the laboratory: a short history of food poisoning in Britain, circa 1850–1950', *Social History of Medicine*, 12 (1999): pp. 293–4.

water.[7] Two types of luncheon were served in the new and scrupulously clean refreshment rooms: the 2/- luncheon in the dining room, and sandwiches—a mix of ham and beef taken from the cold meat section—in the 'engine room'. The clientele in the refreshment rooms was overwhelmingly male; women attending such sales did so for pleasure, in small parties, and generally brought their own refreshments with them. So, when visitors to the sale began to fall ill with griping stomach pain, chills, giddiness, diarrhoea and vomiting, prostration, and cold sweats, the victims were almost all male. Details were obtained of seventy-two cases, but the evidence suggested that there were many more. There were four deaths—and the dead were reported to have looked like cholera victims.[8]

There were many complaints of the ham used by the caterers, which was said to have 'tasted queer' or have been undercooked. Edward Ballard, the investigator sent by the Medical Department, was inclined to think that the meat had been tainted by sewer gas when left overnight in an underground room, but feeling 'very much in the dark', he sought Edward Klein's help. Klein identified a 'living parasitic thing' in the thicker and less well-cooked portions of the ham, and his experiments demonstrated that it was 'capable of spreading by its growth and reproduction through the material in which it was found, and capable of producing disease in animals into whose system it was introduced; capable also of growth and reproduction within the system of those animals'.[9] Although Klein's conclusions were unspecific, Ballard was convinced. He subsequently reported on a similar outbreak at Nottingham in February 1881, which he attributed to the eating of hot baked pork obtained from a cookshop in that town.[10] As a result of these two outbreaks, the Medical Department began recording occurrences of food poisoning reported by local MOHs. During the 1880s fourteen such incidents and outbreaks were detailed, all but one apparently caused by meat, ten of them associated with the consumption of pork.[11] Except for two associated with tinned goods and two family outbreaks, these incidents were linked to bought-in or catered foods prepared in advance.

The inferences which Ballard drew from these fourteen incidents were not such as to incriminate the meat itself. 'The truth of the matter', he noted, seemed to be that 'the accession of the specific bacillus to the food is what we commonly call "accidental"'. 'Accidental' in this case, he continued, only meant 'that it comes from somewhere beyond our present knowledge. We do not know its normal habitat.'[12] In urging cleanliness in preparation and storage, and thorough cooking, Ballard assumed 'an infectiveness of the place where these things were done, in

[7] Edward Ballard, 'On acute specific disease', Medical Officer's Annual Report, Local Government Board, British Parliamentary Papers, 1881, xlvi, Appendix A no 5, pp. 752–60.

[8] Ballard, 'On acute specific disease', p. 752.

[9] Ballard, 'On acute specific disease', p. 765.

[10] Edward Ballard, 'On a series of cases of acute specific disease (similar to that observed in the Welbeck outbreak) following the eating of hot baked pork', MOAR, LGB, BPP, 1881, xlvi, Appendix A no 6, pp. 774–87.

[11] Edward Ballard, 'A summary review of 14 instances reported upon since 1879 . . .', BPP, 1890–91, xxxiv, Appendix 21, pp. 245–58.

[12] Ballard, 'Summary review', p. 257.

association with uncleanliness of air, of soil or of surface'.[13] For Ballard, the blame was external to the animal, to the foodstuff in question: human agency was the factor operating to make the incriminated foods dangerous. His epidemiological gaze was still shaped by his underlying miasmatic convictions: thus he urged the need for light and air to penetrate everywhere—'there should be no corners where refuse matter can lodge and become a centre for the cultivation of morbid micro-organisms in filth'.[14] Nor was Ballard mistaken in one sense: in many cases of food poisoning human agency does operate to make foods dangerous, but he was wrong in assuming that the infective bacteria could not be intrinsic to the food. Just two years earlier, in 1888, a defining moment in the history of food poisoning had occurred, when August Gärtner isolated the organism he named bacillus enteritidis (now *Salmonella enteritidis*) from the meat of an emergency-slaughtered cow, and from the organs of a man who died after eating her meat—the only fatality among some sixty people who fell ill as a result of having done so.[15] It was perhaps significant of the general low level of scientific interest in the issue of food poisoning that news of Gärtner's finding does not seem to have reached the Medical Department by the time Ballard's report was written.

Gärtner's (anglicized as Gaertner's) bacillus, as it was often known into the 1920s, caused a good deal of confusion among bacteriologists. It was very similar to the organism of typhoid and, given contemporary ideas on the fluidity of microbial species and the deficiencies of early bacteriological techniques, the two often proved difficult to distinguish from each other. And the number of similar micro-organisms identified multiplied. Much of the confusion surrounding the typhoid bacillus in the 1890s stemmed from the recognition that it was not a unique and distinct bacterial species, but shared morphological and cultural characteristics with quite a number of very similar organisms.[16] By 1900, bacteria belonging to the 'typhoid' family had been identified in cattle, pigs, mice, and birds, and some had been shown also to cause disease in humans. The broader relationship between these organisms and human disease intrigued a number of researchers and, as had occurred with bovine tuberculosis, they became the subject of study in several European laboratories.

The discovery of this 'typhoid group' of pathogenic organisms also opened up new epidemiological perspectives. During the 1890s, the Medical Department was undergoing difficult times in the face of Treasury cutbacks and internal problems,[17] while the presence of the fifth cholera pandemic in Europe and concomitant renewed sensitivities over endemic typhoid helped to focus the department's energies on investigations into typhoid. With the new century, however, the department began to sponsor research into typhoid's microbial cousins and their

[13] Ballard, 'Summary review', p. 258. [14] Ballard, 'Summary review', p. 258.

[15] Dewberry, *Food Poisoning*, p. 10. See also Anon, 'August Gärtner (1848–1934)', *Nature*, 161 (1948): p. 593.

[16] Michael Worboys, *Spreading Germs: Disease Theories and Medical Practice in Britain, 1865–1900* (2000), p. 265.

[17] Roy M. McLeod, 'The frustration of state medicine, 1880–1899', *Medical History*, 11 (1967): pp. 15–40.

natural habitats. As these organisms were clearly able to cause disease in humans, and it was possible that much endemic gastro-enteritis was due to them, their natural history became a subject of epidemiological importance. As Herbert Durham, a brilliant British researcher who made signal contributions to a field previously dominated by Continental investigators, noted,[18] 'The identification of a given microbe as the cause of a disease is really only the beginning of the knowledge requisite for the proper control of the disease, we must also know its economy in nature.' This, Durham added, 'is extremely difficult to work out in the case of bacteria'. A century or so later, high-powered expert committees were echoing Durham's assessment: 'There is no other zoonosis as complex in its epidemiology and control as salmonellosis'; 'The maintenance of salmonellae in the environment is by complex pathways.' In their turn, they urged the need for epidemiological investigations to improve the identification of the sources and vehicles of *Salmonella* infection.[19]

PATHWAYS IN NATURE

The earliest epidemiological observations of gastric illness associated with particular foodstuffs were almost entirely of meat and meat products. Of the fourteen cases collected by the Medical Department in the 1880s, thirteen were linked to meat, sausages, or meat pies, and just one to salmon from a blown tin.[20] While several of these suspect foods had been submitted to Klein for examination, his conclusions were vague: the bacillus identified at Welbeck (1880) and Nottingham (1881) was not the same as that causing an outbreak at Carlisle (1889), or that in the case of two others isolated from veal and pork pie cases—'It is an altogether different species, as will be clear from my account of its morphological and cultural characteristics'.[21] The limitations of Klein's methodology were typical of much of the work done in this area in the 1890s. It was only with the entry of Herbert Durham to the stage, at the end of the decade, that matters began to move forward.

Durham was a young Cambridge researcher, familiar with the extant European literature and well versed in the new bacteriological methods, having worked with Max von Grüber in Vienna.[22] Durham was called to assist in the bacteriological investigation of an outbreak of food poisoning associated with meat pies, at

18 Herbert E. Durham, 'On infections by unsound meat, more especially with regard to the *bacillus enteritidis* (Gaertner)', *Transactions of the Pathological Society*, 50 (1899): p. 266.

19 Report of the WHO Expert Committee on Salmonella Control (Geneva, 1988), p. 8; Advisory Committee on the Microbiological Safety of Food, *Report on Salmonella in Eggs* (1993), pp. 18, 40.

20 Ballard, 'Summary review', p. 245.

21 Edward Klein, '"Food poisoning". Report on bacteriological investigation ...', BPP, 1890, xxxiv, Appendix B no 3: pp. 333–6. All have retrospectively been identified as *Salmonella*: Tom Humphrey, personal communication, 25 July 1996.

22 Anon, 'Herbert E. Durham', *British Medical Journal* (1945), ii: p. 708; Worboys, *Spreading Germs*, pp. 268–9. Max von Grüber (1853–1927), physician and biologist, a founder of serology, Director of the Institute of Hygiene in Vienna, 1887–1902: see H. Flamm, 'Max von Grüber', *Complete Dictionary of Scientific Biography* (Detroit, 2008), vol 5, p. 563.

Oldham and Chadderton, in 1898. Scientifically, this was a landmark investigation, for Durham introduced the new techniques of serology into the epidemiological inquiry. By his use of agglutination tests, Durham demonstrated that the hitherto indistinguishable bacteria involved in food poisoning outbreaks could be separated into at least two groups, and that the examination of the blood sera of patients suffering from food poisoning was of significant diagnostic value.[23] Epidemiologically, too, Durham's inquiry was important: for the first time in England, investigation pointed to meat itself as the source of infection. It also reinforced Ballard's earlier message of the importance of thoroughly cooking meat and meat products.

The epidemiological story of the Oldham and Chadderton outbreak was presented in the medical press by the MOHs of the two districts; the bacteriological story was presented by Durham. On Thursday 28 July 1898, a confectioner in Chadderton made 268 meat pies: 160 veal and 108 pork. The veal pies were sold between Thursday and Saturday, and many of those who ate them, especially on the Saturday, fell ill with severe and uncontrollable vomiting and diarrhoea. There were some thirty-seven cases in Chadderton, with three deaths, and some thirteen in Oldham, with one death. All were associated with the veal pies only.[24] Typically of many if not most such outbreaks, then and later, nothing of the suspect pies was available for analysis: they had all been eaten, or thrown away, or fed to the dog.[25] This did not, however, discourage Dr Harold Ashton of Chadderton, and Dr J. B. Wilkinson of Oldham, from calling in the services of Herbert Durham. Durham took blood samples from nineteen of the surviving victims and from one lucky consumer of veal pie who had suffered no ill effects. Agglutination tests revealed the guilty organism to be Gärtner's bacillus; the blood of the one unaffected man proved negative.[26]

The conclusions which all three medical observers drew from the evidence available to them was clear: the source of the infection lay in the veal with which the pies had been made, the likelihood being that one batch had been significantly undercooked.[27] Durham noted that only 20 minutes had been allowed for the baking of each batch at a temperature between 200 and 250 degrees centigrade: in domestic cookery, 'so far as I can gather . . . fifty minutes is given as the least time for even a single small raised pie'.[28] All the fatal cases were due to pies kept for more than 48 hours after baking. Unlike Ballard before him, however, Durham linked this episode with similar outbreaks in Europe, and went on to draw a wider lesson than the need for thorough cooking: the evidence clearly indicated that the flesh of cattle and calves could cause food poisoning, and 'mere naked eye inspection' of

[23] Durham, 'On infections by unsound meat'; Herbert E. Durham, 'The present knowledge of outbreaks due to meat poisoning', *BMJ* (1898), ii: pp. 1797–1801. See also Savage, *Food Poisoning*, p. 8.

[24] Harold Ashton, 'An outbreak of food poisoning at Chadderton', *Public Health* 11 (1898–9): pp. 229–33.

[25] Ashton, 'Outbreak', p. 231.

[26] Durham, 'Present knowledge', pp. 1787–8.

[27] Durham, 'Present knowledge', p. 1798; Ashton, 'An outbreak', 235; J. B. Wilkinson, 'At Oldham', *PH*, 11 (1898–99): p. 237.

[28] Durham, 'Present knowledge', p. 1798.

meat was insufficient to guarantee food safety: 'The point of importance is to pay special attention to the animal before it has been slaughtered, if suspicion is thus aroused, bacteriological inquiry should be made.'[29] In this regard, Durham was adding fuel to the controversy over slaughterhouse practices generated by the on-going debates surrounding the transmission of bovine tuberculosis to humans.[30] Indeed, he added the rider that cows were 'notoriously apt' to be tuberculous, and were by no means an ideal source of beef for human consumption.[31] By referring to tuberculosis in the context of food poisoning, Durham was underscoring the danger of a potentially significant range of human infections existing in the flesh of diseased animals.

Thus Durham presented the case for a new field for laboratory investigation. Inaugurating a novel range of Medical Department inquiries around 1900, Klein himself noted that the bacteriological investigation of micro-organisms in food-stuffs had hitherto been limited to tuberculosis.[32] Inquiries now began to be made into the natural economy of the food poisoning organisms, and their presence in foodstuffs, in milk, and in animal intestines. It was in this context that the young William Savage, then MOH for Colchester, began working for the Department. By 1920, Savage had established himself as a leading authority on food poisoning, and especially on *Salmonella*. The research which he undertook for the Medical Department (*c.* 1907–13) was important in establishing his credentials in this field.[33] The series of bacteriological investigations which Savage undertook for the Department included the bacterial and cellular content of milk from healthy and diseased cows;[34] the presence of Gärtner group organisms in animal intestines, prepared meats, and similar foods;[35] and the presence of paratyphoid bacilli in humans–'a natural corollary to the Gaertner investigations'.[36]

29 Durham, 'Present knowledge', pp. 1800–1.

30 Waddington, '"Unfit for human consumption"', pp. 650–60; see also Richard Perren, 'Filth and profit, disease and health: public and private impediments to slaughterhouse reform in Victorian Britain', in *Meat, Modernity, and the Rise of the Slaughterhouse*, edited by Paula Young Lee (2008), pp. 127–50.

31 Durham, 'Present knowledge', pp. 1800–1.

32 Edward Klein, 'Report on the bacterioscopic analysis of various food stuffs', BPP, 1901, xxvi, Appendix B no 2, p. 328.

33 Anon, 'Sir William George Savage', *BMJ* (1961), i: p. 1113. Trained at University College London and University College Hospital, Savage held various posts before becoming MOH and public analyst for Colchester in 1903, and seems to have begun working for the Medical Department in 1906–7. He was appointed MOH for the County of Somerset in 1909.

34 William G. Savage, 'Report on bacterial studies of milk from healthy and diseased cows', BPP, 1908, xxx, Appendix B no 4, pp. 227–74.

35 William G. Savage, 'Report on the distribution of organisms of the Gaertner group in the animal intestine', BPP, 1908, xxx; Appendix B no 5, pp. 275–300; William G. Savage, 'Further report on the presence of Gaertner group organisms in the animal intestine', BPP, 1909, xxviii, Appendix B no 5, pp. 461–80; William G. Savage, 'Report upon the Gaertner group of bacilli in prepared meats and allied foods', BPP, 1910, xxxix: Appendix B no 3, pp. 492–519.

36 William G. Savage, 'The presence of paratyphoid bacilli in man', BPP, 1909, xxix: Appendix B no 4, p. 752.

More particularly, Savage also completed a general investigation into the subject of food poisoning, which summed up the historical background and current state of knowledge.[37] Introducing this report, the CMO to the Local Government Board, Arthur Newsholme, listed three important considerations stemming from current knowledge: first, that some food poisoning outbreaks were associated with actual disease in animals whose flesh was eaten; second, the probability that in other outbreaks, uncontaminated food had been infected by the tissue or intestinal contents of food animals in which infection was present; third, the extent to which, once sources of bacterial infection were present, opportunities for the spread of disease were favoured by lack of cleanliness and care in the handling, preparation, and storage of food. His conclusion was clear:[38]

> Recent additions to our knowledge, in fact, tend to emphasise rather than to lessen the importance of inspection of meat at slaughterhouses, of the experience of adequate control in regard to the suitability of places where food is prepared and stored, and of measures to secure cleanliness in all stages of food preparation.

The accumulating evidence of meat as a major source of food poisoning infections was becoming weighty. The German investigator Robert von Ostertag listed some 85 such outbreaks occurring mainly in Germany between 1880 and 1900; Savage could list 79 British outbreaks occurring between 1878 and 1911. Analysis of the latter showed that nearly all were due to meat from cattle or pigs.[39] Savage himself was clear that food poisoning was best explained as the result of food infected with 'virulent Gaertner Group organisms (or other special bacilli) derived from animals which are either at the time suffering from disease due to the Gaertner group bacilli or acting as carriers of those bacilli'.[40] With the epidemiological thoroughness characteristic of MOH inquiries at their best, Savage took the question beyond the laboratory and related it to circumstances in the local community:[41]

> Under the present system of isolated slaughterhouses in vogue in this country it is impossible to exert any adequate supervision over the slaughter of animals for food, and it is easy for diseased animals infected with Gaertner bacilli to be put upon the market and sold as healthy. No additional bacteriological facilities would prevent this.

By 1913, English investigations into the epidemiology and natural habitat of food poisoning organisms had tracked the pathway of infection from the environment of the kitchen through domestic food animals to the slaughterhouse, and, by implication, beyond again, to the prevailing culture of the country's livestock farming industry. In so doing, as Savage intimated, they met with an intractable problem.

[37] William G. Savage, 'Bacterial food poisoning and food infections', *Reports on Public Health and Medical Matters*, 77 (1913).

[38] Savage, 'Bacterial food poisoning', p. ii.

[39] Savage, 'Bacterial food poisoning', Addendum A, pp. 61–4.

[40] Savage, 'Bacterial food poisoning', p. 54.

[41] Savage, 'Bacterial food poisoning', p. 58.

ANIMALS TO SLAUGHTER

Concern over meat from diseased animals entering the human food chain had existed in England since the 1850s at least, and was sharpened from the 1880s by the new scientific evidence of the transmissibility of bovine tuberculosis to humans through infected meat and milk.[42] The food poisoning issue covered a far larger canvas than did tuberculosis, however, for it focused attention not just on the condition of animals before slaughter, and which parts of the carcase were or were not safe to eat, but on the subject of the hygiene of slaughtering in general. Aside from the 'dirty handling' of prepared meat foods, two possible pathways of food poisoning infection for humans through meat had been established by 1920. The first lay through the use of diseased animal carcasses for human food; the second through the infection of meat after slaughter by the splashing of intestinal contents, blood, and faeces.[43] Even inspection before slaughter to remove sick animals from the food chain was not unproblematic where *Salmonella* infections were concerned: as Savage suggested in 1913, healthy animal carriers of *Salmonella*, as well as diseased animals, were the likeliest channels of meat-borne infection.[44] With this pathway as much as sick animals in mind, the basic hygiene of slaughterhouse practice, previously an issue of nuisance and barbarism, became a subject of public health concern.[45]

The dark subject of animal slaughter had preoccupied a number of MOHs and veterinarians for decades, and the evils of the meat trade had been a concern since at least the 1840s.[46] The killing of animals in British towns and cities took place in two types of establishment: the slaughterhouse and the knackery. The former dealt with animals destined for human food; the latter with the sick, injured, and worn out, beasts considered unfit for human consumption. Unscrupulous practices in both types of establishment were a cause of concern: the eminent veterinary surgeon, George Fleming, noted in 1875 that the flesh of animals killed in knackeries too often found its way on to the butcher's stall or into the sausage-making factory, while slaughterhouses were places 'where every kind of fraud is perpetrated with regard to diseased or objectionable flesh'.[47] The British meat trade, based in small, local, privately owned slaughterhouses, was seen as especially difficult to supervise, and open to bad sanitary and humanitarian practices. Although it has been argued that the meat trade in general was anxious to protect the public (and its own reputation and business) from unscrupulous traders,[48] the

42 Richard Perren, *The Meat Trade in Britain, 1840–1914* (1978), pp. 50–68; Waddington, '"Unfit for human consumption"'; Waddington, *Bovine Scourge*, chapter 1.

43 William G. Savage, *Food and Public Health* (1919), pp. 123–4.

44 Savage, 'Bacterial food poisoning', pp. 54–6.

45 For the slaughterhouse as nuisance see Chris Otter, 'Civilizing slaughter: the development of the British public abattoir, 1850–1910', in *Meat, Modernity, and the Rise of the Slaughterhouse*, pp. 89–106.

46 Perren, *Meat Trade*, pp. 50–68.

47 George Fleming, *A Manual of Veterinary Sanitary Science and Police* (1875), vol 2, pp. 551, 601. See also Keir Waddington, 'The dangerous sausage: diet, meat and disease in Victorian and Edwardian Britain', *Cultural and Social History*, 81 (2011): pp. 51–71.

48 Waddington, '"Unfit for human consumption"', pp. 632–3.

financial incentives for farmers to kill sick animals 'to save their lives' and prevent financial loss remained strong. In the only other British food poisoning cases occurring before 1918 in which Gärtner group organisms were definitely associated with meat, the first resulted from brawn made with a pig's foot, probably with an abscess on it, taken from an animal that had to be taken by cart to the slaughterhouse; the other resulted from beef bought ready-killed by a contractor at an unusually low price, a fact that did not suggest 'sound, healthy meat'.[49] Unscrupulous farmers and traders had little to fear: as late as 1948, diseased animal carcasses were discovered to have been supplied over a period of four months to 250 butchers in twenty-four Lancashire towns.[50]

Significant differences in opportunity for unscrupulous practice existed between Scotland and England and Wales. In England, slaughterhouses had to be registered or annually licensed by the local authorities under the Towns Improvements Clauses Act, 1847.[51] The authorities could only take action against registered houses for selling unsound or diseased meat if the occupier was also the owner or proprietor. A licensed house could, however, be permanently closed after the occupier had twice been convicted, a clause which offered determined local authorities the opportunity to reduce or even eliminate private slaughterhouses from their districts. In practice, however, slaughterhouses were by no means strictly controlled—although, of course, local practices differed—and the general public seemed indifferent: as another eminent veterinarian noted, 'private vested interests in this, as in everything else', were the primary consideration of English law.[52] Moreover, slaughtering in England was by no means a solely urban occupation; many slaughterhouses were located in the countryside and others moved to marginal areas to escape inspection and regulation.[53] In Scotland controls were tighter, since there was no legal distinction between registered and licensed slaughterhouses, and both were required to obtain an annual licence. By 1900, private slaughterhouses were no longer permitted to exist in burghs where a public abattoir had been provided, and private slaughterhouses had vanished from Edinburgh and Glasgow.[54] Although the municipal abattoir was only as effective as its staff were competent in detecting diseased animals and their meat, it was widely recognized as the best available means of controlling the quality of meat entering the human food chain. Moreover, standards of cleanliness both in premises and in handling of meat (so that it did not reach the retail outlets contaminated with blood, faeces,

[49] William G. Savage and C. H. Gunson, 'An outbreak of food poisoning from infected brawn', *Journal of Hygiene*, 8 (1908): pp. 601–8; Edmond J. McWeeney, 'Observations on an outbreak of meat poisoning at Limerick . . . ', *BMJ* (1909), i: pp. 1171–3.

[50] Notes and Comments, 'Unsound meat', *Medical Officer*, 80 (1948): p. 235.

[51] See Peter J. Atkins, 'The Glasgow case: Meat, disease and regulation, 1889–1924', *Agricultural History Review*, 52 (2004): pp. 180–1.

[52] Frederick Smith, *A Manual of Veterinary Hygiene*, 3rd edn (1905), p. 655.

[53] Otter, 'Civilizing slaughter', p. 94. See also Notes and Comments, 'Slaughtering in rural districts', *MO*, 25 (1921): p. 47; Notes of the Week, 'Meat inspection in rural areas', *MO*, 36 (1926): p. 231.

[54] Smith, *Manual*, p. 655. See also Atkins, 'Glasgow case', pp. 180–1. For the rise of the abattoir see Otter, 'Civilizing slaughter', pp. 89–106.

or intestinal contents) were more likely to be maintained under public ownership. Nor did the manufacture of sausages, brawn, and meat pies—a common practice in private slaughterhouses—take place on municipal premises.

The differences in condition and practice between the two types of slaughterhouse were graphically described by R. B. Haines of the Food Investigation Board in the early 1930s.[55] Possible sources of contamination in the slaughterhouse included airborne organisms released during the processes of skinning and gutting; contact with blood, faeces, and intestinal contents on walls and floors; and water and swabs used to wash down carcasses. Observations were made in both types of slaughterhouse; the one described as the small, privately owned establishment, of which there were many in Britain, generally located in a barn or similar outbuilding, where 'as a rule little regard is paid to the elementary principles of hygiene'; the other the large modern abattoir of the big city.[56] In distinguishing between slaughterhouse and abattoir, Haines seems also to have been observing differences between rural and urban practices. He was interested in the bacterial counts to be obtained from carcasses slaughtered in each type of establishment, since bacterial contamination affects the storage life of meat.[57] His account detailed both slaughterhouse conditions and the results of his bacterial counting.

As described by Haines, the typical private slaughterhouse had a cobbled floor, whose interstices were cemented with blood and faeces, and whose walls were covered in mould. Carcasses were frequently dragged through blood and faeces on the floor, and washing down was performed with a single bucket of water and a piece of cloth. As many as ten carcasses would be washed with one bucket of water, and by the end, he argued, they were being 'heavily inoculated' instead of being cleansed. They were then hung above the killing floor overnight to 'cool out', at the mercy of air-borne organisms. In the city abattoir, however, matters were much better. Parallel lines of killing booths with white tiled walls stood on concrete floors, their walls rising short of the roof to ensure ventilation. Ducts and drains carried away offal and dung, each labelled for a different waste product—blood, guts, hides, paunch, general—and the walls were frequently hosed during killing. Comparative bacterial counts were revealing. Private slaughterhouse air yielded 35 per cent soil bacteria and 19 per cent intestinal bacteria, as against 44 and 9 per cent respectively in the abattoir; carcass-swabbing water from the slaughterhouse yielded 2–2.5 million bacteria per cc, and an *E coli* count of 5,000 per cc; at the abattoir the total counts were 15,000 per cc and 5, respectively.[58] Haines ascribed the smaller bacterial load of the abattoir carcasses to the superior ventilation system, but his description clearly suggests the ease with which dead meat could become contaminated with pathogenic organisms by other means.

[55] The Food Investigation Board of the Department of Scientific and Industrial Research was located at the Low Temperature Research Station, Cambridge.

[56] R. B. Haines, 'Observations on the bacterial flora of some slaughter-houses', *Jnl Hyg*, 33 (1933): p. 165.

[57] See also R. B. Haines, 'The bacterial flora developing on stored lean meat, especially with regard to "slimy meat"', *Jnl Hyg*, 33 (1933): pp. 175–82.

[58] Haines, 'Observations', pp. 172–3.

Meat inspection in England took place after slaughter, whether on slaughterhouse premises or in the butcher's shop. During the nineteenth century, the veterinary inspection of animals before and after slaughter, and the establishment of municipal public abattoirs where slaughtering practices could be effectively regulated, had become widespread on the Continent, notably in Germany and Scandinavia.[59] The Continental model was one which many veterinarians and some public health practitioners were anxious that Britain should follow. In England, for the most part, slaughterhouse supervision was performed by nuisance inspectors, and only rarely by qualified veterinarians; the situation was a source of much professional disquiet among veterinarians (who also no doubt could use the professional opportunities and income) and, eventually, of tension between veterinarians and sanitary inspectors. The 1855 Nuisances Removal Act provided for the inspection of articles intended for sale as food, and following the Public Health and Sale of Food and Drugs Acts 1875, local authorities were permitted to destroy food considered unfit for human consumption. Meat inspection was thus deemed a sanitary and medical matter by the law, since meat inspectors were under the supervision of MOHs. The veterinarians, however, considered that only trained veterinarians were qualified to judge whether meat was sound or not, and, looking to the Continental model, emphasized the necessity of inspecting animals for signs of disease before slaughter—a measure which was only implemented with the coming of the single European Market and the BSE crisis in the 1990s. Not surprisingly, the veterinary surgeon Frederick Smith pronounced in 1905 that meat inspection in England, with a few exceptions, among which Manchester was pre-eminent, was 'an absolute farce'.[60] In 1926 it was noted, perhaps rhetorically, that except in the large towns, there was 'strictly speaking' no meat inspection in England: the task was mostly entrusted to men with a few weeks' training.[61]

The situation regarding slaughterhouse provision and practice remained unsatisfactory in England, from a veterinary and sanitary point of view, until the mid-1960s.[62] Under the Public Health Act 1875, local authorities in England and Wales could provide public abattoirs, but could not insist on their use. By 1905, only eighty-four out of 1,083 boroughs had invested in abattoirs. Many of them were said to be little used, and in London there were none, although there were 600 private slaughterhouses.[63] In the 1930s, MOHs still deplored the survival of the private slaughterhouse, complaining of vested interests: 'in this as in all matters concerning food handling, this country is behindhand because the public

[59] Peter A. Koolmees, J. R. Fisher, and Richard Perren, 'The traditional responsibility of veterinarians in meat production and meat inspection', in *Veterinary Aspects of Meat Production, Processing and Inspection. An Update of Recent Developments in Europe*, edited by Frans J. M. Smulders (1999), pp. 7–30.

[60] Smith, *Veterinary Hygiene*, p. 650.

[61] T. Dunlop Young, in discussion following G. H. Wooldridge, 'Some diseases of meat and their relation to public health', *Proceedings of the Royal Society of Medicine*, xix 1–2 (1925–6), Section of Comparative Medicine: p. 62.

[62] Koolmees, 'Traditional responsibility', p. 12.

[63] Smith, *Veterinary Hygiene*, p. 656.

"cleanliness-conscience" is insufficient to overcome trade objection'.[64] As late as 1933, no English municipal abattoir was a paying concern, although it was generally assumed that they would become financially viable were they the sole slaughtering facility on offer.[65] However, small gains only were made in shifting the location of slaughter from private to public spaces: in 1922 it was estimated that there were around 20,000 private slaughterhouses in England and Wales against some 100 public abattoirs; by 1938, the figures were 15,000 and 115 respectively.[66] Between 1875 and 1938, the only improvement in legislative provision for slaughtering lay, from the veterinary point of view, in the 1933 Slaughter of Animals Act, whose sole object was the prevention of cruelty in slaughterhouses.[67] Although several English local authorities adopted a system of veterinary supervision of the meat trade in the years up to 1939, coverage nationally remained fragmentary and incomplete. The establishment of the centralized government Veterinary Inspection Service for the control of animal disease in 1938 to all intents and purposes destroyed the municipal veterinary services, since it drew vets away from municipal service and was concerned with the welfare and economic aspects of animal disease, not with public health issues.[68]

THE BACTERIAL ECONOMY IN NATURE

The identification of the slaughterhouse as a preventive site for food poisoning effectively deflected concerns about the wider environmental sources of animal infections. It created a handy disjunction between the habitats of human and animal infection, setting the latter at a distance from epidemiological and public health interests, which remained focused on the immediate circumstances of human outbreaks. Laboratory researchers, on the other hand, continued to be intrigued by the question of the natural habitats of these organisms. Investigation into the broader ecology of *Salmonella* infections constituted a continuous strand of laboratory-based research in a number of countries through to 1939. Early inquiries centred on whether these organisms were natural inhabitants of the animal gut. William Savage, as we have seen, was investigating the bacterial flora of cattle and pigs in 1905, but much of the research under this head took place in Germany. British attitudes to food safety and issues of animal health were relaxed by contrast with many European countries at this period. Municipal abattoirs and pre- and post-mortem inspection of animals were pioneered in Germany in the 1870s and widely copied elsewhere. By 1930 responsibility for the freedom of all meat and meat products from disease in all other countries was said to rest 'solely with Veterinary

64 Notes and Comments, 'Abattoirs', *MO*, 45 (1931): p. 249.

65 Notes and Comments, 'The abattoir', *MO*, 49 (1933): p. 13.

66 Harold E. Bywater, 'Public and private slaughter-houses in England and Wales', *Veterinary Record*, 60 (1948): p. 219.

67 J. A. Dixon, 'Centralised slaughtering', *Vet Rec*, 52 (1940): p. 767.

68 Anne Hardy, 'Professional advantage and public health: British veterinarians and state veterinary services, 1865–1939', *Twentieth Century British History*, 14 (2003): pp. 18–23.

Officers'.[69] Veterinarians had been respected as scientists in Continental Europe since the eighteenth century, and had early involvement in studying the relationship between human and animal disease—particularly in respect of tuberculosis—whereas in England their professional status was still doubtful, and their involvement in research limited.[70] Nonetheless, England's Medical Department, stimulated perhaps by Durham's findings and by the controversy around tuberculosis, sponsored research into the 'meat poisoning' organisms after 1900.

These early studies marked a watershed in ideas around the causes of food poisoning, displacing ptomaines as an explanatory concept. Two schools of thought emerged.[71] In Germany, Paul Uhlenhuth developed the idea that the *Salmonella* group, and more especially paratyphoid B, were saprophytes which had 'widely colonised the natural world, both living and inert'. From this 'saprophytic foothold' potentially pathogenic strains evolved from time to time, causing infection in animals and humans.[72] In Britain, however, William Savage and Francis Bainbridge, professor of physiology at Durham University,[73] considered the *Salmonella* group as a whole to be essentially pathogenic, depending 'for its indefinite propagation on a more or less closely connected sequence of actively invaded hosts, from which external nature becomes sporadically and abortively contaminated'.[74] By 1930, their views were thought probably to be those of most British workers, 'albeit largely unexpressed and untested'.[75]

Distinctions were increasingly drawn between the natural pathways of different *Salmonella*, between infection in domestic animals, thought to be accidental (with the exception of the pig), and possible endemic infection in rats and mice. The German and British schools could be more or less in sympathy over the latter: Uhlenhuth, for example, declared *Salmonella enteritidis* to be normally and constantly present in rats, while Bainbridge thought the rat intestine might well prove to be the 'true home' of *enteritidis*, with food or bedding contaminated by their droppings infecting other animals. Admitting only that *Salmonella enteritidis* was 'frequently present' in the alimentary canal of grey rats, Bainbridge nonetheless seemed confident that the 'normal habitat' of *Salmonella typhimurium* (*s suipestifer*, as he called it) was chiefly the alimentary tract of pigs, but also of mice and guinea

[69] T. Dunlop Young, 'Meat inspection in England compared with other countries', *Vet Rec*, 38 (1932): p. 1102.

[70] Waddington, *Bovine Scourge*, pp. 30–41.

[71] For the background to these debates see Olga Amsterdamska, 'Medical and biological constraints: Early research on variation in bacteriology', *Social Studies of Science*, 17 (1987): pp. 657–87.

[72] Philip Bruce White, 'The salmonella group', in Medical Research Council, *A System of Bacteriology in Relation to Medicine*, vol 4 (1929), p. 118. Paul Uhlenhuth (1870–1957), assistant professor of hygiene, Griefswald University, specialized in chemotherapy and immunology.

[73] Francis A. Bainbridge, 'The aetiology and epidemiology of paratyphoid fever and "food poisoning"', *PRSM*, 4 (1911): pp. 51–72; Francis A. Bainbridge, 'Paratyphoid fever and meat poisoning' (Milroy Lectures for 1912), *Lancet* (1912), i: pp. 705–9; 771–5; 849–53. For Bainbridge see 'Francis Arthur Bainbridge (1874–1921)', *Oxford Dictionary of National Biography*, vol 3, p. 323.

[74] Bruce White, 'Salmonella group', p. 118.

[75] Bruce White, 'Salmonella group', p. 118.

pigs.[76] The idea of rodents as a natural reservoir for *Salmonella* clearly held some attraction for microbiologists. In 1913, Savage investigated rats collected mostly from refuse tips, concluding that the rat was innocent, although liable to be infected by the Gärtner group.[77] Again in 1918 and 1921 he referred to the potential for rats and mice to spread *Salmonella* infection, noting, in 1918, that 'the question of the infection of rats and mice is obviously of considerable practical importance in view of the frequency with which these animals gain access to food used for man and animals'.[78] He was again investigating rodents under the microscope, on this occasion rats caught in slaughter houses and knackers' yards. From six of ninety-six animals so caught, Savage and his co-worker, Philip Bruce White, obtained a highly virulent strain of *Salmonella enteritidis*, culturally identical to that isolated in food poisoning outbreaks. As they pointed out, these rats would have ample opportunity to infect meat in the environment of the slaughterhouse.[79] A further study conducted on rats by a Liverpool University researcher in 1936 found that 7.3 per cent of 250 animals examined carried *Salmonella* strains, while an American study found an infection rate of 7.5 per cent. The Liverpool study found a marked seasonality of infection, incidence being much higher in the winter months (17.6 per cent) as against spring (4 per cent) and summer (0.4 per cent).[80] In a survey of the *Salmonella* group published in 1933, however, Bruce White remained non-committal on the relationship between animal reservoirs and human infection, noting of human *Salmonella typhimurium* infections: 'of the *epidemiology* of Aertryk food-poisoning we need not speak beyond noting the explosive nature of the outbreaks'.[81]

Despite the suspicions of rodent-borne salmonellosis, reports of incidents associated with naturally infected mice or rats were rare. One was reported from America in 1924, and a second possible case featured among the series of 100 incidents examined by Savage and Bruce White between 1921 and 1923, although these mice were only examined weeks after the event.[82] In 1936, however, a small outbreak of *Salmonella typhimurium* food poisoning was reported from Liverpool, where the source of infection seemed definitely proven to have been food—a dried milk preparation—contaminated with mouse droppings: the organism was retrieved from one of several droppings found in the partially used tin of milk.

[76] Bainbridge, 'Paratyphoid fever', pp. 849, 851–2.

[77] William G. Savage and W. J. Read, 'Gaertner Group bacilli in rats and mice', *Jnl Hyg*, 13 (1913–14): p. 352.

[78] William G. Savage, 'The sources of infection in food poisoning outbreaks', *Jnl Hyg*, 17 (1918): p. 28; William G. Savage, 'Domestic animals as a factor in the spread of infection', *Jnl San Inst*, 61 (1921): p. 289.

[79] William G. Savage and Philip Bruce White, 'Rats and salmonella group bacilli', *Jnl Hyg*, 21 (1922–3): p. 260.

[80] A. M. Khalil, 'The incidence of organisms of the salmonella group in wild rats and mice in Liverpool', *Jnl Hyg*, 38 (1938): pp. 75–8. See also CMOAR (1936), p. 159.

[81] Bruce White, 'Salmonella group', pp. 118–19, 127–38, 128.

[82] O. Salthe and C. Krumweide, 'Studies on the paratyphoid group. VIII. An epidemic of food infection due to paratyphoid bacillus of rodent origins', *American Journal of Hygiene*, 4 (1924): pp. 23–32; William G. Savage and Philip Bruce White, 'Food poisoning: A study of 100 recent outbreaks', Medical Research Council, *Special Report Series*, 92 (1925), case no 51.

The index case here was an eight-month old infant whose diagnosis 'might easily' have been 'summer diarrhoea', had not other features of the case prompted a post-mortem and the finding of *Salmonella typhimurium* infection in the rest of the family.[83] Looking into the past, the authors of the report recalled a 1910 investigation into a group of summer diarrhoea cases (also in Liverpool), where *Salmonella* were isolated from the faeces, heart blood, and abdominal scrapings of the victims.[84] In 1910, bacteriological methods had not permitted the precise identification of the *Salmonella* involved; in 1933 the use of 'specially satisfactory media' played a significant part in establishing the chain of evidence that led to *Salmonella typhimurium* and the mouse droppings.[85]

Rodent reservoirs were not the whole story, however. In 1918, Savage detailed eight different animal diseases caused by Gärtner group members, including swine fever, calf septicaemia, and bovine enteritis. Although a significant number of food poisonings caused by meat from diseased animals were reported from mainland Europe, only four British outbreaks had, at this date, been associated with any evidence of disease in the animal from which the incriminated food came: the two meat outbreaks described above, and two milk-related outbreaks described in 1913 and 1914.[86] In his 1913 study Savage had noted the absence of evidence for Gärtner milk infections:[87] his steady and studious absorption in this literature was paying off. Experimentally, as commonly happened in such studies, Savage was frustrated by his failure to obtain suitable materials for bacteriological examination from diseased animals or animals which had died from one of the diseases associated with the food poisoning organisms. Such research was of extreme importance, he considered, in view of the fact that there appeared to be no recorded outbreaks of Gärtner infections among animals in Britain, apart from the cases traced back to animals because they had caused an outbreak of human disease:[88]

> The prevention of human outbreaks of food poisoning, and possibly a considerable amount of unrecognised disease in animals, can only be attained by an extension of knowledge as to the extent to which these pathogenic organisms are a cause of animal disease.

Given the attention being directed at tuberculous milk and dairy herds, however, and the comparatively minor human death and illness from food poisoning, salmonellosis in animals was not a high research priority in the relevant scientific communities. Thirty years later, an authoritative survey could still note, 'There is

[83] E. R. Jones and H. D. Wright, 'B. aertrycke food poisoning', *Lancet*, 1936, i: pp. 22–3.

[84] R. Stenhouse Williams et al., 'Further researches into the bacteriology of summer diarrhoea', *Lancet*, 1910, ii: pp. 730–52.

[85] Jones and Wright, 'B. aertrycke', p. 23.

[86] Savage, 'Sources of infection', p. 29.

[87] Savage, 'Bacterial food poisoning', p. 44; see also Harold Kerr and H. J. Hutchens, 'An outbreak of food poisoning caused by the bacillus enteritidis of Gaertner in milk', *PRSM*, Epidemiological Section, 7 (1914): pp. 171–2.

[88] Savage, 'Sources of infection', p. 31.

ample scope for a thorough inquiry into the various types of Salmonella capable of infecting domestic animals, and of the type of disease to which they give rise.'[89]

During the 1920s, the pathway of infection through milk assumed greater importance as numbers of milk-borne gastro-enteritis outbreaks began to be recorded, against the background of ongoing concern with tuberculous milk and the pasteurization debate. In 1925, a sudden, widespread gastro-enteritis outbreak (497 recorded cases) occurred in Aberdeen. The city had experienced two previous such outbreaks, both milk-borne: the first in 1919 due to Flexner dysentery infection (nearly 1000 cases, seventy-two deaths), the second in 1923 (110 cases) from a cause undetermined. The 1925 outbreak became apparent to the city Public Health Department on 7 July; cases were reported over a wide geographical area on 7 and 8 July, and then ceased. The circumstances suggested milk as the source of infection, and investigation showed that the suspect milk had been supplied at midday and in the evening of 6 July by a farmer who was also a dairyman and who supplied three other dairies from his own herd.[90] The investigation might have gone no further, for all nine people working on the farm were in good health and admitted no recent history of gastro-enteritis (this was confirmed by serological and bacteriological tests), had Aberdeen not employed a Veterinary Inspector. On 8 July, the veterinarian seized and condemned the carcass of a cow, slaughtered with symptoms of septicaemia, as unfit for human consumption. The carcass was identified as being from the dairyman's herd, and samples of udder and flesh were obtained for bacteriological examination. Under the microscope, *Salmonella enteritidis* stood revealed. It appeared that the cow in question had been ailing for some days, and had been isolated from the rest of the herd, having her milk stripped daily by the farmer and bulked with the rest.[91]

Aberdeen's MOH, John Parlane Kinloch, later to be appointed CMO for Scotland, was an energetic and imaginative man.[92] Aware of the dearth of reliable information on Gärtner infections in animals, and given that *Salmonella* had been isolated from both milk and tissue, he thought it 'advisable' to record the outbreak in detail.[93] Several points of interest can be extracted from this account. Most of the victims were over five years of age, 72 per cent being aged between fifteen and sixty-five. The speed with which the outbreak was uncovered made it possible to obtain three separate samples of infected milk from the homes of patients: in each case milk not consumed at a meal had been left on the table and was still there some twelve hours later, when the family's illness resulted in a call to the Health Department.[94]

[89] Graham S. Wilson and Ashley A. Milne, eds, *Topley and Wilson's Principles of Bacteriology and Immunity*, 3rd edn (1946), vol 1, p. 1261.

[90] John Parlane Kinloch et al., 'The Aberdeen outbreak of milk-borne Gaertner enteritis, July, 1925', *Jnl Hyg*, 25 (1926): pp. 434–43.

[91] Kinloch et al., 'Aberdeen outbreak'.

[92] Notes and Comments, 'John Parlane Kinloch', *MO*, 47 (1932): p. 62; Anon, 'John Parlane Kinloch', *BMJ*, 1932, i: pp. 311–12.

[93] Kinloch et al., 'Aberdeen outbreak', p. 434.

[94] Kinloch et al., 'Aberdeen outbreak', p. 436.

Finally, Kinloch stressed the difficulties inherent in the investigation of milk-borne outbreaks:[95]

> it is our experience . . . that the sense of personal responsibility on the part of the farmer and his financial concern are such that he immediately adopts a policy of reticence which defeats the object of the inquiry. In this connection an educational campaign among dairymen is an urgent requirement, with a view to making them appreciate the fact that *Salmonella* milk infections are liable to occur even in a well-conducted dairy, and that within certain limits the dairymen cannot be censured.

Kinloch's recognition of the part which animal pathology and ecology played in the generation of milk-borne *Salmonella* outbreaks was at once biologically accurate and politically sensitive: the milk of this particular cow had been dangerous only as her illness moved into its acute stage on 6 July, and she had duly been slaughtered on 8 July with a swiftness that was to the farmer's credit. He glossed over the information that the cow had been sent to slaughter rather than to the knacker's, where in theory her carcass would not have been destined for human consumption.

The Aberdeen outbreak provided a significant signpost towards *Salmonella* ecology. Kinloch noted that *Salmonella* infections were commonly regarded as being spread by human carriers, but that this view had no foundation in fact: in just three of the British incidents examined by Savage and Bruce White had any evidence of human source been obtained.[96] Rather, Kinloch argued, the evidence from Aberdeen supported Savage's contention that food-borne *Salmonella* outbreaks were due to active animal infection or to animal carriers.[97] He went on to reason that the presence of 'the typhoid paratyphoid group' in the blood sera of cattle, sheep, and pigs, and its absence in young calves, as demonstrated by Savage in 1918, suggested that these animals either obtained immunity through exposure to non-infective doses of the organisms, or that at some period in their lives they had suffered infections due to them.[98] Since the available evidence indicated that cattle did not commonly harbour *Salmonella* in their intestines, Kinloch suggested that[99]

> the elucidation of the causes of the development of these agglutinins in cattle and other animals may provide fresh information as to the manner in which *Salmonella* infections are transmitted from the lower animals to man, and may eventually show that *Salmonella* infections are essentially and primarily diseases of lower animals occurring only secondarily in man.

For Kinloch, as for Savage, the distribution of *Salmonella* in nature had come to represent the crux of their epidemiology.

The suspicion that the roots of *Salmonella* causation might lie in the animal kingdom was reinforced with the refinement of microbiological techniques and

95 Kinloch et al., 'Aberdeen outbreak', p. 436.

96 Kinloch et al., 'Aberdeen outbreak', p. 443; Savage and Bruce White, 'Food poisoning', pp. 59, 71–2 (case numbers 10, 36, 37).

97 Savage, 'Bacterial food poisoning', pp. 54–6.

98 William G. Savage, 'Further investigations upon the distribution of Gaertner group bacilli in domestic and other animals', *Jnl Hyg*, 17 (1918): pp. 38–45.

99 Kinloch et al., 'Aberdeen outbreak', p. 443.

new bacteriological discoveries in the later 1920s. In particular, methods of identifying and distinguishing different strains of bacteria were greatly improved (Chapter 5). In the van of this research, Philip Bruce White isolated a new serotype, *Salmonella* dublin, which appeared to be especially associated with cattle, four years after the Aberdeen outbreak.[100] The Aberdeen interest in gastro-enteric infections continued, as the city repeatedly experienced a variety of such outbreaks.[101] By 1930 the City Hospital bacteriologist was collaborating with W. M. Scott of the English Ministry of Health laboratory in identifying food poisoning organisms. In 1930, they reported on cases of continued fever associated with *Salmonella* strains of the 'dublin' variety. They noted that dublin's suspected special association with bovines, and hence with cows' milk, was confirmed by its serological identity with the 'paracolon' bacillus previously shown by Danish researchers to cause fatal enteritis in young calves, and by the fact that in most cases where it was isolated from humans, milk could definitely be suspected as the vehicle of transmission.[102]

Throughout the 1930s, investigators chipped away at the links between human and bovine salmonellosis. Further human cases of *Salmonella* dublin were recorded in Aberdeen in 1930 and 1934, and it was recovered from infants with sporadic meningitis in Glasgow.[103] These findings suggested that human infection with the organism was widespread, while concurrent research indicated it to be pathogenic in cattle. For those interested in such questions, these were years in which some of the conundrums of the bacterial origin of gastro-enteritis and food poisoning began to unravel. In a survey of food infections occurring in Dundee between 1923 and 1938, W. J. Tulloch noted three distinct phenomena among incidents recorded. First, most sporadic cases and familial outbreaks were due to *Salmonella typhimurium*, as was one large outbreak; second, there were several limited outbreaks in which the causal organism was one of the 'less frequently encountered' members of the *Salmonella* tribe ('stanley', 'potsdam', 'seftenberg'); and third, two major milk-borne epidemics had been retrospectively determined to be caused by *Salmonella* dublin. These occurred in August 1926 and October 1927, and both had been shown to originate with a cow 'indubitably' suffering from septicaemia.[104] Current bacteriological methods were inadequate to determine the precise nature of the organism involved, but, significant of the level of local medical interest, representative strains of human and bovine origin were retained for future reference. The introduction in 1932 of the Kauffmann–White classification scheme, which classified *Salmonella* into serotypes according to their surface antigens (see Chapter 5),

[100] Philip Bruce White, 'Notes on organisms serologically related to *s. enteritidis* Gärtner. I', *Jnl Hyg*, 29 (1929–30): pp. 443–5.

[101] F. T. G. Bowie et al., 'Paratyphoid fever and aertryke enteritis in Aberdeen—a contrast', *Jnl Hyg*, 26 (1926): pp. 444–52; Andrew M. Fraser et al., 'Sonne dysentery in Aberdeen', *Jnl Hyg*, 26 (1926): pp. 453–60.

[102] J. Smith and William M. Scott, 'Continued fever due to a Gartner-like *Salmonella* type "Dublin"', *Jnl Hyg*, 30 (1930): pp. 32–9.

[103] H. Ross Souper et al., 'Three sporadic cases of infection due to salmonella type Dublin', *Archives of Disease in Childhood*, 5 (1930): pp. 270–4.

[104] W. J. Tulloch, 'Observations concerning bacillary food infection in Dundee during the period 1923–38', *Jnl Hyg*, 39 (1939): pp. 324–33.

made it possible to reinvestigate the organisms involved and determine their precise serological relationships. Both proved to be *Salmonella* dublin.[105]

Tulloch's report seems to have been stimulated by the publication in the previous year of a Ministry of Health investigation into an outbreak of gastro-enteritis in Wiltshire due to raw milk. The source of infection was traced to a single, apparently healthy, cow, whose blood contained antibodies to *Salmonella* dublin and from whose dung the organism was repeatedly isolated.[106] On this evidence, it seemed clear that the animal in question was a healthy carrier, and although no bacilli were found in her milk, it was concluded that contamination with dung had occurred through faulty operation of the mechanical milking plant.[107] As Tulloch implicitly indicated, an appreciable number of bovine carriers might explain the apparently widespread human infection with *Salmonella* dublin being turned up by other researchers.[108]

The further implications of the Wiltshire findings were suggested by the CMO, Arthur MacNalty, in his introduction to the report. Here, he noted, was yet another in the 'long series' of disease outbreaks recorded as a result of drinking raw milk, of the class originating with a diseased cow (and the shadow of bovine tuberculosis can be seen behind his precise words):[109] 'No amount of care in milking and distribution of such raw milk can prevent it from being a danger to the consumer. In other words, a clean raw milk is not necessarily a safe raw milk.' The only practicable way to reduce the risks of such outbreaks to a minimum was, he insisted, by efficient pasteurization.[110]

CLEAN MILK

The question of milk pasteurization was a contentious one in 1930s Britain.[111] Contaminated milk had been known to carry infections such as scarlet fever and typhoid since the 1870s, but it was only with the explosion of concern over tuberculosis around 1900 that the cleanliness and bacterial purity of milk became an issue.[112] Continental models suggested adopting pasteurization as a solution, but the medical profession could not agree on the benefits of the practice. Among the arguments marshalled against pasteurization were a supposed destruction of

105 Tulloch, 'Observations', pp. 328, 330.

106 E. T. Conybeare and L. H. D. Thornton, 'An outbreak of food poisoning due to Salmonella, type "Dublin" and conveyed by raw milk', *Reps on PH*, 82 (1938): pp. 1–8.

107 Conybeare and Thornton, 'Outbreak', p. 5.

108 Tulloch, 'Observations', p. 331.

109 Arthur MacNalty, 'Prefatory Note' to Conybeare and Thornton, 'Outbreak', p. 2.

110 MacNalty, 'Note'.

111 Peter J. Atkins, 'The pasteurisation of England: the science, culture and health implications of milk processing, 1900–1950', in *Food, Science, Policy and Regulation in the Twentieth Century*, edited by David F. Smith and Jim Phillips (2000), pp. 37–51. With raw milk returning to favour as a lifestyle option, this is still the case. The Food Standards Agency is currently reviewing methods of regulation and control.

112 Waddington, *Bovine Scourge*, chapter 9.

important vitamins and trace elements during heat treatment, and that bovine tuberculosis bacilli in milk helped inoculate the population against the human form of the disease.[113] It was, however, recognized that tuberculosis was not the only issue: infected milk continued to produce other human ills, particularly brucellosis, typhoid, paratyphoid, and gastro-enteritis.[114] In 1942, Graham Selby Wilson, Director of the Emergency Public Health Laboratory Service, noted that 113 milk-borne disease outbreaks had occurred in Britain between 1912 and 1937, affecting some 14,000 people. For the same period, he estimated bovine tuberculosis deaths at some 65,000 and deaths among the under-2s from epidemic diarrhoea at around 190,000.[115] These figures, he argued, justified the statement that 'raw milk is probably the most dangerous article in our dietary'.[116]

The persistent danger of intrinsic milk infection constituted the core argument for adopting pasteurization. However clean milk might be, pasteurization alone could protect against the transmission of disease. In the heat of inter-war debates for and against pasteurization, and with government reluctance to enact regulations that would impose additional costs on an industry already struggling to cope with the effects of economic depression, pasteurization and other techniques for securing a clean milk supply made slow progress.[117] In 1924, the MOH for Manchester noted little or no improvement in the quality of milk supplied to the city from Cheshire, and only a slight improvement in that produced in Derbyshire and Staffordshire over the previous 23 years: the involvement of dairy farmers and other dairying interests in local government often produced inertia in implementation of the Dairies, Cowsheds, and Milkshops orders.[118] Although a milk-borne epidemic of 'sore throat' drove Manchester to seek powers to pasteurize the entire city milk supply in 1932, such reaction was rare.[119] In 1939 most British milk supplies were still raw, and in many rural areas and small towns this remained the norm into the 1950s.[120] As with the veterinary supervision of meat supplies, government has been reluctant to interfere with vested interests and with producers' and consumers' right of choice: unpasteurized milk, under the classic Green Top designation, remains available in England in 2014 despite a government threat to ban it following the discovery in 1998 of samples containing cattle dung, *Salmonella*, and *E. coli* 0157.[121] The sale of unpasteurized milk was banned in Scotland in 1983, but

[113] Atkins, 'Pasteurisation', pp. 44, 46–7.

[114] Albert E. Bell, *The Pasteurisation and Sterilisation of Milk* (1900), pp. 15–21; Hugh A. Macewen, *The Public Milk Supply* (1910), chapter 2; Janet Lane-Claypon, 'Milk and its hygienic regulation', Medical Research Council, *Special Report Series* (1916), chapter 15.

[115] Graham S. Wilson, *The Pasteurisation of Milk* (1942), pp. 41, 46.

[116] Wilson, *Pasteurisation*, p. 44.

[117] Jim Phillips and Michael French, 'State regulation and the hazards of milk, 1900–1939', *Social History of Medicine*, 12 (1999): pp. 371–88; Richard Perren, *Agriculture in Depression* (1995), chapter 5.

[118] Editorial, 'Manchester milk cleanliness', *MO*, 47 (1924): p. 153.

[119] Annotation, 'Compulsory pasteurisation of milk', *MO*, 47 (1932): pp. 36–7.

[120] Atkins, 'Pasteurisation', p. 39.

[121] <http://www.naturalfoodfinder.co.uk/unpasteurised-raw-milk-uk>, accessed 25 May 2013; <http://www.readabstracts.com/Retail-industry/Green-top-milk-may-be-banned-Heart-inquiry-to-involve-1000-children.html#b>, accessed 17 June 2014. See also Frank Trentmann, 'Bread, milk and

Salmonella dublin infections have continued to occur among farming families who habitually drink raw milk.[122]

Running parallel to public health concerns around the transmission of disease by milk were concerns over the new technology of milk delivery. Traditionally retailed from open pans in shops or by decanting into customers' receptacles from mobile churns, milk was increasingly being sold in bottles by the 1920s. Bottling spread from America to Britain in the years around 1900; the London Dairy Supply Company is said to have pioneered the production of sterilized bottled milk in England.[123] Bottling was, however, by no means a uniform procedure; nor did it guarantee cleanliness and quality. In St Helens in 1925, milk was either bottled on the farm, or bought in bulk and then bottled. The city's MOH was anxious: if the milk was not bacteriologically clean when bottled, it could prove dangerous.[124] Initially, it seems, bottles were used for higher grade milk, but they were adopted enthusiastically by local distributors of undesignated milks, resulting in some of the dirtiest milks examined by municipal analysts.[125] In Glamorganshire in 1928, a milkman was caught skimming dead flies from his milk churn before filling his bottles by hand on the highway.[126]

The nature of what went into the bottle was not the only problem. Wider issues of cleanliness and standards of food preparation were involved. Although the Milk and Dairies Order 1926 required the thorough cleansing and sterilization of all equipment in contact with milk, the regulations caused trouble in practice.[127] It took time to educate dairymen in the necessity of sterilizing bottles before use. Cleanliness of bottles was described as 'the weakest link in the chain', and housewives were urged to see that bottles left the house as clean as they could make them.[128] In Blackburn, it was said that some of the farmers who had taken up bottling had no clear conception of what was meant by 'cleanliness'.[129] In Manchester, several thousand bottles were retrieved from city graveyards, where they were being used to hold flowers. Despite the retailers' insistence that all would be thoroughly washed before re-use, a leading firm of distributors refused to have anything to do with the 'resurrected bottles'.[130] Huddersfield had problems with dirty bottles; in Salford a third of all bottles tested in 1934 were found to be dirty;

democracy: consumption and citizenship in twentieth century Britain', in *The Politics of Consumption, Material Culture and Citizenship*, edited by Martin Daunton and Matthew Hilton (2001), p. 160.

122 A. Mateus et al., 'Looking for the unusual suspects', *PH*, 122 (2008): pp. 1321–3.

123 Bell, *Pasteurisation*, p. 33. The history of milk bottling is somewhat sketchily examined in Adam P. den Hartog, 'Serving the urban consumer: The development of modern food packaging with special reference to the milk bottle', in *Food and Material Culture*, edited by Martin R. Scharer and Alexander Fenton (1998), pp. 248–67.

124 Notes of the Week, 'Bottled milk', *MO*, 33 (1925): p. 125.

125 Notes of the Week, 'Bottling of dirty milk', *MO*, 35 (1926): p. 239; Notes of the Week, 'Bottled milk', *MO*, 38 (1927): p. 158.

126 Notes of the Week, 'Flies in milk', *MO*, 40 (1928): pp. 178–9.

127 Betty C. Hobbs and Graham S. Wilson, 'The cleansing and sterilization of milk bottles', *Jnl Hyg*, 43 (1943): p. 96.

128 Notes of the Week, 'Cleaning of milk bottles', *MO*, 36 (1926): p. 160.

129 Notes of the Week, 'Bottled milk', p. 158.

130 Notes of the Week, 'Milk cemeteries', *MO*, 44 (1930): p. 9.

and in Hinckley the discovery that milk bottles were being reclaimed from refuse tips decided the council to ask all milk producers to install sterilizing plants.[131] Concern over the condition of milk bottles peaked in the public health literature in the early 1930s and had faded by the end of the decade, even as the battle over pasteurization rumbled on.[132] Nonetheless, the Ministry of Health remained anxious about bottle cleanliness, commissioning a survey of bottle plant effectiveness (undertaken between October 1937 and July 1939) in 1936.[133] Clean milk in the inter-war period was not simply a question of pasteurization versus natural purity. The dairy industry had to be educated in a wider concept of cleanliness, and taught to apply it to the new technologies of milk delivery. Yet despite the evidence for external sources of infection, the core problem remained, as with meat, one of a product infected at source, in the bodies of domestic livestock.

Realization of the critical role played by infected animals in transmitting *Salmonella* infections other than typhoid came slowly through the inter-war period, as epidemiological and laboratory investigations accumulated to underpin William Savage's 1913 suggestion that healthy animal carriers disseminated food poisoning infections to humans. Different strands of scientific understanding fed into the picture of *Salmonella* infections which was built up in Britain between 1900 and 1940. Turn-of-the-century debates around the transmissibility of bovine tuberculosis helped to shape acceptance of the lesser *Salmonella*'s ability to travel in meat and milk, while recognition of healthy human carriers of typhoid led, via recognition of the serological relationship between *Salmonella typhi* and its cousins, to the realization that food products derived from infected animals, whether or not showing signs of clinical disease, could carry infection onwards to humans through the food chain. Laboratory isolation of animal serotypes from cases of human disease assisted in this process. And finally, experience with epidemic outbreaks during these years demonstrated the fragility of food security in existing systems for meat and milk production—in the weakness of supervisory powers over production, in the nature of traditional slaughtering provision, in the new technologies of bulking and bottling in milk production. On the eve of World War II, powerful figures in Britain's public health community prepared to bring their veterinary colleagues aboard in the emerging struggle against *Salmonella* infections.

[131] Notes of the Week, 'Cleaning of milk bottles', *MO*, 48 (1932): p. 29; Notes of the Week, 'Cleaning of milk vessels', *MO*, 55 (1936): p 125; Notes of the Week, 'Milk bottles reclaimed from refuse tips', *MO*, 50 (1933): p. 115.

[132] Editorial, 'Pasteurised milk', *MO*, 59 (1938): p. 115.

[133] Hobbs and Wilson, 'Milk bottles', p. 96. Due to war-time paper shortages, this report was never published, and has since disappeared.

PART II

LABORATORY PURSUITS

5

Pursuing Parasites

The epidemiological discovery of pathways of infection dominated the story of the *Salmonella* between 1880 and the early 1900s. In this discovery, the laboratory had played a part, but rather as a supporting player to the field deductions of outbreak investigators. In the twentieth century the laboratory increasingly emerged as a key contributor to epidemiological investigation, albeit after a period in which much laboratory work seemed to contribute little to the problems of outbreak investigators. It was through the laboratory that the family relationships between typhoid, the paratyphoids, and the food poisoning and other *Salmonella* were elaborated—and for a time disputed—in the first decades of the twentieth century, and it was through the laboratory that the vastly complex natural history and modes of transmission of these organisms were elucidated and mapped in the years after 1920. The laboratory was the critical site within which the power relations between observational epidemiology and microbiology were gradually reversed. By 1950, the detective formula 'When you know how, you know who' had been reversed, and the laboratory identification of the causal organism of a *Salmonella* outbreak generally resolved the question of its origin.

The stages by which this transfer of determinative power took place were uneven: slow for most of the inter-war period, but accelerating rapidly from 1939. The early history of bacteriology was marked, as has been well noted, by a virtual frenzy of discovery, in which the identification of new causal organisms became an end in itself. This process of discovery was not uncomplicated. Knowledge of the great variety of intestinal bacteria identified at this time was, one authority observed, 'very elementary', and the project of identifying, differentiating, and evaluating the importance of the many types found in human and animal excreta must have seemed 'well-nigh hopeless' to many bacteriologists.[1]

Progress was made, however, and by 1920, the discovery of variations of type within bacterial species was engendering a hair-splitting type of minute microbiology whose primary focus was on taxonomy: on the identification and classification of new types of particular bacteria. In practice, this led many laboratory scientists to concentrate on the organisms themselves, rather than on their natural history and public health significance. This pursuit of parasites was to result in rich epidemiological reward, but for much of the inter-war period the interests of laboratory research appeared to diverge from those of public health. Thus *Medical Officer*

[1] J. A. A., 'Arthur Theodore MacConkey', *Journal of Pathology and Bacteriology*, 34, ii (1931): p. 698.

complained in 1920 that 'We are becoming all too petty in our juggling with the micro-organisms that harm us, and the results hardly lead us anywhere at all.'[2] Such research, it was argued, bore little relation to 'the science of epidemiology', and was of little benefit to 'the science of preventive medicine': knowing that there were half a dozen types of dysentery did not help to prevent dysentery. 'The bacteriologists', the complainant continued, 'some of them at any rate, seem to live in little boxes of their own, separated entirely from those who are interested in preventive medicine and epidemiology'.[3] For much of the inter-war period, and for most practical purposes, outbreak investigation and preventive medicine continued as they had done, resorting to the laboratory only for final confirmation of their findings in the field.

Yet an understanding of the natural history of *Salmonella* was essential if the pathways by which enteric infections passed to humans through the food chain were to be elucidated. Although powerful groups within microbiology remained preoccupied with taxonomic matters, the epidemiologists' need to discover pathways of infection ensured that a slender thread of research interest in microbiology with practical applications was maintained through the Ministry of Health, as was shown by, for example, the outbreak survey jointly commissioned with the Medical Research Council (MRC) in the early 1920s, and by W. M. Scott's research, notably into *Salmonella* in duck eggs and live pigs, in the Ministry of Health laboratory.[4] The outcome was effectively the development of two research communities, with some overlapping membership and interests, but with different concerns. Both were laboratory-based, but one was absorbed by the identification and classification of organisms of the *Salmonella* family while the other sought also to track these organisms to their source, to their natural hosts, and to the environmental circumstances that resulted in them gaining access to human digestive tracts. The first community was almost exclusively absorbed by what could be observed under the microscope; the second sought to relate laboratory findings to events in the field and to the economy of these organisms in nature. Although divergent, both communities contributed to knowledge with eventual practical outcomes.

LABORATORIES IN AN EPIDEMIOLOGICAL LANDSCAPE, 1870–1940

Laboratory investigations into bacteria and their habits took place against an established background of epidemiological investigation which pre-dated the effective involvement of the laboratory. Public health officers and outbreak

[2] Notes and Comments, 'Labels and the laboratory', *Medical Officer*, 24 (1920): p. 136.

[3] Notes and Comments, 'Labels', p. 136.

[4] Linda Bryder notes the 1923 delineation of responsibilities between the Ministry of Heath (public health research with practical application) and the Medical Research Council (pure research): Linda Bryder, 'Public health research and the MRC', in *Historical Perspectives on the Role of the MRC* (1989), edited by Linda Bryder and Joan Austoker, p. 59.

investigators thought in epidemiological terms, and it took time for laboratory services to be accommodated within this approach to disease investigation and management. Well into the inter-war period, laboratory investigators were generally brought in as a last, confirmatory, resource by epidemiologists rather than being involved in investigations from the beginning. Moreover, the map of laboratory provision even in inter-war Britain was by no means a planned one.[5] Laboratory work of different kinds was required by hospitals, pharmaceutical companies, manufacturers, general practitioners, local health authorities, and universities. A spectrum of laboratories existed across the country, from the Ministry of Health's small pathological laboratory—which had an active interest in preventive microbiology—at one extreme, through a variety of commercial, hospital, and university facilities which undertook commissioned work not directly related to their principal functions and municipal or county laboratories engaged in practical, preventive-related work, to the independent, research-oriented labs run by the Clinical Association, the Lister Institute, and the Royal College of Physicians of Edinburgh at the other. The powerhouses of research into *Salmonella* at this period were the Ministry and the Lister facilities, but no central co-ordinated research and investigation establishment existed before the creation in England of the Emergency Public Heath Laboratory Service on the eve of World War II. During the inter-war period, the relations between outbreak investigation and laboratory investigation remained for the most part fragile and unsatisfactory.

The involvement of the laboratory in English public health practice predated the emergence of bacteriology. In 1871, John Simon, then Chief Medical Officer (CMO), applied for and received an annual grant of £2,000 from the Privy Council to support laboratory research related to the concerns of the Central Medical Department.[6] In the decades that followed, laboratory research formed an important component of the Department's activities, and accounts of the Auxiliary Scientific Investigations were published annually in the CMO's report. In the years to 1910, these investigations were commissioned from independent scientists, notably from Edward Klein, who had come to England from Vienna at Simon's invitation in 1869.[7] Among the investigations carried out by Klein and others, a significant number related directly to epidemiological problems in the field. In the 1890s, for instance, Klein and others worked on the survival capacities of the typhoid bacillus in different media (soil, water, food),[8] and in the early years of the new century on the economy of food-poisoning organisms in nature. The established tradition of the Medical Department linked field and laboratory investigation closely. The laboratory research was, however, primarily directed to wider scientific issues, rather than providing regular assistance to field investigation.

[5] Bryder, 'Public health research', pp. 61, 67.

[6] Royston Lambert, *Sir John Simon, 1816–1904, and English Social Administration* (1963), chapter 14.

[7] Anon, 'Edward Emmanuel Klein', *Lancet* (1925), i: pp. 411–12.

[8] See Michael Worboys, *Spreading Germs. Disease Theories and Medical Practice in Britain, 1865–1900* (2000), pp. 265–71.

As the new laboratory-based medical sciences developed, more formal arrangements seemed increasingly desirable. In 1910, CMO Arthur Newsholme succeeded in obtaining a small pathology laboratory within the Medical Department, taking over some of the equipment belonging to the laboratory of the Royal Commission on Bovine Tuberculosis and acquiring its principal researcher, Arthur Eastwood, as medical inspector in charge.[9] Initially staffed by Eastwood, Frederick Griffith (who had also been involved with the Bovine Tuberculosis Commission), and two assistants, the number of staff had doubled by 1917 with the addition of William McDonald Scott and three further assistants.[10] The laboratory survived into the Ministry of Health, and came to provide a key research and diagnostic facility during the inter-war period. This laboratory had, however, been envisaged as part of a much larger national facility. Politically speaking, the Bovine Tuberculosis Commission had demonstrated the value of pathology to public health, and the Local Government Board set up a departmental committee to examine the methods by which the work of tuberculosis prevention might be carried forward in the community. In a letter to the committee, dated October 1912, Newsholme argued strongly for the establishment of a national network of large clinical laboratories. Pathological work, he declared, 'forms an important means of ascertaining the distribution and character of disease in a district, and thus of enabling preventive measures to be taken'.[11] He emphasized that inadequate existing laboratory provision 'must represent an enormous economic loss to the community and a great amount of unnecessary sickness'. Newsholme saw this not simply as a clinical facility, but in wider public health terms; elsewhere he commented on the undesirability of separating public health bacteriological work from more general pathology.[12] His arguments were accepted by the committee, and in 1913 he recorded Budget proposals for 'a large extension' of pathological facilities, 'making it hopeful that these will before long be available for any disease to which these facilities are helpful for prevention, diagnosis, and treatment'.[13] The outbreak of war in 1914 put paid to these plans for a cohesive national pathology service. Financial constraint between 1920 and 1937 limited the expansion of the Ministry's facility, and it was only under the shadow of another European war that a national network of public health laboratories was established in 1939.

During the inter-war years, however, the Ministry's small laboratory played an active role both in servicing epidemiological investigations, and in conducting research into selected pathogens. In cramped quarters in Carlisle Place, and later Endell Street, Frederick Griffith and his colleague W. M. Scott offered a unique

[9] John M. Eyler, *Sir Arthur Newsholme and State Medicine, 1885–1935* (1997), p. 226; British Parliamentary Papers, 1910–11, xxxii, p. 59.

[10] Chief Medical Officer's Annual Report (1932): p. 183. The laboratory occupied premises in Carlisle Place near Victoria Station, until 1928, when it moved to Dudley House, Endell Street, Covent Garden. It remained under the direction of Eastwood until his retirement in March 1933.

[11] Departmental Committee on Tuberculosis, BPP, 1912–13, xlvii, Appendix, p. 177.

[12] Departmental Committee, pp. 175–6. See also Graham S. Wilson, 'The Public Health Laboratory Service. Origin and development of public health laboratories', *BMJ* (1948), i: p. 681.

[13] CMOAR, BPP, 1914, xxxix, p. 10.

service, later described as a 'compendium of knowledge, a wealth of experience and, above all, a willingness to help at whatever cost of time and trouble'.[14] Griffith, whose special field was the haemolytic streptococci, provided the driving ethos behind the enterprise. His obituarist noted that his working life 'followed a single star'—he believed that progress in the epidemiology of the infectious diseases would only come with more precise knowledge of their causal micro-organisms.[15] Scott, a world-class expert in the identification of bacterial species by serological methods, was best known for his work on *Salmonella* and dysentery.[16] Both men, it was observed, 'could do more with a Kerosine tin and a primus stove than most others could with a palace'—which was just as well, since the space they inhabited was extremely primitive. As one commentator remarked, the laboratory was 'fantastic in discomfort and lack of good equipment', as indeed were many such spaces at the time. Images of the laboratory too often belie the conditions existing in the practical spaces they occupied.[17]

Conditions notwithstanding, Griffith and Scott maintained the connections between field and laboratory, between bacteriology and epidemiology, and collaborated closely with the Department's medical inspectors in field outbreak investigations. Their services were also available to medical officers of health countrywide, and they maintained an international network of correspondents. Above all, Dudley House offered a free service in identifying causal organisms in disease outbreaks and, as Graham Wilson, Director of the Emergency Public Health Laboratory Service (EPHLS) from 1941, later noted, also acted as a reference laboratory, the prototype of those later established under the Public Health Laboratory Service. Wilson paid warm tribute to the Ministry Laboratory and its staff. They were, he recorded, 'fundamentally interested in epidemiology and collaborated closely with the Ministry's officers in the field':[18] 'This laboratory, almost alone in the whole country, maintained through the long years before the second world war the tradition, established by Simon and carried on by his successors at the Local Government Board, of the intimate relation between laboratory and epidemiological investigation.'

Beyond Dudley House, however, laboratory provision for public health purposes was very much a patchwork affair in England and Wales.[19] London itself was well served, with seven group laboratories run by the London County Council, the Camberwell Borough Laboratory (established 1891), the Lambeth Borough Laboratory (1898), and several large private facilities, including those of the Clinical Association and the Lister Institute.[20] In the provinces, the first municipal

[14] H. D. W., 'A fitting memorial', *Lancet* (1941), i: pp. 588–9.
[15] Anon, 'Frederick Griffith', *Lancet* (1941), i: p. 588.
[16] Anon, 'W. McDonald Scott', *Lancet* (1941), i: p. 588. See also Anon, 'William McDonald Scott', *Public Health*, 54 (1941): p. 169.
[17] Anon, 'W. M. Scott', *BMJ* (1941), i: p. 735. See Chapter 6.
[18] Wilson, 'The Public Health Laboratory Service', p. 678.
[19] Wilson, 'PHLS', p. 678; see also Robert E. O. Williams, *Microbiology for the Public Health. The Evolution of the Public Health Laboratory Service, 1939–1980* (1985), pp. 1–2. For the emergence of this system see Worboys, *Spreading Germs*, p. 263.
[20] Williams, *Microbiology*, pp. 1–2.

bacteriological laboratory had been established at Liverpool in 1897, and Liverpool's example was followed by a number of municipal and county authorities, notably in the North of England. By World War II such labs had been set up by the authorities in Bradford, Birmingham, Cardiff, Derby, Glamorgan, Kent, Hereford, Leeds, Leicestershire, Newcastle, Northallerton, Sheffield, Stafford, Wakefield, West Sussex, and Worcester, among others. An incomplete survey conducted in 1939 recorded 32 municipal or county laboratories outside London, but most local authorities considered bacteriological labs too expensive to be justified, and made use of university, hospital, or private commercial laboratories, as required.[21] The latter found this work a lucrative source of income: the Medical Officer of Health (MOH) for Leicestershire, for example, calculated that the 5,426 specimens dealt with in 1929 would have cost the county £1,350 if performed commercially at an average sample price of five shillings. The increase in the number of specimens examined annually over ten years from 2,449 to 5,426, and the total for the period of 35,290, 'refute the argument that the county laboratory is an expensive and unnecessary luxury'.[22] But Leicestershire did not have a vivisection licence, and so could not do all its own work; the commentator noted specifically that local authorities must pay adequately for university laboratory services, and the latter guarantee a first-class service, since public health tasks were often given scant attention.[23]

The geography of laboratory provision was extended by private, commercial, hospital, and university laboratories, often located a considerable distance from the cities they served. The Lister, for example, examined specimens from Burton-on-Trent, Northampton, and Exeter, while clients of the Birmingham University lab included Hampshire and Southampton. This situation, according to Graham Wilson, exercised a 'profoundly baneful effect' on field epidemiology and local health department investigations.[24] There were certainly a variety of problems with inter-war laboratory services: provision was uneven, there was little co-ordination, services were largely postal (meaning frequent delays and desiccation of specimens through improper packaging), few hospital pathologists had any bacteriological training, and opportunities for personal consultation were rare; by and large, laboratories simply reported on submitted specimens.[25] Rural areas were particularly badly served.[26] It was only with the outbreak of war in 1939 that the country finally achieved a professional network in the EPHLS, regularized into a permanent national service in 1946. Wilson was severe on the consequences of laboratories that found postal bacteriology a useful income stream but left the work to technicians:[27]

21 Williams, *Microbiology*, p. 2; Wilson, 'PHLS', pp. 677–8.

22 Notes and Comments, 'The county bacteriological laboratory', *MO*, 45 (1931): p. 14. The running costs of the Leicestershire laboratory were not noted.

23 Notes and Comments, 'County bacteriological laboratory', p. 15.

24 Wilson, 'PHLS', p. 677. See also Notes and Comments, 'The county bacteriological laboratory', p. 15; Notes and Comments, 'County public health laboratories', *MO*, 4 (1910): p. 269.

25 Williams, *Microbiology*, pp. 2–3; G. H. Gibson, 'Field epidemiology and the health department: practical aspects', *Journal of the Royal Sanitary Institute* (1950): p. 294.

26 Gibson, 'Field epidemiology', p. 294.

27 Graham S. Wilson, 'Presidential Address', *Jnl Roy San Inst* (1948): p. 221.

> The relation between the epidemiologist and the bacteriologist were [*sic*] broken, methods became stereotyped, and examinations were performed without submitting their rationale to continual critical revision. Public health anachronisms grew up, and a great deal of useless laboratory work was carried out . . . little or no research was undertaken, and the numerous problems thrown up by the routine material were left untouched.

The Public Health Laboratory Service (PHLS) resolved these problems and public health, epidemiology, and the laboratory were seen to have entered into a new relationship.[28]

Although the concept of the 'public health laboratory' was well established by the 1920s, the public health community was not unanimous on its nature or function. Some thought such labs should be small, serving small areas; others that that they should be large, serving a group of administrative districts. Many MOH seem to have considered them primarily as diagnostic facilities, although others pointed to their epidemiological potential and their value in providing opportunities for research.[29] In fact local authority labs seem to have provided a wide range of services. In 1934, for example, the most important functions of the Staffordshire County Laboratory were noted to be: providing diagnostic facilities to medical practitioners; veterinary and dairy bacteriology resulting from various acts and orders relating to milk supply; county coroner's work; the bacteriology of water supplies; specimen analysis for other local authorities; bacteriology and pathology for county Poor Law institutions; biochemical and pathological investigations for the General Infirmary; and, finally, 'public health bacteriology'.[30] In offering some of these services, this laboratory too seems to have been generating income.[31] Such an extensive and varied workload meant that local authority laboratories, according to Wilson, were preoccupied with the practicalities of service provision and played little or no part in epidemiological investigation or field work.[32] The laboratory at Bristol (the Bristol Preventive Medicine Laboratory), jointly funded by the city and the university, was perhaps an honourable exception. *Medical Officer* noted in 1935 that its reports always held something of interest: in that year it had investigated the 'reliability' of liquid egg imported from China—an issue that was to become of some moment after World War II (Chapter 7).[33]

At the other end of the spectrum from the Ministry of Health laboratory lay the privately funded Lister Institute of Preventive Medicine, which, like the Pasteur Institute and the Danish State Serum Institute, performed a dual function of research and production of vaccines and immune sera. Founded as the British Institute for Preventive Medicine in 1891, the Lister's interests in disease were

[28] Notes and Comments, 'Emergency Public Health Laboratory Service', *MO*, 62 (1939): p. 124.

[29] Notes and Comments, 'Public health laboratories and preventive medicine', *MO*, 25 (1921): p. 132; see also Notes and Comments, 'County bacteriological laboratory', pp. 14–15.

[30] Notes of the Week, 'The demand for laboratory services', *MO*, 51 (1934): p. 69.

[31] See Steve Sturdy, 'The political economy of scientific medicine: Science, education and the transformation of medical practice in Sheffield, 1890–1922', *Medical History*, 36 (1992): pp. 131–2.

[32] Wilson, 'PHLS', p. 678.

[33] Editorial, 'The Bristol Preventive Medicine Laboratory', *MO*, 56 (1936): p. 191.

wide-ranging.[34] In the period before World War II, it had a strong interest in microbial infections, and Bacteriology was the largest of its departments.[35] The ethos of the Lister was very intense: for its workers, the Institute was 'not merely a place where they were employed, but a way of life, a habit of thought'.[36] In the inter-war period, Lister bacteriologists were increasingly intrigued by the morphology and intimate structure of bacteria which improving microscope technology was beginning to make accessible. It was perhaps no coincidence that, when the MRC decided to establish a national collection of microbial-type cultures, the collection was located at the Lister. Bacteriologists who had previously relied on personal contacts—'upon the kindness of friends'—were now provided with a catalogued resource to assist in their work.[37] While the history of reference collections remains to be written, the British National Collection may have been pioneering: *Medical Officer* noted in April 1920 that it had 'already filled a long-felt want in the scientific world'.[38] It was at the Lister that some of the most significant inter-war research work on *Salmonella* was undertaken, with the discovery of bacterial variation, as well as of the Vi antigen of typhoid in 1934.[39] Lister Institute researchers played an important part in unravelling the scientific riddles of these organisms. Their contributions paved the way for later research which fed directly back into the concerns of epidemiology and public health, but their own focus in this period was centred on that first strand of research interest, the intrinsic character of the organisms themselves.

Despite these developments, the relationship between field epidemiology, public health work, and the laboratory remained fragmented and unsatisfactory from the epidemiologists' point of view throughout the inter-war period. Laboratory research took a clear path away from the immediate concerns of field workers seeking the causes of outbreaks and solutions to the mystery of where and how *Salmonella* existed in the natural world. The need to anticipate epidemic crises generated by civilian evacuation and bacteriological warfare changed the situation when 29 laboratories, ten of them in London, were initially joined in the EPHLS.[40] These gradually began to function as a team, 'co-ordinated epidemiologically', as they were drawn into the investigation of outbreaks that extended beyond their local boundaries.[41] The founding of this service, together with developments in laboratory technique, signally altered the character and function of the 'public health

[34] For the foundation and early years of the British Institute of Preventive Medicine see Worboys, *Spreading Germs*, pp. 257–61.

[35] Harriette Chick et al., *War on Disease. A History of the Lister Institute* (1971), p. 131.

[36] Chick et al., *War*, p. 14.

[37] Notes and Comments, 'The National Collection of Type Cultures', *MO*, 27 (1920): p. 132.

[38] Notes and Comments, 'National Collection', p. 132. For the early history of the National Collection and its predecessors, see R. St John Brooks, 'The National Collection of Type Cultures', *British Medical Bulletin*, 2 (1944): pp. 284–6.

[39] Chick et al., *War*, pp. 136–8.

[40] Williams, *Microbiology*, pp. 9–10. For these labs see *MBEPHLS*, 1 (1941–2): pp. 8–10; MRC, *Report for 1939–45* (1947), pp. 166–71. Changes were made over time, and some of the laboratories identified in these three accounts differ.

[41] Graham S. Wilson, 'The Public Health Laboratory Service', *British Medical Bulletin*, 7 (1951): p. 148.

laboratory' in the years after 1940. In this evolution, Graham Wilson played a crucial part. From being professor of bacteriology as applied to hygiene at the London School of Hygiene and Tropical Medicine, he was appointed Director of the EPHLS following W. M. Scott's death in an air raid in 1941. Wilson was a firm proponent of epidemiology, and it was under his guidance that the new service developed a collaborative, epidemiologically oriented style of operation.[42]

PURSUING IDENTITIES

In the years between *c.*1900 and 1940, the principal concerns of laboratory research into *Salmonella* focused on the identity and identification of these intriguing organisms. As W. D. Foster noted in 1970, early twentieth-century bacteriology was mainly engaged in attempting to develop specific diagnostic methods in clinical bacteriology, and this work 'gradually disclosed' the range of pathogens known as the *Salmonella*.[43] While Keith Vernon has argued that the study of micro-organisms was a marginalized, relatively low-status activity in the first two decades of the twentieth century, the *Salmonella* story suggests that this was not always the case.[44] It was early apparent that this was a vast and confusing field. Herbert Durham observed in 1898 that science was 'but on the threshold of the matter' when it came to knowing which microbes were concerned in outbreaks of meat poisoning.[45] He distinguished between *bacillus enteritidis* and botulism, and recognized that the former comprised a variety of related organisms including, for example, Daniel Salmon and Theobald Smith's hog cholera bacillus and *bacillus typhimurium*.[46] In the early years, however, as was common in early bacteriology, much confusion existed over the identity and nomenclature of these bacilli. The surge in laboratory activity that took place in the 1890s meant that the same organism was often isolated and named by several different workers in different countries.[47] The bacillus now known as *Salmonella typhimurium*, for example, was identified in Griefswald by Friedrich Loeffler in 1890. It was subsequently variously identified and named as Mutton type, Hatton strain, *bacillus aertryke*, Breslau strain, Freiburg type, and *bacillus suipestifer*.[48] It took some 40 years and extensive international research and co-operation before such confusions were resolved.

[42] E. S. Anderson and Robert E. O. Williams, 'Graham Selby Wilson, 1895–1987', *Biographical Memoirs of Fellows of the Royal Society*, 34 (1988): p. 906.

[43] William D. Foster, *A History of Medical Bacteriology and Immunology* (1970), p. 165.

[44] Keith Vernon, 'Pus, sewage, beer and milk: microbiology in Britain, 1870–1940', *History of Science*, 28 (1990): p. 293.

[45] Herbert Durham, 'The present knowledge of outbreaks due to meat poisoning', *BMJ* (1898), ii: p. 1797.

[46] Herbert Durham, 'On infections by unsound meat, more especially with regard to the *Bacillus Enteritidis* (Gaertner)', *Transactions of the Pathological Society*, 50 (1899): p. 266.

[47] Francis A. Bainbridge, 'Paratyphoid fever and meat poisoning', *BMJ* (1912), i: p. 706.

[48] Philip Bruce White, 'The salmonella group', in Medical Research Council, *A System of Bacteriology*, vol 14 (1929), pp. 86–7. For a brief scientific history of the *Salmonella* see Guido Ghyssels, 'Les Salmonelloses: 80 ans d'histoire', in *The World Problem of Salmonellosis*, edited by Eugène van Oye (1964), pp. 9–18.

Two complementary bacteriological techniques helped towards this resolution: immunological methods for the identification of bacteria isolated from patients and the examination of patient serum for antibodies to the bacteria that were causing the illness.[49]

Yet the technical path was by no means straightforward either. National differences in laboratory culture and techniques further complicated the situation. Whereas Robert Koch's 'towering influence' dominated early twentieth-century German bacteriology,[50] the British approach, especially after the fiasco of Koch's pronouncement that bovine tuberculosis did not infect humans, was more flexible. In keeping with the dominant ideology of Robert Koch, the German view was a unified one: there was no distinction between the paratyphoid and the meat-poisoning (*Salmonella)* bacilli—they were all *bacillus paratyphosus B.* In this the Americans followed the German model, being profoundly influenced by German ideas and methods at this time.[51] The British favoured a multiple interpretation, recognizing four 'well defined varieties', if not distinct species, within the *Salmonella* group: paratyphoid A, paratyphoid B, *Salmonella typhimurium,* and *Salmonella enteritidis.*[52] Francis Bainbridge noted in 1912,[53] 'At the present time the term paratyphoid fever has . . . very different meaning for various writers; and as a result the literature abounds in widely conflicting statements, and the whole subject has been rendered obscure to those who have not made a special study of it.'

As F. W. Andrewes observed in 1922, the British position was not unreasonable, since the pathogenic effects of these different bacteria on humans were not in all respects alike, and there was evidence that they did not protect against each other: 'the absorption test offers conclusive proof that each possesses its own special antigen in addition to the group antigen'.[54] The absorption test, adapted in 1906 by A. E. Boycott from serological observations by Aldo Castellani, formed the basis of the British position and was reinforced by the complement deviation method.[55] These techniques were used by Bainbridge in 1912 to argue for the clear distinction between paratyphoid B and the *Salmonella* group, but since

[49] Foster, *History*, p. 177.

[50] James Strick, 'Evolution of microbiology as seen in the textbooks of Edwin O. Jordan and William H. Park', *Yale Journal of Biology and Medicine*, 72 (1999): p. 325. For the divergence of French and German bacteriology see Andrew J. Mendelsohn, '"Like all that lives": biology, medicine and bacteria in the age of Pasteur and Koch', *History and Philosophy of Life Sciences,* 24 (2002): pp. 3–36.

[51] Strick, 'Evolution', p. 326; see also Thomas N. Bonner, *American Doctors and German Universities. A Chapter in International Relations* (1963), especially pp. 110–20.

[52] Bainbridge, 'Paratyphoid', p. 708; Frederick W. Andrewes, 'Studies in group-agglutination. 1. The salmonella group and its antigenic structure', *Journal of Pathology and Bacteriology*, 25 (1922): p. 505. Andrew Mendelsohn has grouped British bacteriologists with the Germans and Americans in their national style of explanations for diphtheria: Mendelsohn, '"Like all that lives"', p. 12. The position on *Salmonella* differed.

[53] Bainbridge, 'Paratyphoid', p. 705.

[54] Andrewes, 'Studies', p. 505.

[55] Foster, *History*, p. 179. Foster provides a clear account of the technical detail of the absorption test. For Boycott, see Charles Martin, 'Arthur Edwin Boycott', *Obituary Notices of Fellows of the Royal Society*, 2 (1936–8): pp. 561–71.

neither of the methods was in use in Germany at the time, his results generated considerable controversy.[56]

Much research work was disrupted with the outbreak of war in 1914, but the importance of gastric infections to the Allied armies in France and elsewhere ensured that some pertinent research continued on the home front. Frederick Andrewes, whose career was spent at St Bartholomew's Hospital, and whose special interest was bacterial variation, had begun by studying the streptococci, but moved on to dysentery bacilli during the war, and then to *Salmonella* afterwards, before returning to the streptococci.[57] Harrie Schütze, Australian by birth, started work at the Lister in 1913 and devoted his career to the antigenic structure of bacteria; his first important work was done on *Salmonella* during and immediately after the war.[58] When bacteriological research was resumed more generally in Britain in 1918,[59] it was focused in a group loosely based around the Lister Institute, which included at various times Harrie Schütze, Joseph Arkwright, Philip Bruce White, Arthur Felix, John Ledingham, and Charles Martin, as well as Scott and Griffith at the Ministry of Health. Together they formed an active and sociable group of workers, whose research findings kept them in constant communication (Chapter 6).[60] Research done by several members of this group laid the base for the path-breaking work which Philip Bruce White performed under the aegis of the Ministry and the MRC in the 1920s.[61] Bruce White's fascination with *Salmonella* went deep. He became absorbed in their taxonomy and classification, and in the relationship between the different species of the genus. He identified many of these, placed them in groups and calculated antigenic formulae for them. His work formed the basis of the Kauffmann–White scheme for the classification of these bacteria which was adopted by the International Society for Microbiology's sub-committee on *Salmonella* nomenclature in 1934.[62]

[56] Andrewes, 'Studies'; Harrie Schütze, 'The paratyphoid B group', *Lancet* (1920), i: pp. 93–7.

[57] 'M. H. G.', 'Sir Frederick William Andrewes', *Obituary Notices of Fellows of the Royal Society*, 1 (1932–5): p. 40.

[58] G. F. Petrie, 'Harrie Leslie Hugo Schütze', *Jnl Path and Bact*, 62 (1950): p. 483.

[59] Many bacteriologists and pathologists served in military hospitals at home and abroad, or with the mobile bacteriological units dedicated to war-related infections, with resulting disruption to civilian research programmes.

[60] Percival Hartley, 'Philip Bruce White', *Jnl Path and Bact*, 62 (1950): p. 472. See also the correspondence preserved in Fritz Kauffmann, *Erinnerungen eines Bakteriologen* (1969). It should be noted that Bruce White was an unhyphenated double-barrelled surname. When on close terms with him, Kauffmann addressed him as Bruce White, never Philip.

[61] Foster, *History*, p. 180; Wilson Smith, 'Philip Bruce White', *Obituary Notices of Fellows of the Royal Society*, 7 (1950–1): p. 284. See also Schütze, 'The paratyphoid B group', pp. 93–7; Joseph A. Arkwright, 'Variation in bacteria in relation to agglutination both by salts and by specific serum', *Jnl. Path. and Bact.*, 24 (1921): pp. 56–60; Frederick Andrewes, 'Studies on the group agglutination of the Salmonella group and its antigenic structure', *Jnl Path and Bact*, 25 (1922): pp. 505–21; Joseph A. Arkwright and P. Goyle, 'The relation of "smooth" and "rough" forms of intestinal bacteria to the "H" and "O" forms of Weil and Felix', *British Journal of Experimental Pathology*, 5 (1924): pp. 104–14.

[62] Smith, 'Bruce White', p. 286. See also Salmonella Subcommittee of the Nomenclature Committee of the International Society for Microbiology, 'The genus *Salmonella* Lignières, 1900', *Jnl Hyg* 34 (1934): pp. 333–50. The taxonomy of bacteria, as a new scientific pursuit, did not suffer from the steep decline of taxonomic interest evident in botany and zoology *c.*1900–40. For the latter

Bruce White was a classic example of the dedicated laboratory researcher. Educated as a biologist, he was interested in experimental approaches to his subject. Debarred from war service by a hand injury, he trained in bacteriology at the Lister, developing sophisticated technical skills and wide-ranging expert knowledge.[63] In 1921 he was appointed, together with William Savage, to investigate the food-poisoning bacteria under the joint sponsorship of the Ministry of Health and the MRC. His investigations clearly established the difference between the food poisoning *Salmonella* and the members of the enteric group (typhoid and para-typhoid), and related these to the toxigenic and invasive properties of the different organisms. Above all, his serological studies were of paramount importance in resolving the vexed question of *Salmonella* taxonomy.[64]

Bruce White's studies were made possible by the work of Polish-born Arthur Felix, who made a number of signal contributions to the unravelling of some at least of the *Salmonella* mystery. Felix was originally a chemist who, like White, came to bacteriology during the Great War: when commissioned in the Austrian Army, he was attached in 1914 to a field hospital laboratory because of his laboratory experience.[65] Working on strains of typhus fever with the distinguished Austrian bacteriologist Edmund Weil, Felix discovered antigenic variations that enabled him to distinguish between two different types of bacteria, the H and O forms.[66] In 1918, Felix and Weil showed that these forms also existed for paratyphoid B—work which was to be important to Bruce White's subsequent research.[67] It may, however, have been significant of the distance between the German and the British researchers, and possibly also of language problems, that Felix, then working in Palestine, complained in 1924 that the work on the enteric organisms had remained unacknowledged for a considerable time.[68] An ardent Zionist, Felix had migrated to Palestine in 1921, where he remained until 1927 as Director of the Hadassah Medical Organisation's bacteriological laboratory in Tel Aviv. In his early career, he published in German but in 1924 he began to publish his work in both German and English. In that year his paper on the application of qualitative receptor analysis to typhoid attracted international attention, including that of Arkwright and Ledingham.[69] In 1927 it was arranged that he should join the Lister on a research contract, and in 1931 he was appointed to the staff of the

see Keith Vernon, 'Desperately seeking status: evolutionary systematics and the taxonomists' search for respectability 1940–60', *British Journal for the History of Science*, 26 (1993): pp. 207–27.

[63] Hartley, 'Bruce White', p. 471. See also Smith, 'Philip Bruce White', pp. 280–1.

[64] Smith, 'Bruce White', p. 283. See also William G. Savage and Philip Bruce White, 'An investigation of the Salmonella Group, with special reference to food poisoning', MRC, *Special Report Series*, 91 (1925); Philip Bruce White, 'Further studies of the Salmonella group', MRC *Special Report Series*, 103 (1926).

[65] Graham S. Wilson, 'Arthur Felix', *Jnl Path and Bact*, 73 (1957): p. 281.

[66] For Weil see <http://www.whonamedit.com/doctor.cfm/3142.html>

[67] Smith, 'Bruce White', p. 284. For the detail of Felix and Weil's work see Foster, *History*, pp. 182–3.

[68] James Craigie, 'Arthur Felix', *Biographical Memoirs of Fellows of the Royal Society*, 3 (1957): p. 55.

[69] Craigie, 'Felix', pp. 62–6; Arthur Felix, 'The qualitative receptor analysis in its application to typhoid fever', *Journal of Immunology*, 9 (1924): pp. 115–92.

Bacteriological Department. He was seconded to the EPHLS during World War II, and stayed on at the PHLS on its civil establishment in 1946 as Director of the Central Enteric Reference Laboratory at Colindale. It was while he was at the Lister that Felix and his co-worker Margaret Pitt discovered in certain strains of the typhoid bacillus the Vi antigen, leading not only to improved methods for identifying typhoid carriers, but to the epidemiologically significant development of phage-typing.[70]

The joint Ministry of Health/MRC investigations into food poisoning and *Salmonella* had been commissioned in 1921, but the first reports were not published until 1925.[71] From its establishment in 1919, the Ministry of Health exhibited a strong interest in the relationship between food, health, and disease, consolidating the various strands of food-related interest developed under the Local Government Board into a specific Health Authority function, designated by the new CMO George Newman as 'the medical supervision of the Food Supply.' Newman introduced a dedicated section on the subject into his annual report from 1920, noting, 'One of the most important medical duties of the Ministry is to investigate outbreaks of food poisoning or disease caused or conveyed by food'.[72] Following up, perhaps, on William Savage's comprehensive 1913 report on food poisoning to the Local Government Board, Newman indicated the necessity of investigation both for effective prevention and for the increase of knowledge. It was a complex problem, he noted, which needed interdisciplinary effort to untangle: 'The etiology is often obscure and requires organised enquiry—clinical, chemical, bacteriological, epidemiological—and unless this can be done by competent investigators *at the critical moment* the opportunity for action and for new knowledge is lost.'

The 1921 project was an attempt at just such an integrated investigation. Savage, now County MOH for Somerset, was, as we have seen, already the leading expert on food poisoning, while Bruce White was the coming expert in bacteriological identification techniques. The three reports which resulted in 1925–6 were landmark publications, especially in relation to the antigenic analysis of *Salmonella*, which Bruce White encoded in a system of symbols and formulae.[73] Bruce White himself insisted that the stage had been set by the contributions of other researchers—that the material was there, simply awaiting 'correlation and summation'. Nonetheless, one obituary writer noted it was his own work that 'unravelled and explained many of the complex problems in this field'.[74] His conviction that any *Salmonella* classification had to be established on the basis of their antigenic

[70] Foster, *History*, pp. 194–5; Arthur Felix and R. Margaret Pitt, 'A new antigen of *B. Typhosus.* Its relation to virulence and to active and passive immunisation', *Lancet* (1934), ii: pp. 186–91.

[71] Savage and Bruce White, 'Investigations'; William G. Savage and Philip Bruce White, 'Food poisoning: a study of 100 recent outbreaks', MRC, *Special Report Series*, 92 (1925).

[72] CMOAR (1920), pp. 122–3; William Savage, 'Bacterial food poisoning and food infections', *Reports on Public Health and Medical Matters*, 77 (1913). Newman's 1920 report covered the control of milk supply, administration of the Food and Drugs Acts, meat inspection, shell-fish, and 'food and disease'.

[73] Smith, 'Bruce White', pp. 283–4.

[74] Hartley, 'Bruce White', p. 472.

relationships was critical to this process. Moreover, he believed that the only satisfactory classification systems were those expressing evolutionary ideas. As a result, he conducted a series of painstaking cross-immunization experiments that eventually enabled him to prove that certain *Salmonella* types derive from a common ancestral source, and to suggest that many if not all had a common origin. By 1929, therefore, he was arguing that all forms of *Salmonella*, including typhoid, are 'inextricably involved in one continuous system of antigenic affinities'.[75] There was no evidence of transmutation between these types: '[they] are seemingly discrete entities, elementary species; a few successful, many abortive; each traversing its little orbit of individual modification along the lines its ancestry has laid down'.[76] The suggestion that typhoid was to be accepted among *Salmonella*, controversial at first, was agreed by the Salmonella Committee of the International Society for Microbiology in 1934 (Chapter 6).[77]

Bruce White was not the only bacteriologist to be intrigued by the diversity of *Salmonella*. Arthur Felix worked on typhoid from his arrival in London, and from 1940 became involved in developing phage-typing techniques for the lesser *Salmonella*. He devoted the later years of his career to organizing the international standardization of phage-typing in collaboration with James Craigie, who had pioneered the technique. They were instrumental in establishing the International Committee for Enteric Phage Typing in 1947, and Felix's laboratory became the International Reference Laboratory for the scheme. By 1953, the total number of national and regional laboratories for enteric phage-typing served by Felix's lab had reached 56, and he was able to produce a comprehensive world survey of typhoid and paratyphoid B types based on data collected from the participating countries.[78] Another major player in this story was Fritz Kauffmann, who began working on *Salmonella* in 1927 while employed at the Robert Koch Institute in Berlin. Removing to the Danish State Serum Institute in Copenhagen in 1933, Kauffmann played a leading part in the international network of *Salmonella* researchers that developed from *c.*1930. He was corresponding with Lister researchers by early 1928 (Chapter 6).[79] An exceptionally talented, dogged, and energetic researcher, Kauffmann became, like Felix and Bruce White, deeply absorbed in the manifold problems of *Salmonella* and devoted the rest of his career to them.

Felix, Kauffmann, and Bruce White were all exemplars of the dedicated laboratory researcher whose world of work lay removed from that of outbreak investigation and the concerns of public health authorities. Like Bruce White, but unlike Felix, Kauffmann manifested little interest in the practical applications of his taxonomic work, and his memoirs reveal minimal concern for the epidemiological aspects of salmonellosis. Felix's talent, however, was for observations that could be developed and applied to the practical business of diagnosis and prevention, and he

[75] Bruce White, 'The salmonella group', p. 88.

[76] Bruce White, 'The salmonella group', p. 110.

[77] Smith, 'Bruce White', p. 286.

[78] Craigie, 'Felix', pp. 74–5; Arthur Felix, 'World survey on typhoid and paratyphoid B phage types', *Bulletin of the World Health Organisation*, 13 (1955): pp. 109–70.

[79] Kauffmann, *Erinnerungen*, pp. 28–9.

clearly relished the epidemiological applications of his research.[80] Nonetheless, he was noted to have 'cultivated a narrow field in his experimental studies . . . he did so systematically, tenaciously and intuitively'; his genius lay 'in an infinite capacity for taking pains'.[81] Those were characteristics common to all three of these researchers. Bruce White was, perhaps, the extreme example. Although greatly respected by and on friendly terms with his colleague William Savage, his behaviour during their collaboration on the MH/MRC project also drove Savage to distraction.[82] Bruce White's gaze was so firmly fixed on his own research trajectory that he had little time to spare for concerns that he regarded as irrelevancies. The epidemiological component of the investigations required close collaboration between field and laboratory: prompt laboratory diagnoses were essential for the elaboration of epidemiological investigations in the field. Bruce White, however, was observed to have 'a constitutional inability to appreciate the just claims of the administrative machine for detailed records and reports. Any outbreak of food poisoning which failed to supply further ammunition for his research was, to him, a trivial incident unworthy of further notice or mention'.[83]

Bruce White's routine disregard for work that did not contribute to his own interests was a 'sore trial' to Savage, who was in charge of the investigation, and to the local authorities, who awaited the results of crucial lab tests in vain. As a result of Bruce White's intransigence, the laboratory work was transferred to the Ministry's own permanent pathological laboratory in 1924, and Bruce White moved to the Lister to pursue his taxonomic studies.[84] In 1927 he was invited to join the MRC staff at the National Institute for Medical Research in Hampstead.

The character of the laboratories in which Felix, Kauffmann, and Bruce White conducted their research was significant of the nature of their interests and scientific dedication. The Robert Koch, the Danish State Serum Institute (DSSI), the Lister, and the National Institute for Medical Research (NIMR) belonged to a small elite of research laboratories, sheltering congenial communities essentially dedicated to pure research, even though they might also have commitments to the practical application of their science. However potentially significant their research would be for field epidemiology and public health in the longer term, their own gaze was focused through the microscope.

From the public health point of view, however, there were drawbacks to this taxonomic industry. The frustrations voiced by *Medical Officer* in 1920 were echoed by Graham Wilson in 1948 when he noted of the broad field of inter-war microbiology that 'a vast amount of bacteriological knowledge had been accumulated, much of which remained academic and unapplied, except on a trivial

[80] See Arthur Felix, 'Experiences with typing of typhoid bacilli by means of Vi bacteriophage', *BMJ* (1943), i: p. 437; Arthur Felix, 'Laboratory control of the enteric fevers', *BMB*, 7 (1951): pp. 153–62; Arthur Felix, 'Phage-typing of *Salmonella typhimurium*: its place in epidemiological and epizootiological investigations', *Journal of General Microbiology*, 14 (1956): pp. 208–22.

[81] Craigie, 'Felix', p. 57. [82] Smith, 'Bruce White', p. 284.

[83] Smith, 'Bruce White', p. 284; see also Hartley, 'Bruce White', pp. 475–6.

[84] Smith, 'Bruce White', p. 285.

scale, to the practical control of disease'.[85] On the eve of World War II, relations between public health, epidemiology, and the laboratory were far from close.

PURSUING HABITATS

The inter-war explosion in minute microbiology did not entirely override interest in the practical application of laboratory findings to questions of disease control and related issues. For much of the period, for example, Graham Wilson, with colleagues at the London School of Hygiene, was engaged in what became known as 'experimental epidemiology'—in studying the behaviour of epidemic infections of *Salmonella typhimurium, Pasteurella muriseptica* and the virus *Ectomelia* in populations of laboratory mice. This work placed the concept of herd immunity, previously suspected but unconfirmed by field observation, on a scientific footing, and as such was welcomed by the public health community.[86] The intense laboratory-based pursuit of *Salmonella* types was paralleled, if not matched in intensity, by a continuing attempt to elucidate their origin and natural history. As we have seen, the Local Government Board's Medical Department had sponsored a number of investigations into this problem before the Great War. Following upon pre-war interests, George Newman's regime at the Ministry of Health initiated a more concerted attempt at investigation. Stressing the importance of inquiring into food poisoning outbreaks in 1920 (without explaining why), Newman noted previous attempts to engage the support of local MOHs in this activity. In 1911, the Local Government Board (LGB) had required local MOHs to inform the Medical Department of outbreaks; in 1915, the Home Office had made a similar request to coroners. There had been a 'substantial failure' to respond to either request. In January 1921, Newman issued a revised circular to the MOHs.[87] The jointly MRC-sponsored investigations undertaken by Savage and Bruce White were a another indication of the Ministry's determination to further understanding of the more obscure features of food-poisoning epidemics, as was its reaction to the general exasperation induced by Bruce White's prioritizing of his own research interests. The MOHs were informed of the new arrangements by letter on 1 April 1924.[88] The transfer of outbreak analysis from Bruce White's laboratory in Bristol to Carlisle Place was symbolic of the difference in research ethos between pure science and public health science: by virtue of its association with public health, Carlisle Place was closely connected with outbreak investigation and the concerns of public health and epidemiology.

[85] Wilson, 'Presidential Address', p. 221.

[86] This work gave rise to many publications, but see the final report: Major Greenwood et al., 'Experimental epidemiology', MRC *Special Report Series*, 209 (1936); Editorial, 'Epidemiology in 1926', *MO*, 37 (1926): p. 53; Notes and Comments, 'Topley's mice', *MO*, 37 (1927): p. 128. For discussion of this work see Olga Amsterdamska, 'Standardising epidemics: infection, inheritance and environment in pre-war experimental epidemiology', in Jean-Paul Gaudillière and Ilana Löwy, eds, *Heredity and Infection: The History of Disease Transmission* (2001), pp. 135–79.

[87] CMOAR (1920), p. 134. [88] CMOAR (1923), p. 155.

The Ministry's public health concerns were reflected in the work undertaken in its laboratory. In 1924, Scott, who had been working on diphtheria bacilli, turned his attention to the food-poisoning organisms. Work on the serological criteria for diagnosis, variability in the antigenic structure of infectious strains, and the specificity of the heat-stable antigenic components was recorded by George Newman for the first time.[89] Interest in serological criteria for diagnosis of the 'enteritis group' of bacteria continued through the 1920s and 1930s, resulting in several publications, often in collaboration with colleagues working in local public health laboratories,[90] and the extension of such typing work to other pathogens, such as the pneumococci and the dysentery groups. Antigenic variation was the critical discovery of these years: as Newman observed in 1931, it was significant epidemiologically, but also scientifically, for its 'remarkable influence on pathogenic activity':[91]

> It has been shown that many groups of pathogenic bacteria are composed of a number of serological races or types, the differentiation of which is dependent on variations in antigenic structure. The outstanding example of the influence of such variations on pathogenic activity is provided by the Salmonella group, different serological types of which are responsible for typhoid and paratyphoid fevers, food poisoning and pyogenic lesions.

The close relationship between the Ministry Laboratory and outbreak investigators distinguished the work done there from research elsewhere. The practical application of antigenic analysis to epidemiological research was a central feature of the laboratory's work. By this means human carriers could be identified, and investigations furthered into the ways in which bacterial infections spread and persisted in communities.[92] In the years around 1930, following the extensive serological studies of the previous decade, Newman began once again emphasizing the lack of progress made in discovering the natural reservoirs of the food poisoning bacteria.[93] Against this background, and encouraged perhaps by his relative success in solving the conundrum of the duck's egg (Chapter 3), in the 1930s Scott developed the ecological aspects of his *Salmonella* research. Analyses of crude sewage, for example, suggested that human carriers probably had a hitherto unsuspected role to play in the dissemination of such types as *typhimurium*, *enteritidis*, and newport.[94] Other investigations involved both vermin and pigs; in

[89] CMOAR (1924), p. 210.

[90] See for example William M. Scott, 'The "Thompson" type of Salmonella', *Jnl Hyg*, 24 (1925): pp. 398–405; William M. Scott, 'Stimulants to bacterial variation', *Jnl Hyg*, 23 (1923): pp. 317–46; S. H. Warren and William M. Scott, 'A new serological type of salmonella', *Jnl Hyg*, 29 (1930): pp. 415–17; J. Smith and William M. Scott, 'Continued fever due to a Gaertner-like salmonella of the type "Dublin"', *Jnl Hyg*, 30 (1930): pp. 32–9.

[91] CMOAR (1931), p. 174.

[92] CMOAR (1932), p. 189. See also W. M. Scott, 'Virulence and antigenic complexity of bacteria in relation to epidemic disease', in MRC, *Bacteriology*, vol vi, pp. 27–30.

[93] CMOAR (1930), p. 182; CMOAR (1931), p. 169.

[94] CMOAR (1931), p. 169; CMOAR (1932), p. 190.

1937 Scott reported significant findings of *Salmonella* infection in healthy pigs slaughtered and passed for human food by meat inspectors.[95]

Besides this research programme, the principal business of the laboratory was to assist the Ministry's medical officers, and local MOHs as required, by identifying causal organisms and providing laboratory confirmation of the field investigator's deduction as to source of infection. Newman's attempts at encouraging the local MOH to report food-poisoning episodes to the Ministry were not entirely successful. Local MOHs had many preoccupations, especially with the post-war development of maternity and child health services and venereal disease clinics, and in many cases responsibility for local authority hospitals after 1929. Reporting food-poisoning incidents to the Ministry commonly proved a bridge too far. Savage complained in 1925 of instances where MOHs showed little interest in co-operating with his *Salmonella* research:[96] 'Their interest being limited to the administrative problem involved, an outbreak which had ceased appeared to them to be an outbreak finished with and of no further significance.'

Many incidents, especially minor ones, were either not investigated or investigated superficially, so that little was known about their causation or potential prevention. Newman, similarly, noted that the difficulties of 'field-work' acted as a disincentive to investigation: outbreaks were often over by the time investigation was begun; suspect food had all been destroyed; special clean-ups had been undertaken; and once the victims had recovered, interest in discovering the source of their misery rapidly waned.[97] By the 1930s, indeed, the MOHs were showing a tendency to use the laboratory resources available to them locally, perhaps for reasons of convenience, rather than calling on the Ministry facility. This shift in practice not only reduced the Ministry's information on the number and nature of outbreaks, but also reduced the research material available to its staff. In 1936 Newman's successor, Arthur MacNalty, pleaded with local MOHs at least to provide the Ministry with details of bacteriological tests made and results obtained if they preferred to make local arrangements.[98]

The Ministry's epidemiological research interests were critically dependent on local MOH input, for without their co-operation field investigation became impossible. The Ministry's inspectors, for example, depended on them both for outbreak information and for the local knowledge and contacts essential to any successful inquiry. Even where such assistance was forthcoming, minute investigation often failed to produce results. Scott's duck egg research provides one illustration. When *Salmonella* poisoning by duck eggs became topical in 1926 (Chapter 3), Scott began work on the pathways by which the eggs became infected. It was not until 1932, however, that it was possible to obtain specific proof of *Salmonella* infection in duck eggs, when the Cambridge County MOH retrieved a flock of nine apparently healthy birds whose eggs had been implicated in a local

[95] CMOAR (1937), pp. 145, 173; see also William M. Scott, 'Salmonella in healthy pigs at slaughter', *Proceedings of the Royal Society of Medicine*, 33 (1940): pp. 366–8.

[96] Savage and Bruce White, 'Investigation', p. 9.

[97] CMOAR (1928), p. 211.

[98] CMOAR (1936), pp. 156–7.

incident, and dispatched them to Endell Street. Post-mortem analyses yielded *Salmonella typhimurium* from the ovaries, oviduct, or intestines of all nine ducks. Eggs about to be laid were retrieved from six, and one of these yielded a rich culture of the pathogen, the others being bacteriologically sterile. Here, however, the trail ended: although the birds' native farmyard was far from clean, none of the pigs or other poultry kept there showed any signs of illness, and faecal swabs taken from the pigs were negative.[99] Despite this disappointment, the breakthrough here was dependent on the action of the local MOH, and demonstrates both how co-operation through different levels of the public health administration was crucial to the furthering of epidemiological knowledge and the degree to which that knowledge could be furthered by work conducted in the laboratory.

Scott's *Salmonella* researches show the inter-war Ministry of Health not simply as a supervisory, admonitory, investigative, and bureaucratic authority, but as one making a genuine research contribution to public health. Scott's personal distinction as a public health bacteriologist and researcher, and his standing in the public health community, was recognized in his appointment as the first Director of the EPHLS in 1939.[100]

JOINING THE CIRCLE

A transforming moment in this story of laboratory divergence and epidemiological frustration took place in 1938. In that year, two Canadian-based researchers, James Craigie and Chun Hui Yen, published a new typing scheme for *Salmonella typhi*. The phenomenon of bacteriophage—microscopic viruses that grow in bacteria—had been identified independently by Frederick Twort and Félix d'Hérelle *c.*1920.[101] Craigie and Yen, studying bacteriophages associated with typhoid bacilli, noted that certain 'phages' only attacked strains of the bacillus containing Felix's Vi antigen. From this observation they developed a practical typing scheme which was quickly demonstrated to be a highly sensitive epidemiological tool, enabling the distinction of different strains of bacteria within a species.[102] Some initial reactions were unenthusiastic. The *BMJ*, for example, found it alarming that an organism hitherto regarded as 'an oasis of simplicity in the desert of complexity' that constituted the enteric group in general had now acquired seven different varieties,

[99] William M. Scott, 'Les empoissonnements par les oeufs de cane contenant de bacilles pathogènes', *Bulletin Office Internationale de Santé*, 5 (1933): pp. 828–33.

[100] Anderson and Williams, 'Wilson', p. 891. Williams earlier recorded that Wilson had noted that he did not think Scott had had the title of Director, nor would have wished it in deference to Griffith, his senior colleague: Williams, *Microbiology*, p. 15.

[101] Foster, *History*, pp. 191–3.

[102] James Craigie and C. H. Yen, 'The demonstration of types of *B. typhosus* by means of preparation of type 2 Vi phage. 1. The principles and technique', *Canadian Public Health Journal* 29 (1938), pp. 448–83; James Craigie and C. H. Yen, 'The demonstration of types of *B. typhosus* by means of preparations of type 2 Vi phage. 2. The stability and epidemiological significance of Vi form types of *B typhosus*', *Canadian Public Health Journal*, 29 (1938): pp. 483–96.

and was pessimistic about the usefulness of the method.[103] It was not long, however, before the value of the technique was recognized. A year later, J. S. K. Boyd, of the Royal Army Medical College at Millbank, London, recorded that the method was far from intricate (unlike the absorption test) and an 'extremely delicate and accurate' means of studying various aspects of the epidemiology of disease.[104] By 1940, 18 different types and subtypes of *Salmonella typhi* had been identified.[105]

The EPHLS provided an institutional context for the further testing and practical application of the new method. Arthur Felix was seconded from the Lister to the EPHLS, with the brief to establish an Enteric Reference Laboratory.[106] Working in close collaboration with Craigie in Canada, Felix developed a phage-typing service, which came on stream in 1940, for the benefit of the new English laboratory system.[107] It was not long before his own and his colleagues' investigations 'amply corroborated' Craigie's expectations for the importance of phage-typing to epidemiology. As anticipated, the new technique greatly facilitated the identification of chronic typhoid carriers; more particularly, it permitted the identification of such carriers as the source of trouble in endemic areas which had suffered series of sporadic and apparently unrelated cases, often over many years.[108] A vivid illustration of this phenomenon was provided by William H. Bradley, one of the Ministry's leading epidemiologists, in a companion paper to Felix's account of the technique.[109] Bradley showed how, beginning with a single recorded case of a typhoid phage-type previously unknown in England, a far-flung series of apparently unrelated sporadic cases scattered through Buckinghamshire and the borders of Hertfordshire over a two-year period could be traced back to a carrier on a farm in Wiltshire that supplied milk to the affected area.

The extraordinary degree of refinement which Vi phage-typing brought to the epidemiological investigation of typhoid, as well as the intrinsic charm of microbiological detection, led Felix and his co-worker Bessie Callow to develop first a Vi phage-typing scheme for paratyphoid B, and then for *Salmonella typhimurium*.[110] The latter, developed and refined over a period of 17 years by Callow, eventually resulted in a highly sensitive typing tool, capable of being widely applied to a much

[103] Annotation, 'Serological diagnosis of typhoid', *BMJ* (1938), ii: pp. 211–12.

[104] J. S. K. Boyd, 'Laboratory methods in the diagnosis and control of the enteric group', *BMJ* (1939), ii: p. 904. For his career see L. G. Goodwin, 'John Smith Knox Boyd', *Biographical Memoirs of Fellows of the Royal Society*, 28 (1982): pp. 27–57.

[105] Craigie, 'Arthur Felix', p. 72.

[106] Williams, *Microbiology*, p. 21.

[107] Arthur Felix, 'Experiments with typing of typhoid bacilli by means of Vi bacteriophage', *BMJ* (1943), i: p. 438.

[108] Felix, 'Experiments', p. 438.

[109] W. H. Bradley, 'An epidemiological study of Bacterium Typhosum type D4', *BMJ* (1943), i: pp. 438–41.

[110] Arthur Felix and Bessie Callow, 'Typing of paratyphoid B bacilli by means of Vi bacteriophage', *BMJ* (1943), ii: pp. 127–30; Arthur Felix, 'A note on bacteriophage typing of strains of Bacterium Typhi-murium', *MBEPHLS*, 2 (1943): p. 99.

greater range of *Salmonella* types than had originally been imagined.[111] Phage-typing provided a solvent that permitted a fusion of laboratory and field concerns to an extent that previously seemed impossible. Felix, for example, was clearly intrigued by the epidemiological results achieved by use of the new technique,[112] while the epidemiologists were thrilled by the possibilities opened up by these laboratory methods. As Bradley concluded in his account of the 1940–2 milk-borne epidemic, phage-typing permitted the identification of the typhoid carrier 'no less precisely than . . . the criminal by his finger-print'.[113] He remained aware, however, of the very intensive nature of such work, and of the effort that had to be maintained if investigations were to be effective: 'The apprehension of the miscreant still depends on the observations and deductions of the field investigators. Without determined field work and the help of what may be a large team of practitioners and medical officers of health, mysteries like [this one] are not easily solved.'[114]

Nonetheless, the development of phage-typing initiated a significant shift in the balance of investigation between field and laboratory. The laboratory assumed an increasingly central role. Whereas outbreak investigation between 1900 and 1939 had largely been a question of field inquiry supported by supplementary bacteriological identification, phage-typing now set the laboratory at the centre of the inquiry. In 1951, Felix published a paper significantly entitled 'Laboratory control of enteric fevers', in which the assumption of the laboratory's centrality to epidemiological investigation was implicit, and that of the PHLS explicit. He set out an emphatic case for the 'necessity for focusing laboratory control of the enteric fevers in a central laboratory and a central bureau serving the whole country'.[115] The argument was based in a review of the impact of phage-typing and associated administrative developments within the laboratory sector. From 1940, the EPHLS laboratory had acted as a central reference laboratory. Public health and clinical labs all over the country could submit cultures of typhoid and paratyphoid B for phage-typing, and records were kept of every patient's occupation and the Vi phage-type of the infecting organism.[116] In 1945, the Ministry of Health initiated a scheme under which recovered enteric victims were routinely screened by Vi test to determine whether or not they had become carriers—a process which was the more possible because detection of the Vi antigen was by blood test, and did not involve the collection of urine and faeces. In January 1948 the PHLS 'assumed the function' of a central enteric reference bureau, collecting all available information about cases and carriers in Britain. MOHs were asked to help make the register as

[111] Bessie R. Callow, 'A new phage typing scheme for Salmonella typhimurium', *Jnl. Hyg.*, 57 (1959): pp. 346–59. See also E. S. Anderson, 'Salmonella food poisoning. The use of bacteriophage typing in the investigation of outbreaks', in William C. Cockburn et al., *Food Poisoning* (1962), pp. 39–40.

[112] Felix, 'Experiments', p. 437.

[113] Bradley, 'Epidemiological study', p. 441.

[114] Bradley, 'Epidemiological study', p. 441.

[115] Arthur Felix, 'Laboratory control of the enteric fevers', *BMB*, 7 (1951): pp. 153–62.

[116] Felix, 'Laboratory control', p. 159.

complete as possible, and in turn were encouraged to make full use of the central records when investigating cases in their own areas. By 1950 the register was sufficiently complete to provide a basis for the epidemiological investigation of isolated cases in widely separated areas.[117] The new laboratory methods had thus, Felix argued, put the investigation of the enteric fevers on 'an entirely new basis'. The public health authorities were now in a position to intensify action against chronic carriers, and he speculated that it might now be possible to engineer 'a long term policy, based on close co-operation between epidemiologist, clinician and laboratory worker, that might in time lead to the complete eradication of enteric infection'.[118] While there seems to have been no direct response to Felix's argument from the local public health services, there was a noticeable falling off in *Salmonella* incidents reported in *Medical Officer* after 1952.

If the prospects for enteric control looked good in 1950,[119] there remained the issue of the lesser *Salmonella. Salmonella typhimurium* lay at the core of the problem, since it accounted for 75 per cent of recorded food-poisoning cases in England and Wales, but the number of new serotypes coming to the attention of the microbiologists continued to increase (Chapter 7). Joan Taylor, director of the PHLS Salmonella Reference Laboratory (established 1945), described an alternative strategy of applied microbiology which emphasized the epidemiological value of the continuing identification of new serotypes: 'By watching the distribution of the different types throughout the country and noting the changes in their time, place and source of origin, [the laboratory] is in a position to help anyone who attempts to investigate a particular outbreak of the disease.'[120]

Within a few years, Felix was providing evidence of the value of phage-typing in *Salmonella typhimurium* outbreaks, and with the publication of Callow's revised typing scheme in 1959, the laboratory shifted the pursuit of *Salmonella* back into the ecological arena.[121]

PHLS researchers took a lead in moving the boundaries of laboratory application outwards into the natural world. In the 1960s, identity and habitat were coming together again. Recognizing that livestock constituted a significant source of infection for humans, E. S. Anderson, who succeeded Felix as director of the Enteric Reference Library in 1954 (and Wilson as Director of the PHLS in 1963), approached the veterinary community, encouraging veterinarians to submit as many cultures as possible for PHLS identification.[122] Anderson and his team were able to establish that of the six *Salmonella typhimurium* serotypes most frequently encountered in humans and livestock, five were common to both groups. Of all animal cultures examined, 97 per cent came from chicks or calves,

[117] Felix, 'Laboratory control', pp. 158–61.

[118] Felix, 'Laboratory control', p. 161.

[119] The prospect of eradication was delusory, given the vast expansion of human travel in regions where enteric infections remained endemic.

[120] Joan Taylor, 'The Salmonella Reference Laboratory', *BMB*, 7 (1951): p. 166.

[121] Arthur Felix, 'Phage-typing of Salmonella typhimurium', *Journal of General Microbiology*, 14 (1956): pp. 208–22; Callow, 'A new phage typing scheme', pp. 346–59.

[122] Anderson, 'Salmonella food poisoning', p. 41.

and although the type distribution for chicks was quite different from that for calves, the combined distribution was broadly similar to that for humans. Anderson concluded, 'the chick and the calf are, directly or indirectly, major sources of human infection with this organism'.[123] In making animal sources of human salmonellosis the focus of systematic laboratory studies, Anderson initiated a new form of epidemiological practice with the potential to extend the scientific understanding of the economy of these organisms in nature.

It is clear from Anderson's writings that he regarded laboratory investigation as an integral component of epidemiological inquiry. The identification of the source of a given food poisoning outbreak could often be achieved only by weaving a web of circumstantial evidence garnered from 'public health workers, medical and veterinary bacteriologists, clinicians, epidemiologists and farmers'. The key part in making sense of all this information was played by the laboratory: the investigation of *Salmonella typhimurium* was now complete 'only if supported by phage-typing'.[124] Phage-typing was the technique which brought taxonomy and public health back into step: together they were essential to outbreak investigation. In the long history of *Salmonella* serotypes that followed, increasingly sophisticated laboratory methods have proved an ever more important tool.

[123] Anderson, 'Salmonella food poisoning', pp. 42–3.
[124] Anderson, 'Salmonella food poisoning', p. 47.

6

Network and Knowledge

The tight world of English *Salmonella* science did not exist in isolation, but operated in relation to a wider international *Salmonella* community located within the rapidly expanding field of microbiology. The developing history of *Salmonella* science in the years after 1920 was one of increasing internationalism, in which private and national reference collections were extended by international exchanges, and an international network was created. The work being done in inter-war Britain formed part of, and was informed by, a global scientific enterprise; the histories of both bacteriology and *Salmonella* fall within the 'knowledge in transit' approach.[1] The speed with which the practice of bacteriology as a laboratory science spread across the world was a remarkable feature of its early history. By 1900, it had moved outward from its heartlands in France and Germany across Europe, to the Americas, India, and Japan, often but not exclusively following imperial and colonial interests.[2] In 1930, at the first meeting of the International Society for Microbiology, it was stated that 30 nations were currently 'adhered' to the Society, each with its national committee.[3] At the Second Congress, in London in 1936, 64 countries were represented.[4] This highly international community was by no means a homogenous one either in terms of its scientific practices or its politics; its history reflects David Livingstone's emphasis on the significance of site, region, and circulation in the production of scientific knowledge and their importance to the ways in which such knowledge was understood and applied.[5]

[1] James A. Secord, 'Knowledge in transit', *Isis*, 95 (2004): pp. 654–72.

[2] This is an underexplored area but see Ilana Löwy, 'Yellow fever in Rio de Janiero and the Pasteur Institute vision (1901–1905). The transfer of science to the periphery', *Medical History*, 34 (1990): pp. 144–63; Stephen Palmer, 'Beginnings of Cuban bacteriology: Juan Santos Fernandez, medical research and the search for scientific sovereignty, 1880–1920', *Hispanic American Historical Review*, 91 (2011): pp. 445–68; Pratik Chakrabati, *Bacteriology in British India: Laboratory Medicine and the Tropics* (2012); Pratik Chakrabati, *Medicine and Empire, 1600–1960* (2013), chapter 9. Japanese methods of acquiring western scientific knowledge are addressed in Masao Watanabe, *Science and Cultural Exchange in Modern History. Japan and the West* (1997); Yoshiyuki Kikuchi, *Anglo-American Connections in Japanese Chemistry: The Lab as Contact Zone* (2013).

[3] Société Internationale de Microbiologie, *Premier Congrès Internationale de Microbiologie* (1930), vol 1, p. xi.

[4] Ralph St John Brooks, ed., *Second International Congress for Microbiology, London 1936, Report of Proceedings* (1937), pp. 563–74. The second meeting of the International Society for Microbiology, scheduled to be held in Berlin in 1933, was hurriedly rescheduled to London in 1936 following political developments in Germany in 1933.

[5] David N. Livingstone, *Putting Science in its Place: Geographies of Scientific Knowledge* (2003); David N. Livingstone and Charles W. J. Withers, eds, *Geographies of Nineteenth-Century Science* (2011).

For bacteriology, James Stark's recent work on anthrax has shown also that locality mattered for the historical actors themselves.[6] Bacteriology—or microbiology—was still a discipline in the making by the 1930s, in terms of agreeing standards and classifications, and into the 1950s actors and locations were contesting forms of knowledge within the world of *Salmonella* science. Tensions inherent to the international political situation added a further dimension of complexity to the internal politics of the discipline.[7]

As a young science, developed simultaneously in several different countries, bacteriology did not exist as a set of standardized practices. Early accounts make it clear that standards of practice were very different from those that evolved as the science matured. The recollections of Thorvald Madsen, Director of the Danish State Serum Institute, as they relate to Paul Ehrlich's laboratory *circa* 1899 and of the Pasteur Institute in the inter-war period are suggestive. Madsen observed that most laboratories of that period were incredibly dirty, and Ehrlich's was no exception. Cleanliness, Madsen reflected, seemed to be thought rather superfluous: 'What I experienced in that direction at the Pasteur Institute even in the 1920s defies description.' His observations of Ehrlich's methods suggests the informality of practice in this young discipline: 'At the back of his lab was a shelf, on which stood various reagents, these he would mix together in glasses—large quantities of cigar ash frequently fell into them—and from time to time he injected some of these mixtures into mice, which were kept on the next shelf.' Ehrlich's little dachschund, Manne, was his invariable companion in the simple little building that housed the laboratory.[8]

Even as common standards of laboratory hygiene became established, other methods and practices were by no means uniform or standardized either locally or internationally. One American survey conducted in the mid-1920s found that performance of the Widal test for typhoid differed in every single one of the 53 laboratories surveyed.[9] Nor was standardization always considered a good thing: in 1955, Fritz Kauffmann wrote to the World Health Organisation's Chief of Section of Biological Standardization:[10]

[6] James F. Stark, *The Making of Modern Anthrax, 1873–1920: Uniting Local, National, and Global Histories of Disease* (2013).

[7] See Anne Hardy, 'Thorvald Madsen, Denmark and international health', in *Of Medicine and Men. Biographies and Ideas in European Social Medicine between the Wars*, edited by Iris Borowy and Anne Hardy (2009), pp. 127–42.

[8] Thorvald Madsen, 'Forskere omkring århundredskiftet: Koch, Ehrlich og Metchnikoff', *Medicinsk Forum*, 18 (1965): p. 142. A more detailed version of the same appears in E. Gottfredson, 'Dr Thorvald Madsen fortæller. 1', *Medicinsk Forum* 6 (1953): p. 205. Translations from the Danish are my own. See also Anne Hardy, 'Questions of quality: The Danish State Serum Institute, Thorvald Madsen and biological standardisation', in *Standardising Therapeutic Agents 1890–1950*, edited by Christoph Gradmann and Jonathan Simon (2010), pp. 139–52.

[9] T. G. Hull, 'The Widal test as carried out in public health laboratories', *American Journal of Public Health*, 16 (1926): pp. 901–4. These labs were 'among the larger institutions in the country with a large personnel and specialization of activities': p. 903.

[10] Fritz Kauffmann, *Erinnerungen eines Bakteriologen* (1969), p. 222.

> *On principle, methods should not be standardised* as this would delate [*sic*] or retard any progress . . . it cannot be our goal to have all laboratories use the same substrates, but to use only such substrates which give the same results in tests with the same standard cultures.

Kauffmann argued that it was important to demonstrate the usefulness of special media, which the World Health Organisation might then recommend—but not impose—for general use. He noted that it was impossible to recommend just one standard method as long as basal substrates such as meat-bouillon, different peptones and agar-agar were being used, rather than chemically defined media. In his view, the impossibility of standardizing substrates meant it was wrong to standardize methods.[11] Just as scientific understandings of bacteria differed between different national communities (Chapter 5), so the global distribution of the practice of microbiology did not result in a global geography of scientific practice.

This heterogeneous world of laboratory practice contained a multiplicity of knowledge networks shaped by both personal and scientific allegiances, the latter relating to specific working methods and practices. Fault lines ran through national scientific communities and the larger international landscape. Practitioners were divided by nationalism and patriotism, and by different scientific methodologies and philosophies. These differences helped to shape the ways in which research was done at different sites and regions, and what was accomplished. Research methods also helped to forge scientific allegiances and influence patterns of factional dominance within different scientific communities. In the years after 1930, a clutch of microbiologists loosely associated with the Lister Institute in London, together with Fritz Kauffmann at the Danish State Serum Institute in Copenhagen, formed a politically dominant and scientifically influential knowledge network within the wider microbiological community. Their activities established the first uniform basis for and practice of nomenclature for the *Salmonella*, which provided the context and impetus for the development of an international network of centres working on *Salmonella*. The resolution of issues surrounding nomenclature made possible international cohesion in the study of the distribution of these organisms, and the post-1940 recognition of their global spread (Chapter 7). Although the next generation of researchers challenged the basis of their assumptions after World War II from within the newly powerful English Public Health Laboratory Service, the 'Lister group' constituted the network that set *Salmonella* science on a modern footing.

CLASSIFYING *SALMONELLA*

The trajectory of research into *Salmonella* furnishes one example of the different factors that shaped patterns of scientific influence and dominance in the years between *circa* 1900 and 1950. As noted in the previous chapter, the years 1900 to

[11] Kauffmann, *Erinnerungen*, p. 223.

1940 were for the *Salmonella* the years of taxonomy—the period in which the microbiologists worked out methods of identifying and classifying this numerous family of bacteria. The identification of the typhoid bacillus, the most virulent of the family for man, in 1880, and August Gärtner's isolation of the bacterium he named *bacillus enteritiditis* in 1888, initiated the emergence of a new field of scientific inquiry. The isolation of a number of similar bacteria during the 1890s led, as we have seen, to a state of some confusion regarding nomenclature and identity, with the same bacteria being identified and differently named more or less simultaneously in different countries. Moreover, it was not easy to tell these different organisms apart—something that was often desirable for epidemiological and public health purposes, quite apart from the pure scientific interest of their complex relationships. As late as 1920, William Hamer, MOH to the London County Council, noted with some exasperation:[12]

> The typhoid, paratyphoid, Gaertner, Aertryke etc etc organisms present every *nuance* within the range of what some would regard as *species*, some as the *family* of organisms; and indeed, it has been maintained that they overflow lines of demarcation so as to make clean-cut distinctions between the various types a matter of practical impossibility.

By the first decade of the twentieth century, two distinct schools had formed, with different opinions on the identity and family relationships of the various organisms so far identified in the *Salmonella* group. As previously noted (Chapter 5), German bacteriologists considered typhoid to be a genus distinct from the paratyphoids and *Salmonella enteritiditis* and its cousins, the food poisoning bacteria. The English by contrast considered them to belong to a family spectrum. The German position derived from results achieved by biochemical analysis, perhaps shaped by their concurrent interests in chemotherapy, whereas the English had adopted the serological techniques initially developed by Max von Grüber and Herbert Durham in Vienna, and translated into English science with Durham's return to England in the mid-1890s.[13] Durham's research contributions, stimulated by his investigation of the veal pie poisonings at Chadderton and Oldham (Chapter 4), were critical in establishing serological techniques as the preferred English method for exploring enteric infections. The papers which he published as a result of this episode demonstrated how serology could link living patient (as opposed to cadaver tissue) and infecting organism, and also distinguish between different types of infecting organism.[14] In the years that followed, serological methods were generally adopted by English researchers working in this area.[15] By 1912, when Francis Bainbridge

[12] William H. Hamer, 'The ultra visible viruses considered from an epidemiological point of view', *Proceedings of the Royal Society of Medicine*, 16(1–2) (1922–3): p. 69.

[13] Anon, 'Herbert E. Durham', *BMJ* (1945), ii: p. 708. See also Michael Worboys, *Spreading Germs: Disease Theories and Medical Practice in Britain, 1860–1900* (2000), p. 268.

[14] Herbert E. Durham, 'The present knowledge of outbreaks due to meat poisoning', *BMJ* (1898), ii: pp. 179–801; Herbert E. Durham, 'On infections by unsound meat, more especially with regard to the *Bacillus Enteritidis* (Gaertner)', *Transactions of the Pathological Society*, 50 (1899): pp. 262–8.

[15] William H. Foster, *A History of Medical Bacteriology* (1970), pp. 179–80.

delivered his Milroy Lectures on paratyphoid fever and meat poisoning, English and German understandings of the nature of the *Salmonella* family had diverged (see also Chapter 5). Bainbridge noted that the close relationship between these organisms 'necessitates the employment of rather laborious methods for their identification': cultural tests were inadequate and must 'invariably' be supplemented by agglutination and absorption tests. The absorption and complement deviation methods were not used in Germany, hence the difference in classification.[16]

The divergence between English and German research methods persisted through the 1920s, while America's adherence to German models brought dissension to the Subcommittee convened to agree an international *Salmonella* classification in the 1930s, as discussed later in the chapter. As William Savage and Philip Bruce White observed in 1925:[17] 'Owing, in our opinion, to faulty classification and terminology of bacterial type, it is very common, especially on the Continent and, to a lesser extent in the USA, to ascribe outbreaks of food poisoning to *B. paratyphosus B*... We entirely disagree with this concept.'

Two sets of issues were involved in this disagreement. The first was purely scientific, relating to questions of taxonomy—that topic of absorbing and all-consuming interest to some researchers.[18] The second had wider implications, since it connected to public health practice. A diagnosis of paratyphoid B rather than *Salmonella typhimurium*, for example, could, depending on country of occurrence, carry very different epidemiological implications and consequences for patients.[19] More broadly, the specific differentiation of the various organisms of the *Salmonella* family was an essential basis for the identification of species pathogenic to humans and/or animals. As the number of serotypes identified increased dramatically and exponentially in the years after 1940, their accurate description became important. Whereas some 90 different serotypes were known in 1940, the number was 2,399 by the end of the century.[20]

THE SALMONELLA CONNEXION: THE 'LISTER' GROUP

In the aftermath of World War I, a number of the scientists associated with the Lister Institute had a common interest in aspects of *Salmonella* serology.[21] They

[16] Francis A. Bainbridge, 'Paratyphoid fever and meat poisoning', *BMJ* (1912), i: pp. 705–6.

[17] William G. Savage and Philip Bruce White, 'Relationship of paratyphoid fever to food poisoning outbreaks', *Journal of Hygiene*, 24 (1925): p. 37.

[18] Jean-Pierre Dedet, personal communication, Paris, 29 April 2006.

[19] In America, for example, a diagnosis of typhoid or paratyphoid often involved monitoring the patient for carrier status, and employment and behavioural restrictions on individuals found to have become carriers.

[20] Thorvald Madsen, *Statens Seruminstitut: Institutets Udvikling 1902–1940* (1940), p. 91; D. C. Old and E. J. Threlfall, 'Salmonella', in *Topley and Wilson's Microbiology and Microbial Infections*, edited by Leslie H. Collier et al., 9th edn (1998), p. 897.

[21] For a brief account of some of this research see Harriette Chick et al., *War on Disease. A History of the Lister Institute* (1971), pp. 136–8.

included Harrie Schütze,[22] Philip Bruce White, Ralph St John Brooks,[23] John Ledingham,[24] and later Arthur Felix.[25] Frederick Andrewes, briefly at the Lister in 1917, was still working on *Salmonella* at St Bartholomew's.[26] Their research informed Philip Bruce White's elaboration of the first classificatory system for *Salmonella*, published in 1926.[27] When W. M. Scott redirected his research interests towards *Salmonella* in 1924, he too adopted these methods and began publishing a series of papers describing new members of the family identified as a result of investigations into food-poisoning outbreaks. Common interests drew both Scott and Bruce White into association with the Lister community, and together they formed the nucleus from which an international network of *Salmonella* scientists developed in the 1930s. The catalyst for the emergence of this group as a power in the international microbiology community was their conversion of an energetic and dedicated German scientist to the serological position.

Fritz Kauffmann was a bacteriologist based at the Robert Koch Institute in Berlin, who began work on *Salmonella* in the later 1920s.[28] Kauffmann later published a volume of memoirs and selected correspondence,[29] as well as a memoir of his scientific work and publications,[30] and through these it is possible to track the emergence of an international power-group in *Salmonella* research. Kauffmann appears first to have made contact with Frederick Andrewes in February 1928 with a view to exchanging publications, strains of *Salmonella*, and views on different *Salmonella* types.[31] At this time, it seems, Kauffmann was still using the traditional

[22] Harrie Schütze, 'The paratyphoid B group', *Lancet* (1920), i: pp. 93–7. For Schütze see G. F. Petrie, 'Harrie Leslie Hugo Schütze', *Jnl Path and Bact*, 62 (1950): pp. 481–8.

[23] See Anon, 'Ralph St John Brooks', *BMJ* (1963), ii: p. 1238.

[24] See S. P. Bedson, 'John Charles Grant Ledingham', *Obituary Notices of Fellows of the Royal Society*, 5 (1945–8): pp. 325–40.

[25] See James Craigie, 'Arthur Felix', *Biographical Memoirs of Fellows of the Royal Society*, 3 (1957): pp. 153–79.

[26] Frederick W. Andrewes, 'Studies in group agglutination. 1. The salmonella group and its antigenic structure', *Jnl Path and Bact*, 25 (1922): pp. 505–21. For Andrewes' career see M.H.G and E.B.P., 'Sir Frederick William Andrewes', *Obituary Notices of Fellows of the Royal Society*, 1 (1932–5): pp. 37–44; Anon, 'Frederick William Andrewes', <munksroll.rcplondon.ac.uk/Biography/Details/102>, accessed 28 June 2014.

[27] Philip Bruce White, 'Further studies on the Salmonella Group', Medical Research Council, *Special Report Series*, 103 (1926).

[28] Fritz Kauffmann (1899–1978) was born into a Jewish family who owned a shoe factory in Stargard, Prussia. During World War I, young Kauffmann worked as a truck driver in munitions, and after the war studied medicine at Hamburg. He was awarded his MD in 1922. From 1923 to 1933 he worked at the Robert Koch Institute in Berlin. Sacked from the Institute in 1933, he emigrated to Denmark following the offer of a post at the Danish State Serum Institute in 1933, and remained there until his retirement in 1969. He became a Danish citizen in 1939. When Denmark's Jews were obliged to flee the country during the Nazi occupation of Denmark during World War II, Kauffmann found his way first to the University of Lund, Sweden, and then to Columbia University, New York, before returning to Denmark in 1946. He died in Copenhagen on 27 September 1978: Donald Jerne, Danish National Library for Science and Medicine, to Sharon Messenger, 20 June 2005.

[29] Kauffmann, *Erinnerungen.*

[30] Fritz Kauffmann, *Erlebte Bakteriologie. Zur Geschichte Der Salmonella-und Escherichia-forschung* (1967).

[31] Kauffmann, *Erinnerungen*, pp. 28–9.

German biochemical methods in his own work. In January 1930, for example, we find W. M. Scott writing to him, in the course of a discussion on the common identity of the German 'paratyphoid C Berlin' and the British *Salmonella* thompson: 'I think you are to be congratulated on detecting the type as you did, it is much easier to do it by serological methods.'[32] At what point Kauffmann adopted serological methods is not clear, but he had certainly done so, and done so with an unshakeable conviction of their superiority, by 1933. His published correspondence shows that he entered into the community of these English researchers on an equal footing, exchanging letters with them frequently and meeting occasionally over the next decade or so. The relationship was perhaps made easier by Kauffmann's relocation outside Germany from 1933. In that year he was appointed to a post at the Danish State Serum Institute (DSSI), where he remained for the rest of his career except for a brief period (October 1943–August 1946) during the German occupation of Denmark in World War II.[33]

Kauffmann and the 'Lister group' came to form a close network during the 1930s, due to their common interest in *Salmonella* and their adoption of serology as the research tool of choice. This was a network based in their common espousal of the serological approach to classification, and rooted in their extensive mutual correspondence. How typical this group was of inter-war microbiology and research is not at present easy to assess. They were not a 'congress elite' in the sense that their relationships were established independently of conference attendance, although they used conferences to extend the influence of their own scientific methodology.[34] Nor was their scientific unity a function of a specific disease—it was a function of their common belief in a specific scientific method.[35] It appears that their allegiance, together, no doubt, with the scientific distinction of their institutional affiliations, enabled them to dominate the international *Salmonella* community that was developing in these years. It seems likely also that the special nature of their institutions, being dedicated research laboratories with world-class reputations, gave them an added sense of community, of operating within a privileged sphere of pure research. As long as their network functioned it managed the space of contest and co-operation provided by the conference, but the conference also provided the space in which the network's hegemony was challenged by a new generation of scientists, based in new facility, after World War II.

The visible envelope for this inter-war community was the International Society for Microbiology. Established in 1927 following discussions at an international meeting on rabies organized by the Health Committee of the League of Nations, the Society held its first international congress in Paris, at the Pasteur Institute,

[32] Kauffmann, *Erinnerungen*, p. 31. [33] Kauffmann, *Erinnerungen*, pp. 118–29.

[34] For congress elites see Chris Leonards and Nico Randeraad, 'Transnational experts and social reform, 1840–1900', *International Review of Social History*, lv (2010): pp. 213–39.

[35] For a disease-oriented international network see Valeska Huber, 'The unification of the globe by disease? The International Sanitary Conferences on cholera, 1851–1894', *Historical Journal*, 49 (2006): pp. 453–76.

in 1930.[36] In its early incarnation, the Society was a remarkable and—like many inter-war international bodies—visionary organization. Its aim was both to improve scientific knowledge by building close relationships between researchers in member countries and, very explicitly, to contribute to world peace. The Society's statutes expressly stated that 'science should unite nations in an ideal of enduring peace and constant solidarity', and it required that each individual member confirm support for this aim in writing.[37]

The published transactions of the Paris meeting are a testament to the spirit of reconstruction and optimism that pervaded this scientific community in 1930. In a notable speech at the opening session of the Paris meeting, the great Belgian microbiologist Jules Bordet spoke feelingly of the role of such international organizations and congresses, and the exchanges they encouraged:[38] 'It is truly a comfort and a support, when one gropes and seeks a way in deepest darkness, to make contact with those groping in the same darkness, to join them on the path so that one may travel more surely with their aid towards the much-wished for light.'

Even more poignantly, Bordet went on to articulate his—and the Society's—vision of microbiology as a force for world peace:

> During the terrible period which we have recently experienced, while other sciences contributed their sophisticated techniques to the work of destruction, there was one, ours, which disregarded hostilities of race, recognising no adversary but suffering, uniquely preoccupied with its helping mission, with never a thought but for preserving life. Our science saved the honour of humanity by proving that even though it did not resist the blast of madness that dragged our society to the cruellest of disasters, it still remained capable of dedication and goodness. To a greater extent than other sciences, microbiology encompasses in its aims the persuasive force that urges co-operation and concord on mankind.

Science's highest mission, according to Bordet, was 'to enjoin the notion of universal solidarity', and in gathering microbiologists together, the International Society was addressing not the specialist, but the man whom science had created: 'We all know well that one cannot ignore disturbing influences, such as economic rivalries which compromise human relations, but the appropriate therapy for this pathology is not barbarous conflict in which the victors emerge as unhappy as the vanquished.'

Against this background of vivid hope and intention, the Congress established a committee to study the questions of nomenclature and taxonomy which had bedevilled international microbiological communications for the past 40-odd

[36] The Society became the International Union of Microbiological Societies in 1980. See Karl-Heinz Schleifer, 'The International Union of Microbiological Societies, IUMS', *Research in Microbiology*, 159 (2008): pp. 45–8; Eric Kupferberg, *A History of the International Union of Microbiological Societies (1927–1990)* (1993): both available on the International Union's website at <http://www.iums.org/index.php/homepage/history>, accessed 1 October 2013.

[37] Société Internationale de Microbiologie, *Premier Congrès* (1930), vol 1, p. xii.

[38] Jules Bordet, 'Allocution', *Premier Congrès*, vol 1, p. 7. This quotation and those that follow are author's translation. For Bordet see C. L. Oakley, 'Jules Baptiste Vincent Bordet', *Biographical Memoirs of Fellows of the Royal Society*, 8 (1962): pp. 19–25.

years.[39] As this task was immense, however, the Commission provided for 'the encouragement of monographing of special groups or genera of bacteria by those best qualified to do the work'.[40] Following on from this provision a *Salmonella* Subcommittee was established early in 1933; the London Congress of 1936 saw the formation of a Subcommittee on the *Protista*.[41] The grounds for the preferential selection of these two groups of bacteria is not clear from the published record but may reflect the advocacy of organized interest groups within the Nomenclature Committee.

The idea for the International Committee on Nomenclature and also, no doubt, for the Salmonella Subcommittee came from Ralph St John Brooks; he and John Ledingham had been the English representatives on the Nomenclature Commission. As Curator of the British National Collection of Type Cultures, based at the Lister since 1920, Brooks was a natural member of the 'Lister group'.[42] Together with the American Robert S. Breed, he was to act as Secretary to the International Committee on Bacterial Nomenclature until 1950. Brooks was something of an *éminence grise* in the bacteriological community: his obituary writer noted him to be 'one of those Irishmen who can make others agree among themselves, and for many years he was the guiding light and inspiration that kept going the International Association of Microbiologists'.[43] The central role of Brooks within the 'Lister' network is evident from the correspondence reprinted in Kauffmann's memoirs.

Brooks was an insider in the *Salmonella* community by virtue of his position at the Lister, and was certainly aware of their particular concerns. These concerns are apparent in Kauffmann's selected correspondence. In July 1930, for example, W. M. Scott wrote to Kauffmann on his return from the Paris Congress, 'We must have a conference some day to settle denominations among the salmonellas'.[44] In April 1932, we find W. W. C. Topley, of the London School of Hygiene and Tropical Medicine, writing to Kauffmann:[45]

> . . . I have been wondering whether it would not be possible to reach some uniformity with regard to the numbering and lettering of various antigenic factors. The numbering adopted by Bruce White has naturally become prevalent in this country, and it is sadly confusing for students, and for junior workers, to find different numbers used to designate the same antigenic components in English and German papers. Personally I prefer your method of grouping . . . but I am sure that it would make things easier for many of us if some international nomenclature could be adopted.

39 *Premier Congrès*, vol 2, pp. 519, 525. In sharp contrast to the confidence of 1930, see Sven Gard's presidential address to the seventh congress held in Stockholm, 1958, in the context of the Cold War: International Association of Microbiological Societies, *Recent Progress in Microbiology* (1959), p. 9.

40 *Premier Congrès*, vol 2, p. 526.

41 St John Brooks, ed, *Second International Congress*, p. 546. *Protista* are unicellular life forms with a nucleus.

42 Anon, 'Brooks', p. 1238. For the establishment of the National Collection of Type Cultures see Chick et al., *War on Disease*, pp. 140–1.

43 Anon, 'Brooks', p. 1238.

44 Kauffmann, *Erinnerungen*, p. 34.

45 Kauffmann, *Erinnerungen*, p. 39.

Eight months later, on 30 December 1932, Brooks, in his capacity as committee Secretary, wrote to Kauffmann inviting him to join in deliberations on a scheme of classification for *Salmonella*. The majority members of this committee—the Salmonella Subcommittee—were, significantly, Lister group associates: Harrie Schütze, W. M. Scott, and Philip Bruce White, with St John Brooks as Secretary. The only outsider (J. Lignières of Brazil having died in post, and A. Senokai apparently not having materialized) to the 'Lister' community was Edwin O. Jordan of the University of Chicago. The composition of the Subcommittee was thus heavily weighted towards the opinions and methods of the serologists: it is perhaps not too much to say that it was a stitch-up. The committee reached agreement on the classificatory scheme, subsequently known as the Kauffmann–White Scheme. It was based on the taxonomic scheme published by Kauffmann in 1931, which was itself a re-examination and amplification of Bruce White's 1926 scheme,[46] which again was based in the fundamental work of Schütze, Andrewes, Bruce White, Scott, and others.[47] With this quality research pedigree, the scheme became the universally accepted 'diagnostic, simplified scheme for routine-diagnosis'.[48]

Agreement within the Subcommittee was not unanimous, however. Jordan only signed after recording his disagreement over the inclusion of the typhoid bacillus in the classification, and afterwards resigned.[49] In this he was following the German research tradition so influential on his generation of American microbiologists.[50] The basis of his objection was that, biochemically, the typhoid bacillus seemed to be as closely related to some of the dysenteries as it was to some of the *Salmonella*, and thus the dysenteries should be included in any genus broad enough to accommodate *Salmonella*. The 'Lister' contingent disagreed 'entirely', pointing out that Jordan's resemblances were purely negative. In their view, the relationship between the typhoid bacillus and the Gärtner family was 'precisely confirmed and mapped out by their antigenic similarities with each other and with others grouped with them on generic grounds'.[51] While *Salmonella* species were defined both serologically and biochemically, serology remained a contentious issue, constituting Britain and Denmark as the region or domain of one understanding of *Salmonella*, Germany and America of another. Concluding the published report, St John Brooks struck a blow for the 'Lister' group position, in an implicit rebuke to the Americans and Germans who took the biochemical approach espoused by Jordan:[52]

> This belief in serology as the ultimate criterion in the taxonomy of the group is the consequence of the experience of the very great practical service serology has rendered, turning a field full of uncertainties and pitfalls into one in which identification has become easy, certain and closely correlated with pathology and epidemiology. It is not

[46] Bruce White, 'Further studies'.

[47] Salmonella Sub-committee, 'The genus *Salmonella* Lignières, 1900', *Journal of Hygiene*, 34 (1934): p. 335.

[48] Kauffmann, *Erinnerungen*, p. 308; Foster, *History*, p. 180.

[49] Kauffmann, *Erinnerungen*, p. 336; Brooks ed, *Second International Congress*, p. 546.

[50] See James Strick, 'Evolution of microbiology as seen in the textbooks of Edwin O Jordan and William H Park', *Yale Journal of Biology and Medicine*, 72 (1999): pp. 321–8.

[51] Sub-committee 1934, p. 338.

[52] Sub-committee 1934, p. 338.

> suggested that the classification of bacteria should be based on serological criteria alone. The true field of serology lies in differentiating between bacteria that are plainly related to each other on other grounds (morphology or general bionomics). Within a group so recognised the serological differences are so definite as to be valid in erecting species.

The establishment of the Kauffmann–White scheme thus marked a disciplinary triumph for the 'Lister' group, so demonstrating that unity and agreement were not necessarily achievable even within the bacteriological community. Members of the group were wry about Jordan: St John Brooks noted, 'I do wish that Jordan hadn't been so "hartnäckig" about *S typhi*',[53] while Schütze expressed regret 'that Jordan was so ridiculous about *S typhi*'.[54]

NETWORK AND POWER

Despite the convictions of the Lister group, serological methods were not universally regarded as easy to use. They were laborious, time-consuming, and required the use of living cultures.[55] While the 1930s witnessed a global diffusion of interest in *Salmonella*, the number of laboratories working in the field of typing and classification remained relatively small. Connections to the Lister group and to Kauffmann, in particular, remained important. Kauffmann had been appointed Director of the DSSI's Salmonella Laboratory shortly after his arrival in Copenhagen in 1933,[56] and he thereafter occupied a central position in the international *Salmonella* community. The Danish laboratory to all intents and purposes functioned as an international reference collection and sample strains were continually in transit by post between Copenhagen and laboratories elsewhere. The DSSI was also a magnet for researchers from all over the globe, a space where personal contacts reinforced scientific links and allegiances.[57] These exchanges represented a transfer of knowledge and expertise on an extensive scale, begun even before Kauffmann went to Copenhagen. In 1929, for example, we find Frederick Andrewes asking Kauffmann for a culture of the new *Salmonella* type 'Berlin' to be sent to the National Collection of Type Cultures at the Lister, 'if you have not already done so'.[58] In 1934, Scott was writing to Kauffmann, 'Yes, I think it is probable Newcastle dysentery will be found in Denmark—or rather that it will be identified with strains that have already been observed. I shall send you 4 strains from different outbreaks and a little agglutinating serum in a day or two'.[59] In December 1939, Kauffmann wrote to Schütze: [60]

[53] Kauffmann, *Erinnerungen*, p. 52.
[54] Kauffmann, *Erinnerungen*, p. 68.
[55] Foster, *History*, 80.
[56] Karl Jensen, *Bekæmpelse af Infektionssydomme. Statens Serum Institut 1902–2002* (2002), p. 173.
[57] Thorvald Madsen, *Statens Seruminstitut* (1940), pp. 14–15; Thorvald Madsen, 'Hideyo Noguchi', *Medicinsk Forum*, 13 (1960): pp. 112–13.
[58] Kauffmann, *Erinnerungen*, photostat inset between pp. 28–9.
[59] Kauffmann, *Erinnerungen*, p. 69.
[60] Kauffmann, *Erinnerungen*, p. 107.

> It will no doubt interest you to learn that I am just working on a new Salmonella type possessing the typhoid Vi-antigen and isolated here in Denmark... As soon as my examinations into this interesting strain have been completed I shall give you further information. This new type will be named *s. ballerup*.

Schütze's reply is suggestive of the international co-operative venture that the classification and naming of *Salmonella* had become. He noted that he had a few days previously received 'a bunch of letters' from Philip Edwards. Edwards, a bacteriologist based at the Agricultural Experiment Station in Kentucky and later Chief of the Communicable Disease Center's Enteric Bacteriology Laboratories in Atlanta, Georgia, had established a National Salmonella Center for the USA in 1934.[61] By 1939, he too had become associated with the Lister network.[62] 'By putting the two of you together', Schütze continued,[63]

> I see that the following types have been agreed upon *S. meleagridis, S. litchfield* and one which has still to be named by Edwards. Then there is under dispute the strain which you respectively call *S. chester* or *S. san diego*. When you have thrashed the matter out between you, I expect I shall be informed of the result of the thrashing...

Such exchanges between the Lister group were replicated on the international scale. Thus Mary E. Caldwell, of the University of Arizona, sent Kauffman a *Salmonella* culture in May 1940, which he was able to identify as a 'distinct new type'.[64] Other requests were for help. In July 1938, for example, S. S. Bhatnagar of the Central Research Institute in Kasauli, India, who had worked with Arthur Felix at the Lister Institute from 1935 to 1937, wrote to Kauffman asking for another subculture of 'the Typhoid Vi-O strain which you kindly gave me... It has now gone sterile and I can not grow anything from it.' He continued:[65]

> Dr Felix writes me to say that it contains H antigen and produces a titre of 2000 in rabbits. I never had any evidence of H antigen in it. I should therefore like to compare the strain I am working with and the original parent strain along with the one I sent to Dr Felix.

Bhatnagar's remarks appear typical of much of this correspondence, but Kauffmann also actively sought information. It was he who initiated the correspondence with Caldwell, writing in January 1940 to Caldwell and her colleague Dwight Ryerson

[61] James H. Steele, 'Salmonella 1885–1962', *Public Health Reports*, 78 (1963): p. 1065.

[62] For Edwards' career see Anon, 'Philip R Edwards': <http://www.ukalumni.net/s/1052/semi-blank-noimg.aspx?sid=1052&gid=&pgid=755>, accessed 28 June 2014.

[63] Kauffmann, *Erinnerungen*, p. 108.

[64] Kauffmann, *Erinnerungen*, p. 114.

[65] Kauffmann, *Erinnerungen*, p. 91. For the origins of the Kasauli Institute, see Pratik Chakrabati, *Bacteriology in British India* (2012), pp. 66–7. Shankar Sahai Bhatnagar (1903–69), FRCP, Indian Medical Service and later Director of Research at CIBA Pharma Ltd, Bombay, is not to be confused with Shanti Swarup Bhatnagar (1895–1955), FRS, distinguished industrial chemist, who was also one of the close coterie of scientists around Jawaharlal Nehru before and after Indian independence: Pratik Chakrabati, personal communication, 8 October 2013; Anon, 'Shankar Sahai Bhatnagar', *Munk's Roll of the Royal College of Physicians*, vol 6, pp. 45–6.

requesting a 'transplant' of a culture mentioned in a paper they had published in *The Journal of Infectious Diseases*, and also a reprint of the paper.[66]

The power networks and politics may also have influenced the choice of journals in which to publish. Cambridge University Press published the *Journal of Hygiene* (now *Epidemiology and Infection*), founded in 1901 by George Nuttall, with John Haldane and Arthur Newsholme, to serve 'as a focus to English-speaking investigators for work in Physics, Chemistry, Physiology, Pathology, Bacteriology, Parasitology and Epidemiology in relation to Hygiene and Preventive Medicine'.[67] By the 1920s, the journal had become a favoured outlet for researchers from the London School of Hygiene and Tropical Medicine, the Lister Institute, and the Pathology Laboratory of the Ministry of Health. Graham Wilson, Topley, Bruce White, W. M. Scott, his colleagues Arthur Eastwood and Frederick Griffith, and Harrie Schütze all published there, as did some of their connections—for example J. Smith, of the City Hospital Laboratory, Aberdeen, published there jointly with Scott, with other colleagues, and also on his own account. Non-British contributors seem to have been uncommon into the 1930s, but Edwards began publishing in the journal in 1936, and S. S. Bhatnagar and colleagues had an article in the volume for 1938.[68] As the political situation in Europe darkened, however, a shift in place of publication can be observed. Many Danish researchers published for preference in German journals, regarding themselves as culturally more akin to that country, and Fritz Kauffmann had continued to publish in German journals even after his departure from Germany. In the years immediately before World War II, however, five papers from DSSI researchers were published in the *Journal of Hygiene*, including two co-authored by Kauffmann.[69] The German occupation of Denmark in May 1940 silenced the DSSI for the duration of the war.

One of Edwards's contributions to the *Journal* offers a glimpse of the workings of the Lister group associates. In 1938, Edwards and his colleague D. W. Bonner published a paper describing two new *Salmonella* types which they had recently identified. They had received 'a group of salmonella cultures' from one Dr B. S. Pomeroy, probably a veterinarian, since his samples were taken from poultry in Minnesota. The two new types were named *Salmonella* Minnesota and *Salmonella* Worthington, the turkey poult from which the latter had been isolated having been obtained from a hatchery in Worthington, Minnesota.[70] A footnote reference to this paper reflects the discussions evident in Kauffmann's published

[66] Kauffmann, *Erinnerungen*, p. 110. The paper in question was Mary E. Caldwell and Dwight L. Ryerson, 'Salmonellosis in certain reptiles', *Journal of Infectious Diseases*, 65 (1930): pp. 242–5.

[67] George Nuttall, 'Introduction', *Jnl Hyg*, 1 (1901): p. 1. See also George S. Graham-Stuart, 'An account of the *Journal of Hygiene*, 1901–1940', *Jnl Hyg*, 49 (1951): pp. 1–12.

[68] Philip R. Edwards, 'Serological variants of Salmonella typhi-murium with special reference to S. typhi-murium var. Binns', *Jnl Hyg*, 36 (1936): pp. 348–54; S. S. Bhatnagar et al., 'A Vi variant of *salmonella typhi* and its application to the serology of typhoid fever', *Jnl Hyg*, 38 (1938): pp. 663–72.

[69] J. Smith and Fritz Kauffmann, 'A new Salmonella type (s.rubislaw)', *Jnl Hyg*, 40 (1940): pp. 84–103; Fritz Kauffmann and Ebba Møller, 'A new type of Salmonella (s. Ballerup) with Vi antigen', *Jnl Hyg*, 40 (1940): pp. 246–51.

[70] Philip R. Edwards and D. W. Bonner, 'Two new salmonella types isolated from fowls', *Jnl Hyg*, 38 (1938): pp. 716–20.

correspondence: Harrie Schütze and Kauffmann were thanked for advice regarding the symbols assigned to the newly identified antigens. Kauffmann was also thanked for cultures of 'certain newly recognised types' of *Salmonella*, which Edwards and Bonner needed for comparison with their own.[71] Similarly, Fritz Schiff and Lotte Strauss of the Beth Israel Hospital in New York City thanked Kauffmann in 1939 for 'rendering their work possible' by providing the sera and test cultures needed to resolve the identity of the organism responsible for an outbreak of serious diarrhoea among newborns in Wichita, Kansas in 1935 (see also Chapter 7).[72]

Knowledge dissemination thus occurred through various routes: personal correspondence, specimen exchange, personal visits, international meetings and publication in internationally read journals. Arthur Felix, another German émigré who made signal contributions to *Salmonella* science, had, like Kauffmann, a worldwide circle of acquaintances, and was a familiar figure at many societies' meetings.[73] Kauffmann and Felix also corresponded: letters to Felix in August 1938 and March 1939 were written in German. Kauffmann's letter to Felix of August 1939 is not included in the collection, but Felix's reply of 23 August is written in English.[74] Travel occurred less frequently than became customary after World War II, with the opening up of commercial air travel, but personal visits were made. Kauffmann travelled to Copenhagen via London in 1933, in order to meet Scott and his colleague Frederick Griffith. He was again in London in 1935, apparently visiting Bruce White.[75] The DSSI being a mecca for microbiologists from all over the world, it was in Copenhagen that Kauffmann personally encountered Bhatnagar and other distinguished scientists, such as Estenio Hormaeche of Uruguay.[76] International conferences as such receive little attention in the published correspondence before World War II, although there was much excitement over the travel arrangements to New York for the Third International Congress of the International Society for Microbiology in 1939, which Kauffmann, Bruce White, Schütze, and Felix, among others were to attend, sailing together on the SS *Acquitania* on 23 August.[77] In the event, with war clearly imminent, the two émigré scientists, Felix and Kauffmann, decided not to venture abroad.

During the 1930s, Kauffmann succeeded in establishing the Copenhagen laboratory as a world-renowned resource for *Salmonella* research. Such was the flood of requests for typing and sample strains that the DSSI began to find its *Salmonella* laboratory a serious financial burden.[78] At a Salmonella Subcommittee meeting in 1937, the English 'Listerians' suggested that an international centre for

[71] Edwards and Bonner, 'New salmonella types', p. 716, fn 2.

[72] Fritz Schiff and Lotte Strauss, 'A new Salmonella type (Salmonella Wichita)', *Jnl Inf Dis*, 65 (1930): p. 125. Schiff was a former associate of Kauffmann's in Berlin, and a recent émigré. He had previously been on the staff of the municipal hospital in Berlin-Friedrichheim (renamed the Horst-Wessel after the Nazi takeover). See <de.wikipedia.org/Fritz_Schiff>, accessed 28 June 2014.

[73] Craigie, 'Arthur Felix', p. 57.

[74] Kauffmann, *Erinnerungen*, pp. 91, 98, 103.

[75] Kauffmann, *Erinnerungen*, pp. 36, 76.

[76] Kauffmann, *Erinnerungen*, pp. 80, 91. For Hormaeche see Ciro A. Peluffo, 'Hormaeche Estenio (1892–1964)': <http://www.smu.org.uy/dpmc/hmed/historia/articulos/hormaeche>, accessed 19 July 2010.

[77] Kauffmann, *Erinnerungen*, pp. 98–105.

[78] Jensen, *Bekaempelse*, p. 175.

the identification of *Salmonella* strains should be created. This enabled the DSSI's Director, Thorvald Madsen, to appeal to the Commonwealth Fund (founded by Mrs Stephen V. Harkness in 1918 'to do something for mankind') for funding to establish the laboratory as a League of Nations sponsored International Salmonella centre. The centre was duly established in 1938.[79] Its remit was to deliver diagnostically essential cultures and sera to some 50 intended local *Salmonella* centres in different countries.[80] Following this development, *Salmonella* centres began to be established across the world. There were 37 by mid-1939, located in the USA, South America, Australia, Africa, Vietnam, India, China, Israel, and Turkey, and in 16 different European cities.[81] Each centre received a starter pack of 115 test cultures and 57 different diagnostic sera.[82] In 1939, the Copenhagen centre sent out more than 4,000 cultures and over 2,000 bottles of serum, and received more than 70 different cultures, for which it provided accurate typing. More than 2,000 rabbits were required for production of the necessary diagnostic sera.[83]

The new centres seem to have been essentially daughter institutions of the Danish hub, possibly established under Kauffmann's patronage. S. S. Bhatnagar, for example, reminded Kauffmann in July 1938: 'I have already written to you in connection with my taking charge of a Salmonella centre.'[84] The patronage element seems clearly present in the case of the Lexington *Salmonella* centre. Kauffmann's correspondence shows that Philip Edwards first made contact in January 1935.[85] He was soon incorporated into the network of Kauffmann's correspondents, exchanging scientific papers and bacterial cultures, and discussing their characteristics. In 1939, a *Salmonella* centre was located with Edwards in Lexington, Kentucky. Edwards, however, working in the area of veterinary bacteriology, was an outsider to the wider medical microbiological community, veterinary microbiology being as yet a distinct branch of the science. Harrie Schütze, attending the Third International Microbiology Congress in New York in August 1939, wrote to Kauffmann: 'The fact that he [Edwards] had accepted a Salmonella Centre seemed quite unknown . . . Schiff was a little huffed at a mere veterinary having a centre, I think.'[86] For the serologists, however, allegiance to that scientific methodology was more important than considerations of professional status.

If we turn to the list of newly identified *Salmonella* species recognized by the Salmonella Subcommittee between 1934 and 1939, the dominance of the Kauffmann connection, and of just a few laboratories worldwide, is again apparent.[87] Of 38 new species listed for that period, 16 were typed by Kauffmann with or

79 Jensen, *Bekaempelse,* p. 175; Kauffmann, *Erinnerungen*, p. 340.
80 Madsen, *Statens Seruminstitut,* p. 91.
81 'Discussion on Salmonella infections', *PRSM*, 33(1) (1939–40): p. 370.
82 Madsen, *Statens Seruminstitut,* p. 92.
83 Madsen, *Statens Seruminstitut,* p. 92.
84 Kauffmann, *Erinnerungen,* p. 91.
85 Kauffmann, *Erinnerungen,* pp. 71–2.
86 Kauffmann, *Erinnerungen,* p. 106. Edwards was qualified as a bacteriologist; his work at the Agricultural Experiment Station was with birds and animals.
87 Third International Congress of Microbiology (1939), *Report of Proceedings,* pp. 836–40.

without assorted colleagues, five were typed by Edwards, and five by Hormaeche, also with or without colleagues. The remaining 12 were variously typed elsewhere. Although Hormaeche does not figure largely in Kauffmann's published correspondence, they had met soon after Kauffmann arrived in Copenhagen in 1933—presumably when Hormaeche was visiting the DSSI. On Hormaeche's death in 1963, however, Kauffmann wrote of him as 'my eldest and best friend', describing him as 'the only "grand-seigneur" in bacteriology'.[88] Significantly, Montevideo, where Hormaeche had his laboratory, was one of the two South American *Salmonella* centres, the other being in Rio de Janeiro. As post-war correspondence also suggests, the centres where taxonomic *Salmonella* research was actively pursued were closely linked to Kauffmann and, before the war, by extension to the Lister group, with whom he had such close and supportive ties.

HEGEMONY CHALLENGED

In the Lister–Kauffmann *Salmonella* connection, defined by their particular scientific approach to the typing of *Salmonella* species, we find a network of influence that, operating both privately and through the authority of an international society and its congresses, shaped the practices of *Salmonella* research in the 1930s. The dominance of this group was rooted initially in the greater delicacy and precision of type definition within the species permitted by serological methods. It was probably also assisted by their location within internationally recognized centres of scientific excellence—the Lister Institute and Ministry of Health lab in London and the DSSI in Copenhagen. The effectiveness of the group was, however, reinforced by its vigorous personalities, and by the close ties of scientific conviction that bound them. Their scientific influence, if not their individual scientific standings, was also closely tied to membership of this group and the place it had carved for itself within the International Society for Microbiology. The importance of individual personalities, however, made the network's influence vulnerable in the event of the loss of any member. Scott, Schütze, and Bruce White all died between 1940 and 1949: Scott in an air raid that destroyed his temporary laboratory at the London School of Hygiene and Tropical Medicine; Schütze tragically by suicide following his wife's death; Bruce White of natural causes. Noting Bruce White's death in his diary for 1 June 1949, Kauffmann recorded sadly that with this tragic death, 'my 3 best English co-workers and friends'—Schütze, Scott, and Bruce White—were no longer living.[89]

By 1950, the serological approach was being seriously challenged within the Society by a new generation of English researchers, who objected to the primacy of serological classification and preferred a biochemical one.[90] Prominent in this dispute were researchers from the new English Public Health Laboratory Service

[88] Kauffmann, *Erinnerungen*, p. 325.
[89] Kauffmann, *Erinnerungen*, p. 133. Author's translation.
[90] Kauffmann, *Erinnerungen*, p. 192.

(PHLS), notably Joan Taylor, head of the Salmonella Reference Laboratory, and K. Patricia Carpenter, head of the Dysentery Reference Laboratory, with Graham Wilson representing Taylor's views when she was unable to be present, as at the International Microbiological Congress at Rio de Janeiro in September 1950.[91] With extensive war-time experience in their specialities, and with the imprimatur of what was already one of the leading research sites for microbiology, Taylor and Carpenter, also supported by J. S. K. Boyd, were a formidable pair.[92] Trouble began brewing in that year, with the English raising issues about the microbial groups included in the category of *Enterobacteriaceae*. Philip Edwards wrote to Kauffmann in June 1950 of a recent British report to the Society on the *Enterobacteriaceae* which suggested the adoption of purely biochemical definitions: 'I found the British report most unacceptable. The trend of the action of the British Subcommittee is a backward step. Frankly I cannot understand the reaction of this group. To me, it is unthinkable that a group of such enlightened persons should go on record with such proposals.'[93] Kauffmann's own comment was both sad and telling: 'It was an other time when Schütze, Scott and Bruce White were living. Such a situation would have been impossible. I am very sorry I have lost the good co-work I had during 20 years with my British colleagues.'[94]

The British *Enterobacteriaceae* Subcommittee was strongly opposed to the proposed separation of the *Escherichia* and *Klebsiella* groups of bacteria from the *Salmonella*, and to the formation of an international Escherichia Centre.[95] In 1952 the British Subcommittee published their Memorandum to this effect in the *International Bulletin of Bacteriological Nomenclature*. Kauffmann wrote out the passages which he found most offensive in his diary.[96] The Subcommittee had expressed the view that the continuing recognition of new species or serotypes, 'though logical, is unjustifiable and is leading to confusion'. And, they continued: 'We believe that the progressive concentration on antigenic structure is having a pernicious effect on bacteriology. It is being used as an end in itself rather than as a tool, and is diverting attention, from much more important problems.'

[91] Kauffmann, *Erinnerungen*, pp. 135–6. See also Kauffmann's letter to Taylor of 8 August 1960, copied to Philip Edwards, pp. 294–5. Women were prominent in the PHLS at this period, as they had been in American microbiology earlier: see Wade W. Oliver, *The Man Who Lived for Tomorrow: A Biography of William Hallock Park* (1941), pp. 455–6, 461–2.

[92] J. S. K. Boyd FRS was a distinguished bacteriologist who made his career in the Royal Army Medical Corps, and served as Director of the Wellcome Laboratories of Tropical Medicine, 1946–55. His special interest was bacteriophage: see L. G. Goodwin, 'John Smith Knox Boyd', *Biographical Memoirs of Fellows of the Royal Society*, 28 (1982): 27–57; Anon, 'Sir John Smith Knox Boyd', <munksroll.rcplondon.ac.uk/Biography/Details/501>, accessed 28 June 2014. I have been unable to trace obituaries for Joan Taylor and Patricia Carpenter.

[93] Kauffmann, *Erinnerungen*, p. 180.

[94] Kauffmann, *Erinnerungen*, p. 180.

[95] Kauffmann, *Erinnerungen*, p. 135. See also *International Bulletin of the Bacteriological Nomenclature Committee*, 1 (1951): pp. 135–7.

[96] Kauffmann, *Erinnerungen*, pp. 135–6. See also *International Bulletin of the Bacteriological Nomenclature Committee*, 2 (1952): pp. 137–9.

This view was echoed almost word-for-word by Wilson and his editorial colleague in the fourth edition of the classic textbook *Principles of Bacteriology and Immunity*.[97] In the fifth edition (1964), Wilson and Miles expressed themselves yet more forcibly. Again, Kauffmann wrote out the offending quotation:[98]

> In our opinion, excessive concentration on antigenic structure is having a pernicious effect on bacteriology, and is diverting attention from the much more general problems of virulence and infection. Serological methods have shown themselves to be useful tools in studying the epidemiology of salmonella infections, but are not an end in themselves.

Reflecting Wilson's 1948 stricture (Chapter 5) on minute bacteriology, the PHLS attack on serology was also an attack on taxonomy—it was deflecting energy from more important public health considerations. Shifts in scientific power were noticeable in the changing management of the International Association. Both Kauffmann and St John Brooks resigned from their positions within the Nomenclature Committee in 1950. By 1958, Hormaeche was Chairman of the International Association's Enterobacteriaceae Nomenclature Subcommittee, with Patricia Carpenter as retiring Secretary, to be replaced by Joan Taylor on 13 September 1959.[99]

In the years after World War II, as *Salmonella* research became increasingly extensive and internationalized, there were continuing problems over methodologies and classification. Kauffmann became increasingly bullish and by 1960 was intransigent. In August that year he responded to a proposal by Joan Taylor by trenchantly stating that the question of serotypes or species was one of classification, and could not be settled by binding international agreement:[100] 'In scientific questions there is no place for compromises like in the United Nations. I cannot agree with you in this point. I admit I have done compromises in the past, but I will not repeat such mistakes.' To Taylor's request that he co-operate and collaborate in this international enterprise, Kauffmann responded stiffly, 'It is absurd to request from me international co-operation and collaboration since I have worked for other laboratories in the world more during 30 years than any other person, perhaps with the exception of Phil [Edwards].'[101]

Although this letter to Taylor was copied to Philip Edwards, it appears that the issue also destroyed the friendship between Kauffmann and Edwards, who seems to have come round to Taylor's point of view. Three weeks earlier Kauffmann had written to Edwards that in regard to classification and nomenclature, he agreed with Dr Rauss of Pecs University Medical School (Hungary), Dr Hofmann (Salmonella Centre, Berlin), Dr Rohde (Salmonella Centre, Hamburg), 'and others'. He added, 'I understand very well that you have another opinion and that you have the right to

[97] Graham S. Wilson and Ashley A. Miles, eds, *Topley and Wilson's Principles of Bacteriology and Immunity*, 4th edn (1955), vol 1, p. 802.

[98] Kauffmann, *Erinnerungen*, pp. 136–7; Graham S. Wilson and Ashley A. Miles, eds, *Topley and Wilson's Principles of Bacteriology and Immunity*, 5th edn (1964), vol 1, p. 867.

[99] International Association, *Recent Progress*, p. 435.

[100] Kauffmann, *Erinnerungen*, pp. 294–5.

[101] Kauffmann, *Erinnerungen*, p. 295.

this, but I cannot change my opinion which is in agreement with the old *Salmonella* Subcommittee'—that is, that the *Salmonella* group was a genus, and all the serotypes were species.[102] This is the last letter addressed to Edwards printed in Kauffmann's memoirs—and there was no reference to Edwards's death, aged only 65, in 1966. Kauffmann continued to correspond with Edwards' colleague, W. H. (Bill) Ewing, but the difference between their positions on classification issues was evidently a cause of bitterness to Kauffmann.[103] Without a deeper exploration of the education and convictions of the young generation of PHLS workers and Kauffmann's remaining allies than is possible here, it is difficult to decode this geographical shift in scientific approaches and power sites after World War II. The PHLS was Britain's premier microbiological research institution by 1950, and its Salmonella Reference Laboratory (under Joan Taylor) was recognized by the World Health Organisation as the reference laboratory for the British Commonwealth in 1949. It also had a clear epidemiological function.[104] Arthur Felix, meanwhile, had removed himself permanently from the Lister to join the PHLS in 1945. Along with the loss of key personnel between 1941 and 1949, the Lister group's institutional base in England was eroded with the arrival of the PHLS. Taylor claimed in 1951 to work closely with both the DSSI and the Communicable Disease Center (CDC), setting the PHLS on a par with those two world-class facilities.[105] The Kauffmann correspondence suggests, however, that the axis of power in *Salmonella* research had shifted towards a British–American alliance and against one in which both (if Edwards is allowed to represent America) were aligned with Denmark. The dispute over the basis of classification was a protracted one: for the rest of his career, Kauffmann remained deeply embroiled in that debate.[106]

CONSTRUCTING THE TIES

Political dominance within the international *Salmonella* community between 1900 and 1950 appears to have been linked both to the perceived superiority of one particular scientific technique by a particular group of researchers, and to specific research clusters whose strength depended both on their particular membership and their collective institutional position within the wider field. Transfers of knowledge within this community in the 1930s took place on a worldwide basis. They occurred through scientific journals and international conferences, but also through postal exchanges of specimens, discussion of types and techniques, and personal

[102] Kauffmann, *Erinnerungen*, pp. 293–4. The views of the old Subcommittee are stated on pp. 258–9.

[103] Kauffmann, *Erinnerungen*, pp. 320–1.

[104] Joan Taylor, 'The Salmonella Reference Laboratory', *BMB*, 7 (1951): pp. 163–6.

[105] Taylor, 'Reference laboratory': p. 163.

[106] See Fritz Kauffmann, *The Bacteriology of the Enterobacteriaceae* (1966), pp. 9–13; Fritz Kauffmann, *Serological Diagnosis of Salmonella Species: Kauffmann–White Schema* (1972), pp. 9–15; Fritz Kauffmann, *Classification of Bacteria* (1975), pp. 9–11.

communications by letter and travel. These exchanges were not straightforward but were complicated by different laboratory cultures and, in the 1930s, by the manipulations of a politically dominant clique which sought to entrench one particular form of identification technique in international practice, and which came to control the international distribution of key approved laboratory facilities.

The emergence of this politically dominant clique, and the construction of an international *Salmonella* community, was crucially shaped by scientific publications, shared scientific interests, correspondence, and travel. In many instances, the first contact between future co-workers was by post: often requests for reprints of scientific papers, or comments on published papers. Thus Kauffmann's earliest approach to the English microbiologists came when he wrote to Frederick Andrewes in February 1928, enclosing a reprint of an article from the *Zeitschrift fur Hygiene*, in which he had confirmed some of Andrewes's results. Andrewes's response to that letter was formal, beginning 'Dear Sir' and ending 'Yours faithfully'.[107] Two years later, he was writing 'Dear Dr Kauffmann', and ending 'Yours very truly'.[108] Once again here, we find Kauffmann endorsing Andrewes's results: 'It is always agreeable to find that other people corroborate one's observations', wrote Andrewes, 'and we seem to be in complete accord'.[109] Mutual respect for each other's work provided a foundation of trust and co-operation. There can be little doubt that the scientific accord between Andrewes and Kauffmann facilitated the latter's acceptance by others of the Lister circle. Similarly, the Kentucky bacteriologist Philip Edwards introduced himself to Kauffmann by letter in January 1935. A previous approach addressed to the Robert Koch Institute had been returned instead of being forwarded; Edwards was in search of reprints of Kauffmann articles published in the *Zeitschrift fur Hygiene*, since the journal was not available in Kentucky.[110] By February 1936, Edwards was writing with further comment on findings of mutual interest and requests for cultures and references: 'Will you send me references to the isolation of *S. oranienburg*? I would like to know how many times the organism has been isolated and whether it has been found in animals.'[111]

The selected nature of the published Kauffmann correspondence makes the exact pinpointing of contact and disentangling of chronologies of developments tricky. Nonetheless, travel and social networking clearly played an important role in the development of closer personal friendships from a basis of scientific contact and esteem. It seems probable that Kauffmann's passage through London in 1933 was significant in establishing personal relations with the Lister group: subsequent letters between them frequently convey greetings also to spouses, as from Harrie Schütze to Kauffmann in April 1934, and from Kauffmann to W. M. Scott in February 1937.[112] The letters also track the gradual abandoning of formalities—by 1939, for example, Kauffmann and Bruce White were addressing each other as

[107] Kauffmann, *Erinnerungen*, pp. 28–9.
[108] Kauffmann, *Erinnerungen*, photostat insert between pp. 28–9.
[109] Kauffmann, *Erinnerungen*, photostat insert between pp. 28–9.
[110] Kauffmann, *Erinnerungen*, pp. 71–2.
[111] Kauffmann, *Erinnerungen*, p. 78.
[112] Kauffmann, *Erinnerungen*, pp. 68, 83.

such, as were Kauffmann and St John Brooks—and by 1946 the latter had become 'Brooks'.[113] Significant too was Kauffmann's residence at Columbia University, New York, in 1945–6, following his years of war-time exile at Lund University, Sweden. From Columbia, he visited Philip Edwards at Lexington, where they discussed the latter's Arizona–Antigen scheme.[114] Previous to this visit Edwards had been 'Dear Dr Edwards' in correspondence; subsequent to it he became 'Dear Phil'.[115]

Beyond the immediate Lister circle, the creation of the wider *Salmonella* community is rather more difficult to elucidate. Once again, publication in internationally known scientific journals was important, and the International Society for Microbiology and its congresses clearly played a part. Visits to the leading institutions by interested researchers were also significant, and here it is clear that the DSSI, and the Lister, and the Ministry of Health laboratory in London, where Scott was based, played important roles.[116] Kauffmann, as we have seen, was encouraged by the Lister circle to visit London in 1933, while there was much excited communication in February 1937 when Thorvald Madsen, Director of the DSSI, wrote to Kauffmann from Geneva (where he was as President of the League of Nations' Health Organisation) to indicate that Hormaeche would be visiting Copenhagen to discuss the problems of the *Salmonella* group.[117] Such personal contacts must have been critical in helping to establish relationships, consolidate scientific respect, and develop knowledge of the field and its participants. In 1955, for example, Kauffmann indicated to the World Health Organization (WHO) that *Salmonella* centres were 'very difficult to establish [and] . . . only successful if the right person is present, and such persons are very rare'. It was only now possible, he continued, to establish Centres in Switzerland and South Africa, and 'the Centre in Colombo is finished as Dr E Schmid has left Ceylon'.[118] Quite how 'the right person' could be identified without personal acquaintance, or mutual personal acquaintances, is unclear. It certainly seems that travel and personal visits were important, and probably became more so after World War II. Kauffmann himself provides some clues when mentioning the conferences he attended and a number of the overseas scientists who had paid longer visits to Copenhagen in the immediate post-war period. These included researchers from America, India, Pakistan, South Africa, Sweden, Germany, Canada, Greece, Israel, Uruguay, Mexico, and England.[119]

By 1950, however, Kauffman's position within *Salmonella* science was changing. Geographies of scientific knowledge and power change with the development of disciplines and the passage of individuals and institutions. Work done on the *Salmonella* in London during and after World War I established *Salmonella* as an independent research field within microbiology, and London continued to be at the

[113] Kauffmann, *Erinnerungen*, pp. 99–101, 104, 149.

[114] Kauffmann, *Erinnerungen*, pp. 125–6.

[115] Kauffmann, *Erinnerungen*, pp. 122–3, 191.

[116] For visiting at the Ministry's lab see Chapter 5; for visiting at the Lister see Leslie Collier, *The Lister Institute of Preventive Medicine. A Concise History* (2000), pp. 36–7.

[117] Kauffmann, *Erinnerungen*, pp. 80 ff.

[118] Kauffmann, *Erinnerungen*, p. 223.

[119] Kauffmann, *Erinnerungen*, pp. 129–30.

centre of that research in the 1920s. The key English sites for this work were the Lister and Ministry of Health laboratories, the one a dedicated research facility, the other addressing practical public health agendas. In the 1930s, researchers based around these institutions were at the cutting edge of their field, united by the belief in a classification scheme using serological criteria. In the 1940s the pattern changed. Key members of the group died between 1941 and 1949, the Lister suffered badly after World War II, and the Ministry of Health laboratory disappeared into the PHLS, which became under Graham Wilson the new powerhouse of British bacteriology, with a commitment to public health-oriented research. A new generation of bacteriologists emerged beyond the Lister sphere of influence, with their own views on classification criteria. The arrival of the PHLS as a professional modern facility is clearly stamped on the publications and reports issuing from it, almost from the moment of its creation. Graham Wilson had been trained in a different school from the 'Listerians', and had spent nearly two decades with colleagues developing bacteriological research and postgraduate education first at Manchester, then at the London School of Hygiene and Tropical Medicine. Described as 'possibly the most influential British bacteriologist of the 20th century', Wilson and his staff brought a new professionalism to the workings of British bacteriology.[120] The arrival of a cadre of professionally trained bacteriologists, such as Joan Taylor and Patricia Carpenter, challenged the existing order as arranged by Kauffmann and his circle.

The disruption and disintegration of the old order, and the pain which accompanied it, is clearly reflected in Kauffman's correspondence from 1950 through to the last published letter to Bill Ewing in 1966.[121] If the taxonomy of the many *Salmonella* micro-organisms was complex, so too was the world of scientific communication, politics, and practice which established itself around them. International scientific networks may be constructed and operate in a way that contributes to knowledge but also potentially privilege particular understandings of that knowledge. In the case of *Salmonella* science, new actors and new laboratories generated competitors who favoured techniques and understandings of the bacteria other than those adopted by the members of the first network established around them.

[120] M. T. Parker, 'Graham Selby Wilson', *Journal of Medical Microbiology*, 36 (1987): pp. 301–4.
[121] Kauffmann, *Erinnerungen*, pp. 332–3.

7

Names and Places

The international scientific networks that established themselves around the *Salmonella* in the 1930s, and the development of increasingly refined methods of identification in the 1930s and 1940s, provided the background and expertise for the uncovering of dramatic changes in the global distribution of these organisms in the years after 1940. In this process of discovery, the findings of the microbiologists led to new understandings of changing bacterial landscapes in Britain and America, and how these related to practices in agriculture and food production, and to patterns of international trade. As a result, the American public health and scientific communities became engaged with salmonellosis on a scale that dwarfed earlier British efforts, while the taxonomists continued to mine a rich seam of discovery. The entry of the Americans, as of the British Public Health Laboratory Service, into *Salmonella* science challenged the positions of London and Copenhagen as leading centres for *Salmonella* research, while the international creation of scientific centres and networks led to an explosive acceleration in the discovery of new *Salmonella* types and to a realization of the global dimensions of the food-poisoning problem and its association with international trade—an association which continues to be a problem in international public health.[1]

NAMING

From the beginnings of bacteriology in the 1880s, the *Salmonella* family emerged as commonly occurring bacteria with a wide geographical distribution. As we have seen, this initially caused considerable confusion, with the same organism being identified and differently named in several places (Chapter 5). Between 1920 and 1939, however, increasing international co-operation among microbiologists led to the convention that a *Salmonella* serotype would be named after the locality from which the first isolate was obtained.[2] Thus, for example, the family came to contain *Salmonella* bareilly (India), *Salmonella* montevideo (Uruguay), *Salmonella* agona

[1] See for example <http://www.dailymail.co.uk/news/article2017350/Health-warning-Spanish-eggs-blamed-for-136-cases-of-salmonella-in-UK>, accessed 1 August 2011; BBC News Europe, 'Salmonella in the Netherlands and US from Dutch smoked fish', accessed 3 October 2012.

[2] This convention still holds: see Michael P. Doyle and Dean O. Cliver, 'Epidemiology of salmonellosis', in *Foodborne Diseases*, edited by Dean O. Cliver (1990), p. 187; Kare Mølbak et al., 'Salmonella infections', in *Foodborne Infections and Intoxications*, edited by Hans P. Reimann and Dean O. Cliver (2006), p. 57.

(Ghana), *Salmonella* arizona (USA), *Salmonella* kentucky (USA), *Salmonella* ballerup (Denmark), *Salmonella* derby (UK), and *Salmonella* heidelberg (Germany), among many others. Various generic names established before this convention also persisted: *typhi* (typhoid) and *typhimurium* (mouse typhoid); *gallinarum* and *pullorum* (chickens); *cholerae-suis* (pigs); *bovis morbificans* (cattle); and *abortus* (cows, sheep, and horses). Occasionally, a personal name figured, as in the naming of *Salmonella* saphra in 1957 (discussed later in the chapter). The naming of most *Salmonella*, therefore, enables us to establish something of a geography of spread for these organisms. The local place of naming may not be the original birthplace of a particular serotype, but the global distribution of that particular organism bears witness to the extent of its travels across the world.

As this history of naming suggests, the story of the *Salmonella* family is intimately connected to that of the development of laboratory techniques. The increasing refinement of serological methods in the inter-war period permitted the differentiation, identification, and naming of a growing number of serotypes, and the introduction of phage-typing added a further layer of complexity to the picture. If the *British Medical Journal* complained in 1939 about the seven phage types of typhoid, there was more distress to come: by 1955 international co-operative efforts had demonstrated a total of 33 types and sub-types of *Salmonella typhi*.[3] The epidemiologists, however, were not complaining, since the new procedure considerably enhanced their ability to track down the sources of outbreaks.[4] The advent of phage-typing also brought epidemiological findings that cast light on the local and global aspects of *Salmonella* ecology. The phage-typing of typhoid, for example, was instrumental in solving a war-time outbreak in London, which was at the time a source of considerable consternation to the military establishment and might, in other circumstances, have had wider ramifications for the final stages of Britain's war effort.

This outbreak occurred in spring 1944, in the fraught months leading up to D-Day. Planning for D-Day had been in train for four years and involved top-secret administrative preparations conducted by selected and high-powered Forces personnel. Suddenly, that spring, a number of important military officers developed typhoid. With the spectres of espionage and bacteriological warfare in mind, the War Office contacted the Ministry of Health requesting an immediate investigation. The Ministry of Health knew that quite a number of well-to-do London residents in several of the city's boroughs were suffering from typhoid at the time—a somewhat unusual occurrence, as the investigating epidemiologist wryly noted. But as they were by no means the only typhoid victims in the city, the epidemiological picture was far from clear.

[3] Arthur Felix, 'World survey of typhoid and paratyphoid-B phage types', *Bulletin of the World Health Organisation*, 13 (1955): p. 110.

[4] J. S. K. Boyd, 'Laboratory methods in the diagnosis and control of fevers of the enteric group', *BMJ* (1939), ii: p. 904; see also Epidemiological Notes, 'Paratyphoid fever in Liverpool', *Monthly Bulletin of the Emergency Public Health Laboratory Service*, 1 (1941–2): p. 7.

It was a case tailor-made to demonstrate the power of phage-typing. The epidemiologists went to the well-to-do residents and 'made sure that the organisms causing their disease reached the central laboratory'.[5] In other words, they persuaded them to provide the necessary samples of urine and faeces, and personally conducted the samples to the laboratory. The laboratory results showed the victims all to be suffering infections caused by the same phage-type, one not previously identified in Britain. Inquiry revealed that all these people, five of whom died, had recently returned from holiday at a 'pleasant and fashionable hotel' in Cornwall, which investigation revealed to have a history of associated typhoid cases. The source of infection was traced to an intermittent carrier on the hotel staff, who had contracted typhoid while serving in the Boer Wars in South Africa 43 years earlier. Since he was able to name the stream from which he had drunk the water that infected him, the investigators contacted South Africa: cases of the same phage-type were still occurring in the vicinity of that African stream.[6]

The translation of an African strain of typhoid to a Cornish well in this instance not only illustrated the obvious significance of human agency in spreading the disease, but also opened up a more complex natural history for the infection. What had appeared as a universal disease with global distribution was now fragmented into a collective of infection within which there existed the possibility of different strains with specific local connections. These strains might accidentally be carried beyond their local ecological niche into the wider world, to establish enclaves of infection thousands of miles from home. If phage-typing established a newly complex international identity for typhoid, bacteriological methods of identification also provided evidence for the consequences of the globalization of trade and transport in the years after 1940 for the distribution of the lesser *Salmonella*.[7] In this respect, nomenclatures reveal the experience of England (and Wales) as a story of changing disease ecologies, of a relatively stable bacteriological environment that came under siege from alien invaders, and of bacteria that, in the course of a few decades, took on a global future.

The history of *Salmonella* infections in England and Wales can be charted with some degree of confidence from the mid-1920s. By this date serological methods of identification had been reliably established, and the Ministry of Health's bacteriological laboratory was undertaking the monitoring of food-poisoning outbreaks, identification of causal organisms, and laboratory research into the natural history of *Salmonella*. At the lab, W. M. Scott's expertise was deployed in elucidating the microbiology of reported food-poisoning outbreaks and confirming the links between outbreaks and specific species of *Salmonella*, often for the first time.[8] As we have seen (Chapter 6), Scott was part of an international correspondence network centred on *Salmonella* taxonomy. Given this background, and with the

[5] William H. Bradley, 'The control of typhoid fever', *Public Health*, 62 (1949): p. 161.

[6] Bradley, 'Typhoid', p. 162.

[7] This point is also made in Frank Fenner, 'Infectious disease and social change', *Medical Journal of Australia*, 2(1) (1971): p. 1044.

[8] See for example William M. Scott, 'Food poisoning due to Bacillus suipestifer (sub-group II)', *Journal of Hygiene*, 25 (1926): pp. 406–14.

reservations that must always surround the reporting of *Salmonella* infections,[9] it seems reasonable to accept as indicative the official record that, prior to 1940, just 14 *Salmonella* serotypes had been identified in England and Wales. These included, besides the generic *Salmonella typhimurim* and *Salmonella enteritidis*, what were termed the 'indigenous' types, isolated for the first time in Britain and Ireland: *Salmonella* thompson, newport, dublin, derby, eastbourne, stanley, london, and aberdeen.[10] In fact, *Salmonella* thompson later turned out not to be British at all, as will be shown shortly.

This baseline of 14 serotypes says something about the nature of Britain's import trade in organic materials before 1940, as well as about the nature of British agriculture, and British eating habits—notably the preference for well-cooked meat, and domestic economies so structured as to make left-over cooked meat dishes a rarity.[11] Although long distance trade in organic materials had existed before World War II, the post-war years saw an explosive increase in the level and complexity of such trade.[12] In this respect, the *Salmonella* record reveals World War II as something of a watershed. Britain's food supply situation had become critical by 1941. European sources were no longer available; shipping losses, especially of vessels with refrigerator space, were heavy; and imports of animal feeding stuffs had been drastically reduced. To maintain food supplies 'at the highest level' it became 'imperative' to achieve maximum efficiency of shipping space.[13] War-time provisioning provided bacterial opportunity. From being islands with a near self-contained *Salmonella* ecology, Britain precipitately entered a global bacterial universe.

PLACES

The Ministry of Food turned to America for supplies of spray-dried egg, which were provided by the British Food Mission under the Lend-Lease programme. Spray-dried eggs well outstripped boneless beef, dried milk, canned corned beef, and shell eggs in terms of nutritional value; they were easy to reconstitute and were thought to have 'good palatability'; unlike shell eggs, they could be shipped without refrigeration; and they were 'most economical' of space and packaging material. Unfortunately, this was virtually a new industry, if a rapidly developing one, and although the heat treatment used was known to be relatively mild, the Ministry deemed the adoption of bacteriological standards for spray-dried egg

[9] See <http://www.epigis.dk/frontpage.html>, accessed 28 May 2009.

[10] Medical Research Council, *Special Report Series*, 'The bacteriology of spray-dried egg; with particular reference to food poisoning', 260 (1947): p. 62.

[11] A. Ginsberg and A. Robertson, 'Meat hygiene', *Veterinary Record*, 61 (1949): p. 9.

[12] Editorial, 'Food spread disease', *Medical Officer*, 80 (1948): p. 225. For these developments see Yrjo Kaukianen, 'Growth, diversification and globalisation: main trends in international shipping since 1850', in *International Merchant Shipping in the Nineteenth and Twentieth Centuries: The Comparative Dimension*, edited by Lewis R. Fischer and Even Lange (2008), pp. 1–56, especially Figs 3, 11.

[13] Medical Research Council, 'Bacteriology of spray-dried egg', Appendix by the Ministry of Food (1947), p. 65.

impracticable.[14] The conditions in which American spray-dried egg was prepared were, however, far from satisfactory, and offered every opportunity for contamination. Still dirty from the farm, eggs were transported to the processing plants, where they were in some cases washed, in others not. They were then broken by hand onto wire netting and spray-dried, the temperature used being insufficient to kill bacteria.[15]

The first consignments of spray-dried egg arrived in Britain towards the end of 1941. Distribution was initially limited to bakers, confectioners, and caterers, but from July 1942 to January 1946, supplies were made available to the general public in monthly issues of five-ounce packets, each containing the equivalent of 12 eggs.[16] From July 1942, there was a sudden and unprecedented rise in the number of food-poisoning outbreaks. A total of 428 incidents had been reported between 1923 and 1939, but in 1944 the number reached 454. Most of the isolations made from the latter part of 1942 were of *Salmonella* types new to Britain. In 1942 ten new serotypes were recorded in the country's laboratories; in 1943 a further eight; and in 1944 another six, making 24 in all. The commonest occurring in descending order were *Salmonella* oranienburg, *Salmonella* montevideo, *Salmonella meleagridis* (an avian serotype), *Salmonella* anatum (usually a sub-clinical infection of waterfowl), *Salmonella* tennessee, and *Salmonella* bareilly. *Salmonella* oranienburg had previously been recorded just once in Britain, in 1935.[17] As the Medical Research Council noted, 'the suggestion is very strong that during the latter part of 1942 some new source of infection was introduced into this country'.[18] In fact problems had already been reported to the British Food Mission early in 1942.[19] By 1948, the public health community was finding the spread of food-borne infections 'highly disquieting', describing them as 'escapes' from sanitary control.[20]

In the post-war world, this pattern continued. By 1960, the number of *Salmonella* types reported in England and Wales was getting on for 200, although only a few of the imported ones succeeded in establishing themselves—notably *Salmonella* heidelberg, *Salmonella* anatum, *Salmonella* oranienburg, and *Salmonella* montevideo, each of which had caused more than 200 outbreaks. Of the rest, 50 had been isolated from just one food-poisoning incident, and a further 50 from fewer than five incidents.[21] As the local Medical Officers of Health (MOH) noted, their task was often complicated by not knowing which of all these newly introduced varieties

[14] MRC, 'Appendix'.

[15] P. S. Waters and S. Mander, 'An investigation into the incidence of salmonellae in South Australian eggs and egg pulp', *MBMH*, 12 (1953): p. 127.

[16] MRC, 'Bacteriology', p. 61. Imports ceased when the Lend-Lease arrangement came to an end in 1946, and it became important to economize on dollar imports: see Ina Zweiniger-Bargielowska, *Austerity Britain* (2000), p. 214.

[17] T. V. Cooper, 'A case of fever due to infection with bacillus oranienburg', *MBEPHLS*, 3 (1944): p. 40.

[18] Cooper, 'A case of fever', p. 62.

[19] Mathilde Solowey et al., 'Microbiology of spray-dried whole egg. II. Incidence and types of Salmonella', *American Journal of Public Health*, 37 (1947): p. 971.

[20] Editorial, 'Food spread disease', p. 225.

[21] A. McGregor et al., 'A family infection due to salmonella abony', *MO*, 102 (1959): p. 329.

were pathogenic to man, although from the perspective of global spread this is less of a consideration. More interesting is the speed with which some of these invaders became established, and the routes by which their incursions were made.

It did not need to take long for 'foreign' *Salmonella* to become well established in new territory, although with some it may have taken persistent introductions over a period of time to establish a viable indigenous base for individual bacteria in the community. Thus *Salmonella* thompson, which had first been recorded in 1924 in England, was deemed by the Medical Research Council in 1947 to be one of the country's indigenous varieties, although it subsequently appeared to have been introduced from China. *Salmonella* heidelberg, introduced in 1953, entered the table of top ten isolated varieties in England and Wales within two years, and by the later 1960s was established in breeding flocks of British poultry.[22] In March 1970, *Salmonella* agona entered Britain in imported fish-meal. By early June human infections linked to the consumption of ready-roasted chickens and contact with day-old chicks had been recorded; in July there was a milk-borne outbreak, and turkey poults sold on from a hatchery were dying in several rearing units; it was now being isolated from broiler chickens, turkeys, cattle, and pigs. *Salmonella* agona was isolated from just one further consignment of fish-meal, but rapidly established itself in the breeding flocks, where, it was observed, it might be expected to maintain itself indefinitely.[23]

By contrast with the history of *Salmonella* heidelberg and *Salmonella* agona, the case of *Salmonella* thompson illustrates how the foothold of some *Salmonella* could be more tenuous. Once again, eggs played a critical part in the *Salmonella* thompson story. At the time when *Salmonella* thompson was identified, England was importing considerable quantities of frozen tinned egg from China—some 40,000 tons of Chinese frozen liquid egg and 1,000 tons of Chinese egg albumen found their way to British markets every year, primarily for use in the baking and catering trades.[24] From 1924 to 1941, *Salmonella* thompson was the third most frequently isolated of English food-poisoning *Salmonella*. Between 1941 and 1945, incidents dropped away, but the serotype resumed its position in the league tables in 1946. At this period, although *Salmonella* infection in duck eggs had been established, it was generally thought not to be a problem in hen eggs and the source of the *Salmonella* thompson infection was regarded as a mystery. Despite its indigenous status, it was very rarely met with in cattle, sheep, pigs, rats, or mice, and only very occasionally in Britain in poultry.

Throughout the inter-war period, however, outbreaks of food poisoning were regularly associated with the consumption of bakery products filled with synthetic cream. During the war there was a lull in such incidents; after the war they resumed. In 1952 series of eight outbreaks of paratyphoid fever in South Wales,

[22] John H. McCoy, 'Trends in salmonella food poisoning in England and Wales 1941–72', *Jnl. Hyg.*, 74 (1975): pp. 277–9.

[23] McCoy, 'Trends', p. 280.

[24] Public Health Laboratory Service, 'The contamination of egg products with salmonellae, with particular reference to salm. paratyphi B', *MBPHLS*, 17 (1958): p. 48.

all caused by a single phage-type, were associated with bakeries selling cream cakes. The firm supplying the cream was also sending it to other parts of the country where no paratyphoid was occurring, and the search was on for another ingredient commonly used by all the bakeries. By a painstaking process of elimination in Public Health Laboratory Service (PHLS) labs, processed egg and egg products were identified as the source of infection. It was only then realized that a great deal of food poisoning and many recent outbreaks of paratyphoid fever had been directly or indirectly associated with contaminated egg products.[25]

The alert on egg products threw fresh light on the source of *Salmonella* thompson. As the third most frequently isolated serotype in the 1950s, *Salmonella* thompson was the most successful of the bacterial invaders at this time, and bacterial analysis linked it to frozen Chinese egg. Displaced in the *Salmonella* hierarchy when its medium of transmission ceased to be imported during the war, it returned in force with the resumption of trade in Chinese egg products after 1945. It was circumstantial evidence, but it was strong enough to be incriminating.[26]

The *Salmonella* thompson case raised issues of prevention, but also illustrated the negative influence of political priorities on public health activity. Diplomatically, the PHLS made no attempt to indicate the administrative measures 'that might be taken on the basis of these findings' to prevent illnesses caused by contaminated egg products.[27] Although the MOH of the great seaports would, it seems, have taken action with alacrity, since the episode produced 'convulsion' in their food inspection systems, they found no political support for action. On the one hand, the product was of 'urgent commercial use', since the bakery trade found pasteurized egg unsatisfactory; on the other there was a clear political steer that Chinese egg products 'should have a special place in our favour'—they represented the opening of trade between Communist China and Great Britain.[28] And so, the Port Medical Officer for Liverpool, Andrew Semple, noted, 'statesmen and salmonellas were to compete for our attention'.[29] The issue was far from settled, however. Questions were asked repeatedly in the House of Commons, and as late as May 1963, the Ministry of Health representative answered 'No' to a direct query from MP Dick Taverne as to whether the Ministry would ban imports of frozen liquid egg until regulations had been made for their compulsory pasteurization.[30] As a pasteurization technique resulting in a satisfactory product was developed around that time, however, regulations were made later that year, to come into force on 1 January 1964.[31] After this, outbreaks and concerns appear to have died away.

Egg products were by no means the only imports carrying significant bacterial loads in these early years of resumed and globalizing peacetime trade. Two other foodstuffs raised concerns around 1960: imported shell-fish, and dried coconut.

[25] PHLS, 'Contamination', pp. 36–7.
[26] PHLS, 'Contamination', p. 44; Table 6, p. 45.
[27] PHLS, 'Contamination', p. 51.
[28] Andrew B. Semple, 'Some recent problems of imported foods', *MO*, 104 (1960): p. 101.
[29] Semple, 'Recent problems', p. 101.
[30] Parliament and Public Health, 'Paratyphoid and imported liquid egg', *MO*, 109 (1963): p. 339.
[31] Anon, 'Pasteurised liquid egg', *MO*, 110 (1963): p. 185.

Japanese prawns and Chinese shrimp were not specifically associated with *Salmonella* but they supplied another instance of the problem 'of deciding the most effective point of compromise between the needs of commerce and the needs of public health', a point of special difficulty where the infective significance of certain bacteria to the human organism was not fully known.[32] Japanese prawns first attracted attention in January 1959, when samples taken by the MOH for the Port of London were found to be 'very unsatisfactory'.[33] The Ministry of Health was advised, and their response, again to quote Semple, 'very delicately [summarised the problem] in the phrase '"the difficulty of basing executive action on provisional bacteriological standards"'. This was another new area of trade, and was clearly not to be actively discouraged. Further investigation confirmed that the health authorities were dealing with 'a very carelessly prepared commodity', with bacterial plate counts generally exceeding 250,000 per gram. Liverpool, at least, worked out its own effective methods for managing the problem, and the only consignment of prawns received at the port in the first five months of 1960 gave a plate count of just 15 organisms. But just as the problem of Japanese prawns seemed to be 'resolving' nicely, it metamorphosed into a problem of Chinese shrimp.[34] Keeping up with the development of new global trading opportunities presented significant problems to port health authorities in the 1950s and 1960s.

On the face of it, dried coconut seemed an unlikely vehicle for food poisoning. This was an old established luxury trade run out of Ceylon (modern Sri Lanka) by English merchants, with a very well-organized trading association. In this case, policing of the operation was made easier by the co-operation of the trade, who accepted a system of coding packages of the product to help identify contaminated consignments.[35] The problem proved extensive, however, and involved a great range of *Salmonella* types. As Semple observed—and his phraseology is telling in its recognition of the wider problem: 'We have detected *Salmonellae paratyphi-B, typhimurium, thompson, bareilly, hvittingfoss, waycross, Newport, muenster, Poona, angoda, perth* and *seftenberg*, quite a global assembly!'[36]

In all, 33 different serotypes were identified in dried coconut, their nomenclatures suggesting origins from Norway and Scotland to Africa and south-east Asia.[37] The question of how all these serotypes arrived in Ceylon, which presumably had once had a contained *Salmonella* ecology, goes unanswered, but it was clear how they were enabled to continue on their travels. Once harvested, the nuts were collected and stored on the ground for a month or so before being delivered to the mills. The palm trees were fertilized with farmyard manure, and domestic cattle grazed among them. Contaminated husks could infect workers and contaminate equipment and broken nuts. Tank-washing water could be infected at source, or by the men who went into the tanks to clean them.[38] The problem was compounded, as

[32] Semple, 'Recent problems', p. 102.
[33] Semple, 'Recent problems', p. 102.
[34] Semple, 'Recent problems', p. 102.
[35] Semple, 'Recent problems', p. 103.
[36] Semple, 'Recent problems', p. 103.
[37] Andrew B. Semple et al., 'A review of the sampling of imported dessicated coconut', *MO*, 105 (1961): pp. 59–60.
[38] Semple, 'Review', p. 60.

in bakeries, when infected raw material became lodged or deposited in the processing machinery, allowing the contamination of clean supplies. Despite the coding system, the health authorities were forced to conclude that they should only accept consignments in which repeated sampling had not detected any contamination.[39]

At much the same time as dried coconut was demonstrating the ability to carry a global assembly of *Salmonella*, a rather different product was opening up another trajectory of microbiological expansion. The establishment of the international network of *Salmonella* centres devoted to the isolation and study of these organisms, which had taken place just before World War II, meant that the pace of identification and investigation quickened globally in the post-war world. Partly as a result of the spray-dried egg affair, the question of how the *Salmonella* got into the egg, or into the chicken that produced the egg that contaminated the spray-dried egg, attracted scientific attention. The large-scale commercial production of eggs and poultry had been developed in America during the inter-war years, and part of the regime of these programmes of intensive production was the feeding of birds with high-protein feedstuffs. The use of such feeds in animal husbandry provoked popular disgust and dismay in Britain and elsewhere when the blaze of publicity surrounding bovine spongiform encephalitis broke in the mid-1980s, but the use of these feeds dated back into the nineteenth century. Feeds of bone-meal, dried meat residue, blood and bone, and fish-meal were being advocated by animal feeds experts from the later nineteenth century, and were increasingly used in America from around 1920.[40] In Britain their use was more limited before 1940; it was only with the feedstuff shortages of World War II that British farmers began using fish-meal.[41]

Concerns about the use of high-protein feeds, from a microbiological point of view, began to surface in the mid-1950s. In 1957, for example, Fritz Kauffmann noted that the Scandinavian countries had a problem with *Salmonella* infantis in bone-meal and fish-meal, and advised that they be autoclaved before distribution.[42] A total of 11 different 'American' type *Salmonella* were identified in Angolan fish-meal at the Hygiene Institute in Hamburg in 1958. Kauffmann wrote to his friend Philip Edwards, now at the US Communicable Disease Center, to ask when imports of African fish-flour to the USA began, and whether American turkeys were fed on it.[43] In an additional note he further observed: 'the Angolan product is terrible, it is the greatest reservoir of *Salmonella* types in the world. A German

[39] Semple, 'Review', p. 60.

[40] Emil T. von Wolff, *Farm Foods or the Rational Feeding of Animals*, translated Herbert H. Cousins (1895), pp. 203–6.

[41] James C. B. Ellis, *The Feeding of Farm Live Stock (*1937); James A. Kerr, 'Fish inspection and modern development', *MO*, 34 (1935): pp. 165–6. Research on the nutritional (mineral) value of fish meal as an animal feed was being undertaken at the Rowett Institute, Aberdeen, in the mid-1920s: Notes and Comments, 'Fish meal as a feeding stuff', *MO*, 31 (1924): pp. 177–8.

[42] Fritz Kauffmann, *Erinnerungen eines Bakteriologen* (1969), p. 240.

[43] Kauffmann, *Erinnerungen*, p. 251. The Communicable Disease Centre became the Center for Disease Control in 1970.

colleague who wanted to isolate new *Salmonella* types bought a sack of fish-meal and had a new type at once.'[44]

Edwards's response confirmed that the trade in Angolan fish-meal had existed before World War II, and that there was a 'distinct possibility' that it might have been responsible for many outbreaks of disease among fowls in America. Fish-meal was one of the prime sources of vitamin E, and was heated as little as possible during manufacture to avoid damaging the vitamin content.[45] Edwards observed that American-manufactured fish-meal also contained *Salmonella*, 'although it is entirely possible that the African meal contains much larger numbers'. A member of CDC staff had found one or more *Salmonella* types in every sample of American fish-meal which he had personally collected in the production plants. Edwards considered the *Salmonella* content of fish-meal to be 'entirely a problem of plant sanitation, which I understand is really horrible'.[46] As with American spray-dried egg, Chinese and Japanese crustaceans, and Ceylonese coconut, the conditions in which Angolan fish-meal was manufactured ensured a simultaneous manufacture of *Salmonella* infections.

Ominously and presciently, Edwards noted that there had been an intensive search for sources of protein, especially animal protein, in America, and substances were now being added to animal feeds 'which were never thought of when I was an agricultural student'. He had recently received a number of *Salmonella* cultures isolated from a feed additive composed of the feathers and entrails of fowls. Within the preceding two years, he noted,[47] 'I have been quite concerned about the continuous seeding of our animal population with *Salmonella*. So long as present feed producing practices prevail, and until such time as plant sanitation is enforced, I cannot see how the reservoir of *Salmonella* infections in domestic animals can be reduced'.

Edwards' concerns about the raw materials and practices used in the animal feedstuffs industry foreshadow the later issues around BSE, of course. But below the surface of the Angolan fish-meal problem—which was, essentially, that it was responsible for distributing a wide range of *Salmonella* serotypes among populations of domestic fowl—lay further evidence of global interconnection. These were *Salmonella* types originally designated as 'American', having been identified by American researchers, and (mostly) being named for American places. In April 1958, Kauffmann wrote to Edwards, advising him that 20 so-called American serotypes were being isolated in Africa, especially in the Belgian Congo.[48] Like *Salmonella* thompson, originally considered English but revealed as Chinese, the American *Salmonella* kentucky, *Salmonella* pomona, *Salmonella* california, *Salmonella* saint-paul, *Salmonella* georgia, *Salmonella* richmond, *Salmonella* miami, *Salmonella* waycross, *Salmonella* berkeley, and *Salmonella* urbana, among others, seemed after all to have originated in Africa. The cycles of export trades in fish-meal from Africa to America, and in egg products from America to England, had equally promoted the export and global voyaging of a host of microbial parasites.

[44] Kauffmann, *Erinnerungen*, p. 254. [45] Kauffmann, *Erinnerungen*, p. 255.
[46] Kauffmann, *Erinnerungen*, pp. 255–6. [47] Kauffmann, *Erinnerungen*, p. 256.
[48] Kauffmann, *Erinnerungen*, p. 252.

Edwards's own experience in America revealed a further twist in the story. In September 1957, the serotype which came to be known as *Salmonella* saphra was identified almost simultaneously by the Louisiana state laboratories and by Ivan Saphra of the *Salmonella* Center at the Beth Israel Hospital, New York, together with his colleague Joseph J. Winter and their collaborator, Charles Wild of the Baton Rouge General Hospital. Communicating this to the Director of the Louisiana laboratories, Edwards noted, 'It really is surprising how often new serotypes appear in more than one place simultaneously.' Such occurrences in widely separated areas 'must indicate their distribution through items of food that are distributed nationally'.[49] Two years previously, the CDC laboratories had received cultures of *Salmonella* blockley from many different sources in the space of a few months: the first isolations had been made simultaneously in Philadelphia and California.[50]

The global voyaging of *Salmonella* bacteria had, as the observations of Kauffmann and Edwards suggest, another dimension, although one that did not immediately evoke a public health response. Once established in bird and animal populations, these continued to act as reservoirs which could disseminate the bacteria as the opportunity arose. The situation already existed in American poultry flocks, and was shortly to be replicated in poultry flocks elsewhere. By 1963, for example, it was noted in England that 'there is much published evidence showing that imported foodstuffs (egg products, desiccated coconut, meats, and animal feeding stuffs) have given rise to a vast reservoir of *Salmonella* infection in this country'.[51] The newly established reservoirs included humans, but the sheer numbers of *Salmonella* now being discovered argued for a very widespread distribution of reservoirs of these bacteria in disparate animal and bird populations around the globe.

In the years after 1920, microbiologists gradually uncovered and explored numerous potential and actual reservoirs of *Salmonella* infection; some plausible, some apparently unlikely. As we have seen, rats and mice were initially popular suspects for endemic infections, although the significance of rat infections proved harder to substantiate.[52] Cattle were known to harbour *Salmonella* from the 1880s, and pigs also were quickly fingered. Other species were more unexpected. In 1930, the American veterinary bacteriologists Mary E. Caldwell and Dwight L. Ryerson showed that reptiles were also implicated in *Salmonella* infection.[53] A British

[49] Kauffmann, *Erinnerungen*, pp. 247–8. Ivan Saphra died in October 1958, and the serotype was named in his memory. He was a German émigré, and had been part of Kauffmann's correspondence network.

[50] Kauffmann, *Erinnerungen*, p. 248.

[51] Wilfrid H. Parry, 'The problem of salmonella food poisoning', *MO*, 110 (1963): p. 31.

[52] William G. Savage and W. J. Read, 'Gaertner group bacilli in rats and mice', *Jnl Hyg*, 13 (1913–14): pp. 343–52; William G. Savage, 'The sources of infection in food poisoning outbreaks', *Jnl Hyg*, 17 (1918): pp. 8–9; A. M. Khalil, 'The incidence of organisms of the salmonella group in wild rats and mice in Liverpool', *Jnl Hyg*, 38 (1938): pp. 75–8; M. T. Bulman et al., 'Incidence of members of the salmonella group in rats', *Jnl Inf Dis*, 68 (1941): pp. 125–7.

[53] Mary E. Caldwell and Dwight L. Ryerson, 'Salmonellosis in certain reptiles', *Jnl Inf Dis*, 65 (1930): pp. 242–5.

investigation in 1953 found that tortoises—which were then imported into the country in substantial numbers as pets (about 300,000 a year at this period), largely from the Mediterranean—carried at least 17 different types of *Salmonella*.[54] Thus when in July 1958 a family in Kingston upon Hull were found to be infected with the uncommon *Salmonella* abony (Hungary), the family tortoise, the children's school tortoise, and that belonging to a neighbouring family which was said to be 'a frequent visitor' to the family garden, fell under suspicion. All three were taken to the Public Health Laboratory for bacteriological investigation. The family tortoise and the school tortoise were innocent of *Salmonella*, but the neighbours' tortoise was excreting both *Salmonella* potsdam and *Salmonella* rubislaw (Scotland). The source of the *Salmonella* abony infection remained obscure, although it had been found in the 1953 tortoise investigation and was thus known to exist in these creatures.[55] Reptile infections, from tortoises, turtles, snakes, geckos, iguanas, horned toads, lizards, and chameleons, remain a frequent source of human salmonellosis to this day—to the extent that the American Centers for Disease Control devote a whole feature to them on their Features website.[56]

The twentieth-century reporting of the *Salmonella* thus reveals a global canvas of habitats, and multitudinous strands of migration, transportation, and exchange. In the years after World War II, changes in technology, and in levels of human trading and transport activity, resulted in the opening up of multiple transit routes for this group of organisms. The evidence suggests that, for England at least, hitherto stout borders against minor microbial invasion crumbled. Within the dizzy constellation of international *Salmonella* exchange that then emerged, nothing was stable. Different serotypes dominated in different parts of the world, and their dominance too could change over time.[57] In 1958, for example, it was noted of Britain that *Salmonella typhimurium* had been responsible for 75 per cent of cases of human salmonellosis since 1945, with *Salmonella enteritidis* and *Salmonella* thompson running second and third respectively. Since *circa* 1950,[58] however, *Salmonella* heidelberg had been bidding fair to displace both *Salmonella* thompson and *Salmonella enteritidis* as important causes of infection in humans.[59] The factors determining these shifts in dominance are not always clear, or easy to tease out, but it was noted before World War II that *Salmonella typhimurium* was the dominant infection in Britain, while *Salmonella enteritidis* reigned on the Continent of Europe—a difference thought to originate in the continental preference for lightly

[54] J. A. Boycott et al., 'Salmonella in tortoises', *Jnl Path Bact*, 65 (1953): pp. 401–11.

[55] A. Mcgregor et al., 'A family infection due to salmonella abony', *MO*, 102 (1959): pp. 329–30. *Salmonella* abony had first been isolated in 1939 in Budapest from the faeces of normal humans. No cases were recognized in England before 1952.

[56] CDC Features, *Reptiles, Amphibians, and Salmonella*: <http://www.cdc.gov/Features/SalmonellaFrogTurtle/>, accessed 28 June 2014.

[57] See also Mildred M Galton et al., 'Epidemiology of salmonellosis in the United States', in *The World Problem of Salmonellosis*, edited by Eugène van Oye (1964), pp. 425–8, and Table III, pp. 428–9.

[58] Since 1953, in fact: McCoy, 'Trends', pp. 277–9.

[59] V. D. Allison, 'Crowd diseases', *PH*, 72 (1958): p. 52.

cooked meats as against the British for meat extremely well done.[60] In the post-1945 world, things became more complex, as agriculture commercialized, transport networks facilitated speedy long-distance movements of goods, animals, and people, human foodways changed, and hundreds of *Salmonella* took to the road. Between 1968 and 1998, of the top 100 reported isolates of *Salmonella* serotypes in America, *Salmonella typhimurium* and *Salmonella enteritidis* ranked numbers one and two, but *Salmonella* heidelberg came in at number three.[61] By 2007, *Salmonella* heidelberg was down to sixth position in the American league table.[62] In the European *Salmonella* Atlas published in May 2009, *Salmonella enteritidis* and *Salmonella typhimurium* came in at numbers one and two respectively (in reverse order to the United States) as the serotypes most frequently notified; *Salmonella* heidelberg came in at number ten.[63] Laboratories today are still telling the story which they began to tell in Britain during World War II.

The widespread identification of new *Salmonella* serotypes, the tracking of their distribution, and the investigation of their means of travel which began in the 1940s was made possible by the skills which the *Salmonella* experts had developed in their laboratories after 1920, and by their international co-operation in establishing a globally accepted classificatory scheme. The ground work for this enterprise was laid by European researchers working in Germany, England, Denmark, and Canada (see Chapter 6).[64] In the years after 1940, while European researchers continued to be involved in the power politics of the discipline, those of their American colleagues interested in human as well as animal health surged into the research domain and established their own presence in, and contribution to knowledge of, the world of *Salmonella* science.

AMERICA WAKES

The history of food poisoning in America took a dramatically new turn in the mid-twentieth century. Before the outbreak of World War II, interest in the problems of salmonellosis in America was essentially veterinary and, with respect to human populations, clinical. The two principal centres of interest lay with Philip Edwards in Kentucky and at the Beth Israel Hospital in New York, where the expatriate German Fritz Schiff, like Estenio Hormaeche, was investigating the role played by *Salmonella* in human gastroenteritis (for Schiff and Hormaeche see Chapter 6).[65] Edwards's own interest seems to have been sparked by the publication of the

[60] A. Ginsberg and A. Robertson, 'Meat hygiene', *Vet Rec*, 61 (1949): p. 9.

[61] Centers for Disease Control, *An Atlas of Salmonella in the United States 1968–1998* (2001), CD-Rom version.

[62] <http://emedicine.medscape.com/article/228174-overview>, accessed 19 August 2009.

[63] <http://www.epigis.dk/frontpage.html>, accessed 28 May 2009.

[64] James Craigie was a Briton working in Canada. See Christopher Andrewes, 'James Craigie', *Biographical Memoirs of Fellows of the Royal Society*, 25 (1979): p. 233.

[65] See for example Fritz Schiff and Lotte Strauss, 'Occurrence of several unusual types of salmonella in human infections', *Jnl Inf Dis*, 65 (1939): pp. 160–2; Estenio Hormaeche et al., 'Los salmonellas en Patalogia Infantis', Third International Congress of Microbiology, *Report of Proceedings* (1940), p. 631.

Kauffmann–White scheme in the early 1930s.[66] The public health authorities, although much concerned with typhoid, were not very interested in the food-poisoning *Salmonella* at this time.[67] During the 1920s and into the 1930s, botulism was America's main food-poisoning concern, with paratyphoid a poor second. In 1925, *The American Journal of Public Health* noted botulism as 'our national problem', the cause of nine out of ten outbreaks of food poisoning in the United States; in England, by contrast, Savage and Bruce White's investigation for the Medical Research Council had shown that nine out of ten outbreaks were caused by *Salmonella*. 'As far as evidence goes', the *AJPH* editor continued, 'B. aertrycke has never played such an important part in food poisoning in this country.'[68] The general ignorance of *Salmonella* science among the American public health community is illustrated by the observation made during a 1942 discussion by the American Public Health Association of 'Serological and bacteriologic procedures for the diagnosis of enteric fevers', in which it was suggested, without apparent contradiction, that there was a need for a *Salmonella* centre 'in this hemisphere' to provide diagnostic sera and 'to study the possibility of standardising the nomenclature of the Salmonella group'.[69] Yet at this date Philip Edwards's National Salmonella Center in Kentucky was eight years old, the Center at the Beth Israel two years old, and the Kauffmann–White scheme had been in operation for nine (see Chapter 6). Representative of veterinary, clinical, and European interests, they lay beyond the knowledge landscape of American public health.

The indifference of the American public health community to human salmonellosis was undermined during World War II as recorded outbreaks and incidents of *Salmonella* food poisoning began to rise under the stresses of war and the health authorities discovered for themselves that the problem of controlling *Salmonella* infections was 'at best an exceedingly difficult one', and their epidemiological investigation by no means simple.[70] The complexity of the problem, it was noted, 'is aggravated by the steadily increasing number of newly discovered Salmonella types'.[71] Food poisoning also proved problematic for the American military.[72] Between 1941 and 1944, powdered dried egg was being associated with *Salmonella* by American, Canadian, and British researchers, to the extent that the

[66] Galton et al., 'Epidemiology of salmonellosis', p. 421.

[67] For American concern with typhoid see Anne Hardy, 'Strategic science and ad hoc response: Typhoid in England and America, 1900–1950', *Journal of the History of Medicine and Allied Sciences*, 69 (2014): pp. 1–37.

[68] Editorial, 'The problem of food poisoning', *AJPH*, 15 (1925): p. 896; see also J. C. Geiger and J. P. Gray, 'Food poisoning—a public health problem', *AJPH*, 23 (1933): pp. 1039–44. Bacillus Aertryke is an obsolete name for *Salmonella Typhimurium*.

[69] *American Journal of Public Health Yearbook 1941–43*, Part III, 'Diagnostic procedures and reagents', Report of the Chairman of the Standard Methods Committee, p. 155 in *AJPH*, 32 (1942), Supplement 3.

[70] A. D. Rubenstein et al., 'Salmonellosis as a public health problem in wartime', *AJPH*, 34 (1944): p. 841.

[71] Rubenstein et al., 'Salmonellosis', p. 841.

[72] William S. Stone, 'Food handlers in the Army and their relationship to Salmonella food poisoning', *AJPH*, 33 (1943): pp. 706–8.

US Army Quartermaster Corps wrote 'tentative specifications' for the heat treatment of processed egg in December 1944.[73] Discomfort seems to have been complete when the English Medical Research Council's 1947 report pointed to the part which imported American spray-dried egg had played in introducing new *Salmonella* infections into Britain.[74] As a result of this accumulated evidence of the problems of human salmonellosis associated with animal foodstuffs, Philip Edwards's expertise came to the fore. Following the establishment of the Communicable Disease Center (CDC) at Atlanta in July 1946, Edwards's National Salmonella Center moved to the CDC in 1947. In 1949, the CDC cooperated with the Florida State Board of Health and the Armed Forces Epidemiological Board in setting up a veterinary public health laboratory; in 1959, the CDC set up its own veterinary public health laboratory in Atlanta.[75]

The work of the new veterinary public health laboratories revealed extensive problems of *Salmonella* infection in human and animal foods and led to the establishment in 1962 of the National Salmonella Surveillance Program at the CDC in co-operation with the state health departments.[76] A Salmonella Surveillance unit was established within the Epidemiology Branch's Investigations and Veterinary Public Health Sections, staffed by two Epidemic Intelligence Service Officers, a statistician and a public health veterinarian.[77] This integration of human and veterinary public health interests distinguished the American approach from the British, where matters human and veterinary continued to operate independently, and may point to differences in veterinary culture between Britain and America, as well as between Britain and continental Europe. In 1953 the *American Journal of Public Health* welcomed the increasing numbers of veterinarians registering for the Masters in Public Health in schools of public health, noting that this group had been actively represented at the American Public Health Association meetings in St Louis and Cleveland. 'The veterinarian', the editor concluded, 'from the start has been accustomed to the concept of the protection of populations against crowd diseases and malnutrition. He fits with special facility into the family of public health.'[78] The management of large herds of cattle and horses on the spacious plains of the American West and on large farm estates elsewhere, together with the early introduction of modern methods of mass food production, may have engendered a very different veterinary approach from that associated with the small-scale agriculture that persisted in pre-1945 Britain, the emphasis on specimen animals (stud and show stock, working and racing horses), and an increasing focus on small animal practice. Certainly the American tradition of scientific

[73] A. R. Winter et al., 'Pasteurization of liquid egg products III. Destruction of Salmonella in liquid whole egg', *AJPH*, 36 (1946): p. 451.

[74] James L. Steele, 'Salmonella 1885–1962', Symposium, Epidemiology of Salmonellosis, *Public Health Reports* 78(12) (1963): pp. 1065–6 (hereafter Salmonellosis Symposium).

[75] Steele, 'Salmonella', p. 1066. For the history of the CDC see Elizabeth W. Etheridge, *Sentinel for Health: A History of the Centers for Disease Control* (1992).

[76] Steele, 'Salmonella', p. 1066.

[77] Eugene Sanders et al., 'Surveillance of human salmonellosis', Salmonellosis Symposium, p. 1080.

[78] Editorial, 'The zoonoses', *AJPH*, 43 (1953): p. 477.

veterinary research suggests difference in approach to the management of the diseases of animals.

The establishment of the CDC marked a critical development in American public health, being in some respects a similar facility to England's PHLS. Discussing the Center's Division of Laboratory Services in 1947, the *American Journal of Public Health* described it as a 'public health laboratory service'.[79] Developed out of the success of the war-time Office of Malaria Control, its principal emphasis was initially to be 'in the field where insect vectors or animal reservoirs' were important, although its scope was to be broadened to include 'any or all' communicable diseases.[80] Given existing American interest in rickettsial disease and rabies, veterinary public health was on the programme from the beginning.[81] The transfer of Edwards's National Salmonella Center to the CDC was, in these circumstances, a natural inclusion, as well as recognition that salmonellosis now presented a serious problem for both animals and humans. Like the PHLS, the CDC's services included the provision of investigative and consultative services for communities (and states) where communicable disease outbreaks occurred or presented a continued threat. Epidemiologists and mobile laboratories could be dispatched on request to determine the cause, sources, and extent of epidemic outbreaks. The CDC laboratories undertook research, but also provided consultation services to individual laboratories, including advice and the loan of laboratory personnel to help with technical or administrative problems or to improve techniques and practice.[82]

The integration of a specific veterinary public health interest into the CDC, and the well-established American tradition of scientific veterinary research, meant that the new American interest in salmonellosis was from the beginning a joint scientific enterprise. The benefits of such close linkage had been clear earlier, as when a somatic antigen discovered in cultures of animal origin by Edwards in 1938 proved to be that present in the organism responsible for an outbreak of diarrhoea among newborns in Kansas in 1935, whose identity Schiff and Strauss had been wrestling to unravel at the Beth Israel. It turned out to be a new *Salmonella* type, and one with unusual cultural characteristics.[83] The rapid meshing of the human and veterinary aspects of *Salmonella* research in the United States contrasted with the situation in England, where the strand of human-related public health and laboratory research into the *Salmonella* going back to the 1880s only managed to link up with the few veterinarians interested in aspects of animal salmonellosis in 1940

[79] Editorial, 'A national nerve center for public health laboratory service', *AJPH*, 37 (1947): p. 745.

[80] Editorial, 'National nerve center', p. 745.

[81] Editorial, 'The Communicable Disease Center at Atlanta', *AJPH,* 38 (1948): p. 1578. The Rockefeller Foundation was then funding a rabies research laboratory in Birmingham, Alabama: Editorial, 'National nerve center', p. 746. For American rickettsial diseases see Victoria A. Harden, *Rocky Mountain Spotted Fever: A Twentieth-century Disease* (1990).

[82] Editorial, 'National nerve center', p. 747.

[83] Fritz Schiff and Lotte Strauss, 'A new Salmonella type (Salmonella Wichita)', *Jnl Inf Dis*, 65 (1939): p. 125.

under the auspices of the Royal Society of Medicine, and conceivably at the instigation of William Mcdonald Scott in his capacity as Director of the EPHLS.

Although deeply engaged with the taxonomic aspects of their work, the American *Salmonella* researchers also considered the wider epidemiological implications of their findings. In the early 1940s, the research teams at both the Beth Israel and at the Kentucky Agricultural Experiment Station were studying the occurrence and distribution of *Salmonella* species through North American material. In the first 20 months of the New York Center's existence, cultures from 261 human infections were received, from which 26 different *Salmonella* types were isolated. Two cultures of human origin, 12 from animals, and one from foodstuff came from abroad.[84] The analysis performed in Kentucky was more extensive and elaborate, being based on 3,090 cultures isolated from humans and animals in America and its possessions, studied between 1934 and 1941.[85] Edwards and Bruner found 'a rather wide variety of types' in fowls, pigs, and humans, and fewer in horses, carnivores, rodents, and ruminants.[86] Of 492 human cultures, 118 were paratyphoid, and among the 38 *Salmonella* varieties recorded, *Salmonella typhimurium* was the type most frequent (61 isolations).[87] The results presented offered, the authors noted, 'an excellent example' of the global distribution of *Salmonella* types, and showed the frequency of occurrence of the various types in humans and animals to be strikingly similar.[88] In passing, they noted that although certain rare types of *Salmonella* were dominant in particular locations, 'eventually they are almost invariably found in other places'. The inference was clear: *Salmonella* types travelled. In all, Edwards and Bruner found 59 *Salmonella* serotypes present in North America between 1934 and 1941, in a pattern that differed markedly from that established for England and Wales by the Ministry of Health laboratory. Concluding their paper, Edwards and Bruner observed that the large number of *Salmonella* types might be confusing,[89] 'But their very multiplicity emphasizes the need for accurate identification of the bacilli if the epizoology, epidemiology and control of salmonellosis are to be the subjects of serious study.' The research published from Edwards's Center, supported by that from the Beth Israel, provided a solid indication of the need for American public health authorities to take salmonellosis seriously.

Not all American health personnel agreed with the CDC's acceptance of the importance of *Salmonella*. Discussing the reports of gastrointestinal disease

[84] S. Bornstein et al., 'Frequency of occurrence of salmonella species', *Jnl Inf Dis*, 69 (1941): pp. 59, 64.

[85] Philip R. Edwards and D. W. Bruner, 'The occurrence and distribution of salmonella types in the United States', *Jnl Inf Dis*, 72 (1943): p. 58.

[86] Edwards and Bruner, 'Occurrence', p. 59; Table 1, p. 64.

[87] Edwards and Bruner, 'Occurrence', Table 2, p. 65.

[88] Edwards and Bruner, 'Occurrence', p. 66.

[89] Edwards and Bruner, 'Occurrence', p. 67. Curiously, given his earlier career in agricultural bacteriology, Elizabeth Etheridge notes that Edwards, 'a giant in the field of salmonella research and possessive about his specialty, was interested only in the human aspects of salmonella', although he co-operated 'beautifully' with Mildred Galton: Etheridge, *Sentinel*, p. 95. Her source appears to have been Galton.

outbreaks made to the US Public Health Service for the years 1945–7 in 1950, a Wisconsin District Health Officer, Milton Feig, suggested discreetly that the amount of attention being paid to *Salmonella* was excessive. Within the 'vaguer epidemic groups of bacterial enteric disease' that involved ever-increasing numbers of Americans, *Salmonella* were not of prime significance. The many species of *Salmonella* and their distribution in nature had resulted in an excessive response: 'though a fascinating study to the bacteriologist and epidemiologist', the attention given to these organisms was not justified when their incidence was compared to that of staphylococcal intoxication.[90] Looking perhaps to the dominance of *Salmonella* in European food-poisoning outbreaks as well the numbers of new types being discovered, their distribution pathways, and likely global distribution, the bacteriologists and epidemiologists persisted. The laboratory monitoring of animal infections and the reporting of cases of human infection both indicated a growing problem in America through the 1950s. The number of cultures identified from cattle rose from 0.7 per cent of the total in 1934–47 to 7 per cent in 1957–61. Somewhat ironically, given Feig's scepticism, the Wisconsin Department of Agriculture recorded in 1962 that salmonellosis was being reported in cattle with increasing frequency. The highest incidence appeared to be in October, when the creatures were brought into barns to be housed during the winter months.[91] Over the same period there was a 7 per cent increase nationally in cultures identified from poultry; and the number of human cases of non-typhoid *Salmonella* rose from 1,733 in 1951 to 8,542 in 1961, although the reporting of such infections in America was known to be 'incomplete and inadequate'.[92]

The symposium on salmonellosis organized by the Conference of Veterinarians, American Public Health Association, at the annual meeting held at Miami Beach, Florida in October 1962, echoed the 1940 Royal Society of Medicine meeting in that it brought together the human and animal interests in *Salmonella*. The enormous escalation in knowledge concerning *Salmonella* which had accumulated over the intervening 22 years, was reflected in the meeting's whole approach to the topic. After a brief introductory history (covering the years 1885–1962),[93] papers followed on salmonellosis in livestock and in poultry.[94] Staff from the Georgia Department of Public Health described five outbreaks of human salmonellosis

[90] Milton Feig, 'Diarrhea, dysentery, food poisoning, and gastroenteritis. A study of 926 outbreaks and 49,879 cases reported to the United States Public Health Service (1945–47)', *AJPH*, 40 (1950): p. 1390. The predominance of staphylococcal infections over *Salmonella* in America was confirmed in 1958: see Carl Dauer, '1957 summary of disease outbreaks', *Public Health Reports, Washington*, 73(8) (1958): pp. 681–6; Notes and Records, 'Food infections in the United States', *MO*, 101 (1959): pp. 3–4.

[91] Mildred M. Galton, 'Salmonellosis in livestock', Salmonellosis Symposium, p. 1068. Galton now headed the CDC's Veterinary Public Health Laboratory.

[92] Galton, 'Livestock', pp. 1066–7; see also Galton, et al., 'Epidemiology of salmonellosis', in van Oye, ed, *World Problem*, pp. 422–4.

[93] Steele, 'Salmonella', pp. 1063–4. James Steele was Chief of the Veterinary Public Health Section of the CDC.

[94] Galton, 'Livestock', pp. 1064–71; Kenneth D. Quist, 'Salmonellosis in poultry', Salmonellosis Symposium, pp. 1071–3. Quist was Chief of the CDC's Zoonoses Investigations Unit, Veterinary Public Health Section.

related to poultry, including one resulting from the practice of giving small children chicks and ducklings as Easter presents.[95] Most interestingly, the last two papers in the series moved on from the local situation to position the American experience within the global *Salmonella* picture. First up was Kenneth W. Newell, professor of epidemiology at Tulane University, who argued the case for the international reporting of *Salmonella*.[96] He was followed by Glenn G. Slocum, director of the US Food and Drug Administration's Division of Microbiology, who noted the slender evidence that foods traded inter-state had resulted in outbreaks of human salmonellosis, but also discussed the international problems caused by spray-dried egg and dried coconut.[97]

Newell's discussion of the need for international reporting suggests that American epidemiologists, coming new to the *Salmonella* problem, tended to a greater extent than the Europeans to address it in global context.[98] Although Newell's background was in the British public health system, he went on from Tulane to pursue a successful career with the World Health Organization, and may have learnt this internationalist approach from his American colleagues.[99] Newell set out four separate factors—which, he noted, had occurred simultaneously—as generating the 'recent' marked increase of interest in *Salmonella* (one might argue that the 'recent' applied largely to the United States). First, recognition of food poisoning as an important cause of illness even in developed countries, *Salmonella* infections constituting a large proportion of these cases; second, awareness that a large number of 'new' serotypes had appeared in human populations in the West; third, that *Salmonella* were 'true zoonotic infections'; fourth, that food, food products, and animal food products that had crossed national boundaries were increasingly identified as causing *Salmonella* outbreaks in humans and animals.[100] Suddenly, he concluded, it had become 'urgent to find out what is happening on an international scale, to assess the significance of this transfer of known pathogens across national boundaries, and to try to do something to stop it'.[101] The benefits of the international pooling of information, Newell argued, had already been demonstrated by the war-time dried-egg episode, while the post-war rise of *Salmonella* heidelberg was now recognized as an international phenomenon. Had an international clearing house for *Salmonella* data existed in the early 1950s,

[95] John E. McCroan et al., 'Five salmonellosis outbreaks related to poultry products', Salmonellosis Symposium, pp. 1074–5.

[96] Kenneth W. Newell, 'Value of international reporting of salmonellae', Salmonellosis Symposium, pp. 1083–5. Newell was qualified MD DPH, and pursued a distinguished career in public health, from the PHLS in 1954–6 to the WHO (1958–61, 1967–77): see Anon, 'Kenneth W. Newell', *BMJ*, 300 (16 June 1990): p. 1581.

[97] Glen G. Slocum, 'Control by the FDA of foodborne salmonellae', Salmonellosis Symposium, p. 1086.

[98] This inference is supported by the respective American and European contributions to the 1964 survey of the world salmonellosis problem. Compare Galton et al., 'Salmonellosis in the United States' with H. P. R. Seeliger and A. E. Maya, 'Epidemiologie der salmonellosen in Europa, 1950–1960 (ausgenommen Osteuropa)', in van Oye, ed, *World Problem*, pp. 245–94. British commentators also seemed largely focused on the local problem.

[99] See Anon, 'Newell', p. 1581.

[100] Newell, 'Value', pp. 1083–4.

[101] Newell, 'Value', p. 1084.

it might have been possible to identify the 'vehicle of intercountry transfer', and take steps to counter it.[102] As might be expected, Newell warned that such co-operation would not be easy to achieve; it was also evident from his continued discussion that achieving these aims would take time and perseverance.

If Newell's proposals were an attempt to initiate American hegemony over *Salmonella* science, the existing state of European *Salmonella* science, with its worldwide connections, was strong enough to resist take-over.[103] Newell's proposals appear either to have fallen on stony ground or to have foundered on problems of achieving uniform and consistent practice in global public health. An international survey of current scientific understandings of *Salmonella* and of their global epidemiology, published in 1964, offered no reflective discussion of the possibilities for their international surveillance and control.[104] However desirable international co-operation over the tracking and control of these ubiquitous organisms might be, there were limits to the possible. A global survey of *Salmonella* infections conducted by CDC staff among the 191 WHO member states in the early twenty-first century found that just 76 of 101 responders conducted public health surveillance for *Salmonella*, while 69 undertook serotyping as part of that surveillance.[105] Recognition of salmonellosis as an international problem also demonstrated the limits of international co-operation. Even with the muscle of the American scientific community behind it, global co-ordination of surveillance was beyond the capacities and interests of international public health. While scientific interest in *Salmonella* grew exponentially in the years after 1945, and the identification of new serotypes continued, the resolution of local problems continued effectively to be managed at the local level. In England and Wales, efforts at *Salmonella* control continued to stumble forward with little reference to the wider international context, while the global dimensions of the food-poisoning problem and its association with international trade developed into a serious problem in international public health.

[102] Newell, 'Value', p. 1085.

[103] See the model proposed in John Krige, *American Hegemony and the Postwar Reconstruction of Science in Europe* (2003), chapter 1.

[104] Van Oye, ed, *World Problem*.

[105] H. Herikstad et al., 'Salmonella surveillance: a global survey of public health serotyping', *Epidemiology and Infection*, 129 (2002): pp. 1–8.

PART III

SITES OF INFECTION

8
Field and Farm

Some 20 years before the American symposium on *Salmonella* was convened in 1962, a similar combination of veterinary, epidemiological, and public health interests assembled in war-time London. On 21 February 1940, the first-ever joint discussion session took place between the Section for Comparative Medicine and that for Epidemiology and State Medicine of the Royal Society of Medicine. The subject of discussion was *Salmonella* infections, and the occasion marked the first formal coming together of medical men and veterinarians on a topic of mutual interest. Four speakers contributed papers to serve as the basis for debate. William Savage reviewed the literature linking *Salmonella* to disease in animals; R. Lovell discussed the topic of animal reservoirs; R. F. Gordon spoke on *Salmonella* infection in birds; and W. M. Scott detailed his own research on *Salmonella* infection in pigs appearing healthy at slaughter.[1] Some months later, the meeting was reported in the *Veterinary Record*—the first mention of *Salmonella* infections since the journal began publication in 1888.[2] The year 1940 marked a significant upswing of interest in salmonellosis among British veterinarians. For some decades the profession had been more or less in transition, from the horse-dominated case-load of the nineteenth century towards acceptance of wider interests in livestock, poultry, and small animals, while at the same time prominent figures in the profession urged a shift in focus from general practice to research and a more scientific approach to veterinary problems.[3] Both these factors influenced the growing veterinary interest in *Salmonella,* which was also supported by the recent establishment of the Veterinary Investigation Service (1938), the Emergency Public Health Laboratory Service (1939), and the Animal Health Trust (1942).[4]

[1] Joint Meeting, 'Discussion on salmonella infections', *Proceedings of the Royal Society of Medicine*, 33(1) (1940): pp. 351–70.

[2] Editorial, 'Salmonella infections', *Veterinary Record*, 52 (1940): p. 556.

[3] See Anne Hardy, 'Professional advantage and public health: British veterinarians and state veterinary services, 1865–1939', *Twentieth Century British History*, 14 (2000): pp. 1–23; Abigail Woods and Stephen Matthews, '"Little if at all removed from the illiterate farrier or cow-leech". The English veterinary surgeon c. 1860–1885 and the campaign for veterinary reform', *Medical History*, 54 (2010): pp. 29–54.

[4] See Robert E. O. Williams, *Microbiology for the Public Health: The Evolution of the Public Health Laboratory Service 1939–1980* (1985); Anon, 'The Veterinary Investigation Service in England and Wales: Half a century of development', *Vet Rec*, 91 (1972): pp. 565–70; Richard Onslow, *A History of the Animal Health Trust* (1993). The Animal Health Trust now focuses on companion animals (cats, dogs, and horses), but it had a wider remit in its early years. For the Poultry Research Station see Onslow, *History*, pp. 5-6; for the work of the Trust see also Royal College of Veterinary Surgeons, *Registers and Directory* (1967), pp. 474–6.

The meeting at the Royal Society of Medicine (RSM) was important for establishing the links between human and animal *Salmonella* ecology in the veterinary consciousness. From this beginning, veterinarians and public health personnel began to find common ground regarding food infections associated with animal carriers and the hygienic production of food, and the difficulties of preventive action within modern food production systems. The *Veterinary Record*, commenting on the meeting, drew particular attention to the connections between human and animal salmonellosis and to the role of *Salmonella* in causing animal disease; Gordon's emphasis on the importance of *Salmonella* infections in birds was 'of special interest'. The journal noted that 'we have a long way to go before we can effectively control the pathological manifestations of these bacteria', and further that there was a very general ignorance of the reservoirs of *Salmonella* infection. The latter was, the editor observed, 'largely a problem for workers in the veterinary field'.[5] In the event, it was only in the years after World War II, and in the course of the transition from traditional farming practices to modern agriculture, that the nature and extent of animal reservoirs of *Salmonella* infection began to be realized. In this period, however, interest shifted from the elucidation of pathways of infection that had marked the previous half century, and towards the identification of reservoirs of infection and the means by which the damage they caused to human and animal health might be controlled or contained.

SALMONELLOSIS AND THE MODERNIZATION OF FARMING SYSTEMS

The emergence of salmonellosis as a problem in livestock management and veterinary practice was due to several factors. The economic costs of animal diseases began to be recognized in the 1930s, resulting in the establishment of the Veterinary Investigation Service (VIS) under the auspices of the Ministry of Agriculture in 1938. VIS staff held a brief for researching and controlling the sources of disease in domestic livestock, and they were backed up by laboratory facilities.[6] Second, the Public Health Laboratory Service (PHLS) became increasingly interested in foodborne infections, and in the links between animal foods and human food poisoning, as notified cases of the latter developed an exponential upward curve during the 1940s.[7] The increasing sophistication of laboratory methods also played its part. As microbiologists began to identify bacteria by their antigenic structure, the specific nature of individual *Salmonella* and their association with specific hosts became clear. Thus *Salmonella* dublin was known from 1930 to have its reservoir in cattle,

[5] Editorial, 'Salmonella infections', p. 556.

[6] Hardy, 'Professional advantage', pp. 20–1. The Board of Agriculture and Fisheries had established a bacteriological laboratory *c.*1909: Notes and Comments, 'Bacteriological laboratory of the Board of Agriculture and Fisheries', *Medical Officer*, 4 (1910): p. 257.

[7] Williams, *Microbiology*, pp. 21–2.

but to be pathogenic to humans when consumed in raw milk.[8] These associations had important epidemiological and public health implications in tracing the sources of human infections, as began to be realized in the 1930s. At the RSM meeting in 1940, William Savage, long the established British expert on food poisoning, admitted that although he had for 30 years emphasized that animal diseases were the source of human food-poisoning infections, he had 'not so readily appreciated' that the differential distribution of various types was important to their effective control.[9]

The transformations that were taking place in British farming also helped to shape a new veterinary and public health awareness of the problems of *Salmonella* infection in animals. By the 1930s, livestock had become the most important agricultural sector in terms of both land occupied and production levels.[10] At the same time, however, financial pressures led to deterioration of the agricultural environment: the well-kept farms and tidy landscape characteristic of Victorian 'high farming' largely disappeared.[11] Dairying became an important sector: the number of dairy cows increased by 15 per cent between 1924–5 and 1934–5, while milk production increased by 24 per cent, with a healthy demand sustaining its price in a period of generally falling prices.[12] Pig farming also expanded significantly: the number of pigs in England and Wales increased by 51 per cent between 1921 and 1936.[13] Until World War II, however, farming practices remained largely traditional, and this was particularly true of the fat stock and store animal market, which remained locally based and 'even chaotic'.[14] Multitudes of small markets designed to meet the local needs of producers and consumers persisted, and even animals intended for immediate slaughter were usually bought by local butchers using their own small slaughter houses and traditional, if outdated, techniques.[15] In 1938, despite the best efforts of concerned central and local authorities, there were still some 15,000 private slaughterhouses in England and Wales, as against just 115 public abattoirs.[16] In general, therefore, the structure and practices of British farming remained essentially unchanged during the inter-war period.

The outbreak of World War II forced significant changes to the structure of British farming. Government began to manage food supplies, manipulating

[8] Philip Bruce White, 'Notes on an organism serologically related to S. enteritis Gartner. 1. The Dublin and Tokyo types of Salmonella', *Journal of Hygiene,* 29 (1929–30): pp. 443–5; J. Smith and William M. Scott, 'Continued fever due to gaertner-like *Salmonella* of the type "Dublin" ', *Jnl Hyg,* 30 (1930): pp. 32–9.

[9] Joint Meeting, 'Discussion', p. 361. For the veterinary background see Abigail Woods, 'A historical synopsis of animal diseases and public policy in twentieth century Britain', *Philosophical Transactions of the Royal Society,* series B, 366 (2011), doi: 10.1098/rstb.2010.0388.

[10] John Martin, *The Development of Modern Agriculture: British Farming since 1931* (2000), p. 12.

[11] Martin, *Modern Agriculture*, p. 9.

[12] Jonathan Brown, *Agriculture in England; A Survey of Farming, 1870–1944* (1987), pp. 93–4.

[13] Brown, *Agriculture*, pp. 96–7.

[14] Martin, *Modern Agriculture*, p. 27.

[15] Martin, *Modern Agriculture*, p. 27.

[16] Harold C. Bywater, 'Public and private slaughter houses in England and Wales', *Vet Rec*, 60 (1948): p. 219. In 1920 the numbers had been 20,000 and 100 respectively.

agriculture and encouraging tillage at the expense of livestock.[17] In order to organize an equitable system of food distribution on the Home Front, the Ministry of Food instituted collecting centres for fat stock and the centralization of slaughtering. By 1941, the number of slaughterhouses had been reduced to some 500.[18] The Ministry did not, however, introduce an equivalent meat inspection service: the examination of both animals and meat was left almost entirely in the hands of the local authorities.[19] The effect of these changes in the fat stock market was two-fold: first, a decrease in efficiency of inspection, and second, an increase in *Salmonella* infection rates among cattle and pigs awaiting slaughter. The reduction in the number of slaughterhouses now meant that animals had to travel sometimes considerable distances to slaughter, and they were generally penned in lairages for longer periods before slaughter took place. Tired and distressed by travel, often overcrowded in the lairages, unwatered and unfed, livestock, especially calves and young pigs, suffered a heightened vulnerability to *Salmonella* and other infections (Chapter 9). The situation deteriorated further with the return of peace. The introduction of the single intradermal tuberculin test in 1946 led to a campaign against bovine tuberculosis, and the Attested (confirmed tuberculosis-free) Herds scheme for dairy cattle became increasingly popular. Where there had been a mere 58 attested herds in England and Wales in March 1936, their number had swollen to 59,000 by November 1952.[20] There was a potential drawback to this apparent success, however: the establishment of so many new attested herds involved a great increase in cattle movements, which it was feared would extend other infections into new areas of the country.[21]

The impact of the new organizational practices was the subject of several studies from the 1950s.[22] The spread of infection in animals as they passed from farms through markets to abattoirs was described in 1954. One survey found that whereas 7 per cent of pigs on farms excreted *Salmonella*, the rate was 78 per cent among pigs from the same farms in holding pens at abattoirs.[23] Another study found that rates of *Salmonella* infection in calves held for only a few hours before slaughter was 0.6 per cent, but rose to 35.6 per cent when they were held for between two and five days.[24] Just one infected calf could spread infection to an entire group.[25] Transport of any kind, but especially long-distance transport, also distressed the creatures and made them susceptible to infection, loss of condition,

[17] Martin, *Modern Agriculture*, p. 65. [18] Bywater, 'Slaughter houses', p. 219.

[19] Editorial, 'Inspection of food animals and meat', *Vet Rec*, 52 (1940): p. 304.

[20] John D. F. Tutt, 'Changes in veterinary practice and in the incidence of certain diseases during the last 30 years', *Vet Rec*, 65 (1953): p. 618.

[21] Tutt, 'Changes', p. 618.

[22] For the broader animal disease context see Woods, 'Historical synopsis'.

[23] Betty C. Hobbs, 'Contamination of meat supplies, part 1: *Salmonella* and *Shigella*', *Monthly Bulletin of the Ministry of Health*, 28 (1965): p. 123.

[24] E. S. Anderson et al., 'An outbreak of human infection due to Salmonella typhimurium Phage-type 20a associated with infection in calves', *Lancet*, 1961, i: pp. 855–6.

[25] P. J. Wormald et al., 'An epidemic of salmonella typhimurium infection in calves', *MBMH*, 24 (1965): pp. 58–61.

and heightened excretion of *Salmonella* bacteria.[26] In the years after World War II a whole new ecology of *Salmonella* was being established across Britain's agricultural economy, but the process was by no means complete in the first decade after the war.

During the 1960s a new livestock speciality emerged to service the increasingly well-to-do and demanding consumer market: the intensive rearing of beef cattle. This enterprise involved the collection of surplus bull calves from dairy farms—the dairy sector was now principally located in the west of the country—and transferring them in large batches, usually in the first week of life, to rearing units in the east and north. Calves from many sources were collected together.[27] A typical beef unit might take 20–50 calves every fortnight from a large number of farms. One unit in Essex, for example, held 525 calves born on 434 different farms.[28] As this new form of husbandry spread, the yearly total of *Salmonella* incidents in calves recorded by the Veterinary Investigation Centres in England and Wales rose from 123 in 1958 to 1,902 in 1967. In discussion following papers at a symposium on animal salmonellosis held at the annual Congress of the British Veterinary Association at Brighton in 1967, T. W. Heard, a practitioner in Wiltshire, gave a succinct analysis of the problem in the beef industry, and pointed to the difficulties in remedying the situation:[29] 'Finance and economics ruled the day, and agriculture had for many years been placed at the forefront of the economic squeeze. Legislation of the calf dealer, the marketing organisation, and the transport people would be a slow, resentful and tedious business . . . ' Summing up, Heard concluded that disease was being given 'a golden opportunity' by rapid long-distance travel and mass marketing. Clear evidence supporting the role of long-distance transport was provided, if needed, during the 1968 foot-and-mouth outbreak, when the import of calves into Scotland from south of the border was temporarily suspended. While the suspension lasted, no *Salmonella* isolations were made from pathological material received from north-east Scotland, yet within days of trade being resumed with the south of England, *Salmonella* dublin was again being isolated from calves after transit.[30]

Research undertaken in the veterinary community after World War II led to a significant change in perception of the likely reservoirs causing human *Salmonella* infections. In 1963 the pathologist to Belfast City Hospital, V. D. Allison, was stressing the 'paramount importance' of animal reservoirs in *Salmonella* infection.[31] By 1969 H. Williams Smith of the Animal Health Trust could write that where once the emphasis in human food-poisoning incidents had been on the role of

[26] Hobbs, 'Meat supplies'.

[27] H. Williams Smith, 'Salmonella food poisoning in human beings: the part played by domestic animals', *Royal Society of Health Journal*, 89 (1969): p. 275.

[28] Williams Smith, 'Salmonella', p. 275.

[29] Congress Symposium, 'Salmonellosis: The present position in man and animals', *Vet Rec*, 80 (1967): p. 164. For the traditional opposition to control and lobbying strength of the meat sector see Peter J. Atkins, 'The Glasgow case: Meat, disease and regulation, 1889–1924', *Agricultural History Review*, 52 (2004): pp. 180–1.

[30] Notes and Comments, 'Salmonellosis in North East Scotland', *MO*, 124 (1970): p. 146.

[31] V. D. Allison, 'Clean food: The laboratory's role', *RSHJ*, 83 (1963): p. 47.

human carriers and vermin, humans were now regarded as victims of an infected environment, with food animals believed to be the main sources of infection. This conclusion reflected epidemiological investigations undertaken since the war, and the fact that the *Salmonella* usually causing food poisoning were those commonly found in food animals, their feedstuffs, and their products.[32]

SALMONELLA ON THE FARM

In the immediate aftermath of World War II, Britain's veterinary community became aware of unsettling developments in *Salmonella* incidence among livestock. Alarm over the increasing incidence of salmonellosis in cattle was initially sounded by F. V. John, a veterinary surgeon practising in Llandeilo, South Wales, in 1946. John recorded the occurrence in recent years of frequently fatal acute enteritis in adult cattle, associated with *Salmonella* dublin. The condition was usually sporadic but occasionally infected more than one animal in a herd. All recovered cows became carriers and excreted *Salmonella* dublin in large numbers in their faeces for long periods.[33] Later that year, D. W. P. Bythell, of Harper Adams Veterinary College, reported similar outbreaks on two dairy farms in the West Midlands.[34] Despite a number of human outbreaks of *Salmonella* dublin infection associated with milk, it had generally been assumed that bovine *Salmonella* infections were of minor importance in Britain.[35] Although a 'somewhat voluminous literature' then existed on *Salmonella* in both adult cattle and calves in most parts of the world, only a handful of references had appeared in the British literature by 1948—two on infections in calves in 1931 and 1947, and three on adult cattle from 1946.[36] John's observations and those that followed suggested the existence of a more widespread problem than had hitherto been realized.

The alarm sounded by John and Bythell led H. I. Field, of the VIS at Cardiff, to undertake an investigation into the presence of bovine salmonellosis in West Wales in 1946–7.[37] Infection was diagnosed on 70 farms, specimens from affected animals yielding *Salmonella* dublin on 66 farms and *Salmonella typhimurium* on four. Of these farms, 53 lay in Carmarthen.[38] The great majority of cases occurred between June and October; most affected animals were female and over one year old; the mortality rate was estimated at around 70 per cent. Local observation indicated that the carrier state could persist for at least two years in survivors, that infection from parent to calf took place, and that cattle apparently normal at slaughter were

[32] Williams Smith, 'Salmonella', p. 271. See also Joan Taylor, 'Salmonella II: Public health aspects', *Vet Rec*, 80 (1967): p. 47.

[33] F. V. John, 'A preliminary note on Salmonella dublin infection in adult cattle', *Vet Rec*, 58 (1946): pp. 211–12.

[34] D. W. P. Bythell, 'Two outbreaks of Salmonella dublin infection in adult cattle', *Vet Rec*, 58 (1946): pp. 425–6.

[35] Editorial, 'Salmonellosis in cattle', *Vet Rec*, 61 (1949): p. 113.

[36] H. I. Field, 'A survey of bovine salmonellosis in Mid and West Wales', *Veterinary Journal*, 104 (1948): p. 251.

[37] Field, 'Survey', pp. 251–66, 294–302, 323–39.

[38] Field, 'Survey', p. 336.

carrying both *Salmonella* dublin and *Salmonella typhimurium*. As Field noted, it was important that a small number of *Salmonella* might be found in the milk of carrier animals.[39]

Field published two further studies of bovine salmonellosis in 1949. The first was a survey paper, in which he noted that the sporadic nature of most cases in Britain had meant the problem did not attract the attention it deserved; the public health records suggested it had been present for several decades at least. Cases of bovine salmonellosis causing food-poisoning outbreaks had occurred in widely dispersed areas, indicating that infection was not confined to any one part of the country.[40] Field thought it likely that clinically infected and carrier animals played an important part in maintaining infection on individual farms and in given areas. He advocated employing the measures of isolation and sanitary supervision used against brucellosis in an attempt to reduce the number of active carriers: a recent outbreak in Glamorgan caused by calves bought at Carmarthen illustrated the important role played by carrier animals in spreading infection both within an area and beyond it, into 'clean' areas.[41] Field's second paper reported a knackery survey conducted in 1947 and 1948. This enabled him further to refine his geographical map of the distribution of bovine salmonellosis in South Wales.[42] In both Carmarthen and Glamorgan, where most infections were reported, the affected animals came from the lowland dairying districts, while the hilly northern areas were relatively free. *Salmonella* dublin was by far the dominant strain isolated (257/276), while *typhimurium* (nine), derby (eight), *enteritidis* (one), and brancaster (one) were also found. Discussing the suggestion that infected dried-egg powder in feedstuffs might account for the increased range of *Salmonella* types recently found in poultry, Field noted it as significant that 'types of salmonella not recorded in stock in this country before 1946 have now been demonstrated in poultry, pigs and cattle'.[43]

Although Field's studies and methodologies offered a model for surveys of *Salmonella* distribution in Britain, and a mapping of reservoirs of infection, there is little evidence that his work was followed elsewhere. It may be that the role of *Salmonella* dublin in human infection was too slender to attract significant attention, or that such studies were perceived as too labour-intensive. Instead, both veterinary and public health attention shifted towards the suggestion that animal feedstuffs were responsible for the upsurge in new *Salmonella* types being recorded in the late 1940s. New studies in the 1950s also suggested that pathways of infection and cross-infection were not confined to cattle alone. In 1953, an outbreak of *Salmonella typhimurium* infection in young shorthorn cows was reported from the Veterinary Investigation Centre (VIC) at Leeds. The herd was milked in a shed opening onto a collecting yard where the cows gathered both before and

[39] Field, 'Survey', pp. 337–8.

[40] H. I. Field, 'Salmonella infection in cattle', *Vet Rec*, 61 (1949): p. 109.

[41] Field, 'Salmonella infection', p. 112.

[42] H. I. Field, 'The examination of bile samples as a means of assessing the incidence of Salmonella infection in cattle', *Vet Rec*, 61 (1949): pp. 275–8.

[43] Field, 'Examination', p. 277.

after milking. A duck house and a pigsty both opened into the same yard, and poultry and ducks also ranged the neighbouring stack yard and field, having open access to all the farm premises. Pigs, hens, and ducks were all found to be carrying *Salmonella typhimurium*, although none showed signs of ill health. As there had been no previous outbreaks on the farm, and the poultry were only recently introduced, it seemed plausible that they had brought the infection with them.[44] As this case demonstrated, farmyard infections were not necessarily confined to one species.

If mixed farming carried risks of inter-species infection, the new intensive methods of calf and poultry production—the latter by the 1960s predominantly kept on deep litter—brought additional problems of farm management and hygiene which had implications for the wider environment and for the natural economy of *Salmonella* organisms. Intensive farming produced vast quantities of waste in the form of dirty litter, droppings, and manure, which were frequently recycled. Poultry litter, for example, was used as bedding for calves.[45] The financial constraints of intensive farming were such that the disposal of waste had to be achieved without involving additional staff costs. As a result, droppings were used as manure, often in the form of slurry—mixed with water and pumped or sprayed onto land grazed by other animals. Potential nuisances associated with intensive farming included flies, rodents, the pollution of rivers and sewers, and the further dissemination of bacterial infection to 'clean' animals through pastures contaminated by infected slurry or other fertilizers.[46] Scrupulous farm hygiene and management practices were important: even in large, well-managed dairy herds, a high level of infection could be maintained over many months through intensive housing, highly stocked pasture, and failure to segregate excreters.[47]

The particular concern around cattle arose because once the VIS began recording incidents of animal salmonellosis, it quickly became clear that infections were most frequently reported in cattle. From 1958 to 1967, *Salmonella* dublin and *Salmonella typhimurium* accounted for 97.6 per cent of recorded incidents, from 1968 to 1973 for 96 per cent. The aggregate figures masked an ominous shift. *Salmonella* dublin infections reached a peak in 1969 at 89.2 per cent of recorded incidents, and thereafter declined, to 54.6 per cent in 1973. *Salmonella typhimurium* incidents on the other hand rose to 30.6 per cent of total in 1973, while the number of 'exotics' leapt from 3.5 per cent in 1972 to 14.6 per cent in 1973, encompassing 63 serotypes—a proportion which the VIS reporters found 'disturbing'.[48] In November 1975, the VIS noted that bovine salmonellosis had dominated reports from all regions except the West Midlands in September that year: 20 new outbreaks of

[44] K. C. Sellars and W. B. V. Sinclair, 'A case of *Salmonella typhimurium* infection in cattle and its isolation from other sources', *Vet Rec*, 65 (1953): pp. 233–4.

[45] D. J. H. Payne, 'Salmonellosis and intensive farming', *Public Health*, 84 (1969–70): p. 7.

[46] Payne, 'Salmonellosis', p. 7; W. J. Sojka et al., 'Incidence of salmonella infection in animals in England and Wales, 1968–73', *Vet Rec*, 96 (1975): p. 282.

[47] T. W. Heard and Nada E. Jennett, 'Changing patterns of salmonella excretion in various cattle populations', *Vet Rec*, 90 (1971): pp. 359–64.

[48] Sojka et al., 'Incidence of salmonella', p. 281.

Salmonella typhimurium had been diagnosed in the south-east, and at Penrith in Cumbria one third of cows in a large dairy herd had been found to be infected with the organism.[49] The significance of the shift in dominance from dublin to *typhimurium* lay in the greater risk of human infections arising from the latter. As early as 1954, at least 252 human cases were recorded in an explosive outbreak in County Durham transmitted in unpasteurized, tuberculin-tested milk.[50]

Unpasteurized milk continued to pose a significant food-poisoning risk to humans well into the 1970s. Buxton had noted in 1957 that it was common for milk to become infected by the faeces of carrier animals, and that poor hygiene and handling practices in the distribution of milk in rural areas facilitated contamination. *Salmonella paratyphi* B, for example, had been found to survive for seven months in sour milk and in dried milk crusts in the seams of unwashed milk cans.[51] Although 96 per cent of milk consumed in England and Wales was pasteurized by the mid-1960s, milk-borne outbreaks continued to occur as a result of the sale of 'Green Top', unpasteurized farm milk. Following one such outbreak in 1965, the Medical Officer of Health (MOH) for Midhurst in West Sussex expressed his surprise that 'so many' members of the public should still choose to buy raw milk, believing it to be a better product. He found it even more 'strangely irrational and a quite unjustifiable arrangement' that farmers should be encouraged to sell farm-bottled, unpasteurized milk by being paid more for it.[52] The economics of farming in the modern world, and the tastes of a significant rural lobby, continued, however, to support the production of Green Top, and it was still causing occasional milk-borne outbreaks into the 1970s. More than 300 cases of *Salmonella typhimurium* phage-type U65 were notified in an outbreak resulting from unpasteurized milk in and around Penicuik, Midlothian, between December 1972 and February 1973.[53]

The veterinary emphasis on bovine salmonellosis from the 1940s onwards was only partly due to its implications for human health. *Salmonella* infections in calves, the dreaded 'scour', were a long-standing and economically significant problem, while *Salmonella typhimurium* infection in adult cattle also had severe consequences. Although pigs were the domestic animal most frequently found infected with *Salmonella*, and suffered similar patterns of enhanced infection during transport and lairage as calves,[54] they attracted less agricultural or veterinary attention because infection seldom seemed to affect the animals' own health. The evidence suggests that, until the 1960s at least, both farmers and vets habitually ignored the

[49] Veterinary Investigation Service, 'Salmonella in cattle widely reported', *Vet Rec*, 97 (1975): p. 423.

[50] R. Norton and E. C. Armstrong, 'A milk-borne outbreak of due to salmonella typhi-murium', *MBMH*, 13 (1954): pp. 90–5.

[51] A. Buxton, 'Public health aspects of salmonellosis in animals', *Vet Rec*, 69 (1957): p. 108.

[52] V. P. Geoghegan, 'A milk-borne outbreak of food-poisoning due to salmonella typhimurium', *MO*, 114 (1965): p. 74. The cow concerned had become infected by calves with 'scour' bought in as a result of the farmer's new venture into intensive calf-rearing.

[53] J. Maclachan, 'Salmonellosis in Midlothian and Peebleshire', *PH*, 88 (1974): pp. 79–87.

[54] V. P. McDonagh and H. G. Smith, 'The significance of the abattoir in salmonella infection in Bradford', *Jnl Hyg*, 56 (1958): p. 273.

large numbers of potentially dangerous organisms carried by pigs as long as the stock showed no evidence of illness or disability on inspection.[55] Post-World War II scientific research into bovine salmonellosis undermined belief in the relative innocence of bovines: in 1968, E. S. Anderson concluded that most human infections with *Salmonella typhimurium* were due to meat consumption, especially from bovines.[56] The VIS surveys of *Salmonella* infection in animals certainly suggested that infections in pigs were falling by the mid-1970s, even while the number of infections with exotic serotypes was rising.[57] Increasingly, at least as far as meat was concerned, beef and veal seemed to pose more of a public health risk than pork.

An ongoing source of frustration for both veterinary and medical investigators of *Salmonella* incidents associated with food animals and farm conditions lay in the fact that salmonellosis was not a notifiable animal disease under the Diseases of Animals Acts. Neither farmer nor attending vet was under any obligation to inform the District Veterinary Surgeon, or the VIS, let alone the local MOH. Even where infection had been traced via contaminated milk to a particular dairy herd, there were no powers to enforce eradication in that herd, and the farmer remained free to retain recognized excreters, or to sell them on to others.[58] Nor could action be taken to detain the carcasses of healthy animals found to be positive for *Salmonella* at slaughter, even while informed observers frequently asserted that carrier animals healthy at slaughter constituted the greatest risk of transmitting infection to humans.[59] Although there was considerable insistence from the meat trades that emergency- and casualty-slaughtered animals did not enter the human food chain, outbreak investigations repeatedly showed that casualty animals did, at least occasionally, still end up as human food, and act as sources of human infection.[60]

Whichever group of animals constituted the main source of human food-poisoning incidents, the extensive research into animal salmonellosis conducted in the years after 1945 served to locate the principal sources of human *Salmonella* infection in food animals, and to implicate modern agricultural practices associated with intensive farming in the creation of contaminated environments through which infection could be transmitted within resident animal populations and beyond, to other, 'clean' animal populations. In this configuration, domestic

[55] Kenneth W. Newell et al., 'Salmonellosis in Northern Ireland, with special reference to pigs and salmonella-contaminated pig-meal', *Jnl Hyg*, 57 (1959): p. 101.

[56] A. R. Miller et al., 'Salmonella typhimurium phage type 52 infection in Glasgow and the West Central area of Scotland', *MO*, 121 (1969): p. 225.

[57] Sojka et al., 'Incidence of salmonella infection', p. 282.

[58] Geoghegan, 'A milk-borne outbreak', p. 74; J. R. Baker and W. B. Faull, 'An outbreak of salmonellosis in sheep', *Vet Rec*, 88 (1971): pp. 270–7; M. E. Harris, letter, 'Salmonellosis and public health', *Vet Rec*, 88 (1971): pp. 375–6.

[59] Miller et al., 'Phage-type 32 infection', p. 227; Buxton, 'Public health aspects', p. 107; Williams Smith, 'Salmonella food-poisoning', p. 272.

[60] R. E. A. Hughes, 'The epidemiology of salmonella infections in man', *Roy Soc Hlth Jnl*, 77 (1957): p. 4; J. R. Baker and W. B. Faull, 'An outbreak of salmonellosis in sheep', *Vet Rec*, 88 (1971): pp. 270–7; G. W. Thomas and J. F. Harbourne, 'Salmonella paratyphi B infection in a dairy cow', *Vet Rec*, 91 (1972): pp. 148–50.

animals and wildlife were victims, and humans both victims and perpetrators.[61] Domestic pets too figured as casualties of this system: dogs and cats fed on raw meat were closely linked to the lowest end of the meat trade and with the disposal of animals sick or dead of disease, and might in turn transmit infection back to their owners.[62] In this scenario of perpetuated infection, financial pressures on farmers and continuing difficulty in controlling the meat trades played a critical part.

POULTRY

The post-1945 veterinary realization of the *Salmonella* problem in livestock and its public health implications was matched by a parallel recognition of the dangers of *Salmonella* in poultry. Despite the discovery of human infections acquired through eating duck eggs in the 1930s, other types of poultry product had generally been regarded as innocuous. As with livestock, however, the introduction of intensive farming methods after World War II brought new problems of infection and disease. Veterinary concern initially focused on the dire effects of infection among chicks, and on the economic losses incurred by poultry farmers, but the associated risks to human health were soon receiving attention.

Poultry was another sector of the agricultural industry which was transformed during the course of the twentieth century.[63] In the traditional mixed farming economy, hens were kept to clean up household and farmyard waste, and to provide the farmer's wife with eggs and 'pin money'.[64] The inter-war years saw the beginnings of a movement towards specialist poultry-keeping, and by 1939 the poultry industry had become the third most important agricultural sector after the livestock and dairy industries, with an annual value of over £30 million.[65] At this date general farmers remained the largest poultry owners, although a complex network of related enterprises had grown up: pedigree breeders who maintained and distributed foundation stock, commercial breeders, hatcheries, rearers, and commercial egg and table poultry producers.[66]

[61] Williams Smith, 'Salmonella food-poisoning', p. 271; A. C. Ghosh, 'An epidemiological study of the incidence of salmonella infection in pigs', *Jnl Hyg*, 70 (1972): pp. 151–60.

[62] H. Williams Smith, 'The isolation of Salmonellae from the mesenteric glands of pigs, cattle, sheep, dogs and cats and from other organs of poultry', *Jnl Hyg*, 57 (1959): pp. 266–73; N. S. Galbraith et al., 'Pet foods and garden fertilisers as sources of human salmonellosis', *Lancet*, 1962, i: p. 372; W. R. Cockrill, 'International problems and practices in meat hygiene', *Vet Rec*, 75 (1963): p. 882.

[63] Andrew C. Godley and Bridget Williams, 'The chicken, the factory farm and the supermarket: The emergence of the modern poultry industry in Britain', in *Food Chains: From Farmyard to Shopping Cart*, edited by Warren Belasco and Roger Horowitz (2009), pp. 47–61; Andrew C. Godley and Bridget Williams, 'Demarcating luxury and the contentious "invention of the technological chicken" in Britain', *Business History Review*, 83 (2009): pp. 267–90.

[64] Peter Biggs, 'The veterinary profession and an intensive poultry industry', *Vet Rec*, 103 (1978), p. 251.

[65] Editorial, 'The veterinarian and the post-war problems of the poultry industry', *Vet Rec*, 57 (1945): pp. 388–9.

[66] Editorial, 'The veterinarian', p. 388.

The veterinary community had long despised chickens—'Many practitioners, faced with a poultry problem, exclaim that they know nothing about "hens"!', it was noted in 1949—but as the industry expanded it began to encounter serious disease problems. Leaders of the profession began to nudge their colleagues in the direction of hens.[67] The *Veterinary Record* noted the rising public demand for eggs and table birds in 1945, and set out the advantages that an increased poultry population would bring once the normal importation of poultry feeds (then restricted under war-time rationing provisions) was again permitted: human food 'of excellent quality' would be supplied, healthy rural employment would increase because poultry required a greater number of skilled workers than general farming, and the milk and specialized feed industries, as well as the metal and timber trades, would all benefit from rising demand. Birds, it seemed, were a potential economic miracle.[68] But attention was also drawn to the economic hazards of poultry disease (a cost of some £4 million a year in 1935–8) and the readership was admonished:

> The time has therefore come to call the veterinary profession to awaken to its responsibilities to the community in this important matter, for they are responsibilities which in duty bound it must prepare itself to shoulder. The poultry industry has tremendous capital invested in stock and equipment, greatly exceeding, indeed, that of the other small-animal industry, namely, the dog and cat . . .

The journal's call was not unfounded. The link between an expanding industry and rising disease costs had in this case been marked. Britain's poultry population increased from 15 million birds in 1918 to 85 million in 1938; in the same period mortality rates rose from 5 per cent in 1920 to 10 per cent in 1930, to 21 per cent in 1936.[69]

Problems in poultry rearing were not confined to Britain in the 1940s, but had not yet attracted adverse public health publicity. At the eighth World Poultry Congress, held in Copenhagen in 1948, the 'Disease Section' was reportedly the best attended, the papers provoking serious discussion.[70] R. F. Gordon, Director of the Animal Health Trust's Poultry Research Station, reported on the event in the *Veterinary Record*, observing that the egg and poultry industry had 'a remarkably clean record regarding food-poisoning cases traceable to the consumption of eggs and poultry meat products'. Although there was as yet no indication of a problem, and no public concern, he warned of the importance of producing *Salmonella*-free products if public confidence was to be maintained.[71] Gordon emphasized the potential hazard represented by *Salmonella*—of 60 serotypes found in birds, 56 were known to be pathogenic for humans—and he urged that all branches of the industry co-operate in eliminating these bacteria from poultry farms. He reiterated Buxton's observation that before 1939 only four *Salmonella* types had been found

[67] R. F. Gordon, 'The poultry industry and the veterinary profession', *Vet Rec*, 61 (1949): p. 724.
[68] Editorial, 'The veterinarian', p. 388.
[69] Gordon, 'The poultry industry', p. 724.
[70] R. F. Gordon, 'VIIIth World Poultry Congress, Copenhagen. Review of Disease Section', *Vet Rec*, 60 (1948): p. 626.
[71] Gordon, 'Poultry Congress', p. 627.

in British poultry (*pullorum*, *gallinarum*, *enteritidis*, and *typhimurium*) but since 1943, following the importation of spray-dried egg, another ten had been identified, including thompson, now a serious problem in chicks, as well as a number of exotics.[72]

That Gordon's concerns were not without foundation was demonstrated by a paper delivered by the veterinarian W. F. Blount at the Royal Sanitary Institute Congress at Brighton in May 1949.[73] Addressing the public health aspects of poultry disease, Blount noted that *Salmonella* were 'certainly' the largest 'genus of pathological significance' involving poultry, and that the 'paratyphoid type' (*typhimurium*, thompson) must be regarded with 'considerable suspicion' in domestic poultry where spread to humans was concerned.[74] He demonstrated the potential for public health hazards inherent in the existing nature of the table poultry market. Unlike meat, most poultry escaped any regular inspection except in a few cities. Any butcher, fishmonger, or poulterer could offer game or poultry for sale without any inspection; there was no law of any sort to make the killing or eating of poultry an illegal act, although meat inspectors could examine exposed fowls if they wished.[75] Discussion of Blount's paper opened up other problems, notably in respect of culls and birds slaughtered as carriers or contacts of disease. Poultry farmers, it was said, not only killed unthrifty birds but, faced with a disease outbreak, vigorously culled for the table both contacts and birds showing early clinical symptoms.[76] At this date, however, the problem of *Salmonella* in poultry meat was thought less acute than in eggs and egg products, although, as Gordon noted in discussion, the eradication of 'such ubiquitous organisms' from poultry flocks was impracticable, and damage limitation lay in the hands of the egg producers and processors.[77]

The early discussions of *Salmonella* problems in relation to the poultry industry reflected a considerable amount of ongoing research into the public health aspects of avian salmonellosis in both Britain and America, where poultry plant inspection was somewhat more advanced than in Britain.[78] According to Blount, carrier hens harboured *Salmonella* in the bowel, so that eggs absorbed infected faecal material through the shell material at or after laying. He claimed that improved hygiene had been shown largely to reduce shell contamination, but that the wiping of dirty eggs was inadvisable, since it spread the area of shell inoculation and hastened the rate at which bacteria penetrated the shell. Cloths and water, too, rapidly became heavily contaminated. It had been shown that 5 per cent of clean eggs contained *Salmonella*, as against 15 per cent of slightly dirty eggs and 20 per cent of washed dirty eggs. *Salmonella* were more frequently found in cracked and low-grade eggs than in high-grade eggs.[79] Since there was no sanitary regulation of egg-packing stations in

[72] Gordon, 'Poultry Congress', pp. 627–8. The exotics included bareilly, anatum, montevideo, and oranienburg.

[73] W. F. Blount, 'Public health aspects of the poultry industry', *Royal Sanitary Institute Journal*, 69 (1949): pp. 359–71.

[74] Blount, 'Public health', p. 361.

[75] Blount, 'Public health', p. 359.

[76] Blount, 'Public health', p. 367.

[77] Blount, 'Public health', p. 369.

[78] Blount, 'Public health', p. 367.

[79] Blount, 'Public health', pp. 369, 380.

Britain, the onus of producing clean eggs lay with the suppliers. Yet dirty and cracked eggs did not go to waste: in this era of rationing they were graded as 'seconds' and distributed by the Ministry of Food as 'off-ration' eggs.[80]

Questions of management and hygiene were thus central to health risks in the poultry industry, as perceived by the experts who studied its relationship to human disease. Management and hygiene were also critical to maintaining the health of the birds themselves. R. F. Gordon, an expert on avian salmonellosis, regarded hygiene as essential to sound economic farming. He was, however, both astounded and dismayed to discover that 'otherwise enlightened' poultry farmers regarded hygiene as 'something entirely associated with disease and only to be brought into use when disease is encountered'. Invoking the textbook definitions of hygiene as 'the principles of health' and sanitation as 'conditions designed to obviate influences deleterious to health', he argued that these two terms were synonymous with good husbandry. They were especially important in poultry farming, where large numbers of birds were kept in close proximity under artificial conditions.[81]

Poultry producers were concerned about *Salmonella* chiefly in relation to young birds, among which *Salmonella pullorum* (non-pathogenic to humans) in particular could and did wreck substantial havoc; adult birds are generally unaffected by *Salmonella* infections, although they may become carriers. So much was recognized by 1960, and the potential risks were signalled by the state of the American poultry industry, which was by then regarded as the world's largest natural reservoir of *Salmonella* infection.[82] As dramatic changes developed in the British industry after 1953, concern emerged about the continuing resilience of adult birds.

For some years after World War II, the development of the British poultry industry was constrained by rationing, and by regulation of the import trade in feeding stuffs. The end of rationing in 1953 brought a vast and 'alarmingly rapid' expansion.[83] The highly successful American broiler industry (intensive rearing of young chickens suitable for barbequing) had set an example which British producers were ready to follow. In 1954, some five million table chickens of a live weight of 3.4lb were produced; by 1959, production was 75 million. It was calculated that this allowed for about two chickens per person a year, enabling the average family to eat a chicken every two months. The American example showed the potential market to be much greater: whereas Britons ate about 3lb of chicken per head in 1959, the average American ate more than 27lb.[84] British production reached 174 million birds in 1966 and 377 million a decade later. The size of chicken houses and farm sites grew steadily: by the mid-1970s it was common for farms to have up to 100,000 birds of a single age, located in houses containing from 10 to 20,000

80 Blount, 'Public health', p. 369.

81 R. F. Gordon, 'Hygiene in relation to poultry management', *Vet Rec*, 61 (1949): p. 593.

82 J. H. C. Walker, 'The broiler industry—Transmission of Salmonella infections', *Roy Soc Hlth Jnl*, 80 (1960): p. 142.

83 D. L. Haxby, 'Poultry production: From backyard to batteries', *Vet Rec*, 110 (1982): p. 605. See also Godley and Williams, 'Demarcating luxury', p. 289.

84 A. R. Pendry, 'The production, processing and packing of broilers', *Roy Soc Hlth Jnl*, 80 (1960): p. 132.

birds each.[85] By 1971, annual average per capita consumption of chicken in Britain was estimated at 23.6lb.[86]

The rapid expansion of the British broiler industry was achieved largely by importing fertile eggs and day-old chicks, and with these imports came a number of *Salmonella* serotypes. Fowl salmonellosis being egg-transmitted, these quickly established themselves in British breeding flocks.[87] Yet other serotypes (agona, indiana and S4,12:d:- [sic]) were introduced in contaminated feedstuffs, for example, in fish and meat meals.[88] Like intensively farmed pigs, intensively farmed poultry received all their protein requirements in prepared feeds, which included animal protein. The economic pressures on the industry were such that feathers and poultry offal were recycled into feedstuffs, so helping to maintain infection in the flocks—the seeding of flocks with *Salmonella* that Philip Edwards had deplored in 1958 (Chapter 7).[89] The establishment and maintenance of *Salmonella* infection was integral to the whole process of mass-producing chickens for the table.

The enormous growth of the broiler chicken sector in the 1960s generated a whole new dimension to *Salmonella* ecology. Although there was little direct evidence of poultry causing human *Salmonella* infection in the early 1960s, the risks were already being recognized.[90] Only one outbreak associated with poultry was recorded between 1953 and 1958, but with the example of America before them, PHLS investigators were quickly on the case. A study of birds in a newly erected British factory over a period of 23 weeks found that 13.8 per cent of all specimens examined contained *Salmonella*, while inspection of two turkey farms revealed infection rates of 19.3 per cent and 7.8 per cent. The figures were not as high as in America, but nonetheless gave cause for concern.[91] And concern was justified: by 1967, significant outbreaks of human salmonellosis were being associated with spit-roast and frozen chicken.[92] Frozen chicken legs, for example, were the source of outbreaks at the Liverpool Tennis Club in July 1968 and among staff at the Royal Manchester Children's Hospital in January 1969.[93] Between 1968 and 1973, 1,255 incidents of salmonellosis were reported in domestic poultry, largely in chickens.[94] As with cattle and pigs, the continuing source of infection in table birds

[85] Biggs, 'Veterinary profession', p. 252.

[86] J. A. Lee, 'Recent trends in human salmonellosis in England and Wales: the epidemiology of prevalent serotypes other than *Salmonella typhimurium*', *Jnl Hyg*, 72 (1974): p. 192.

[87] John H. McCoy, 'Trends in salmonella food poisoning in England and Wales, 1941–72', *Jnl Hyg*, 74 (1975): pp. 278–9.

[88] Microbiological precision led to increasingly refined bacterial definitions. S4,12:d:- is a subspecies of *Salmonella enterica*.

[89] Lee, 'Recent trends', p. 193.

[90] Walker, 'Broiler industry', p. 144.

[91] J. M. S. Dixon and F. E. Pooley, 'Salmonellae in a poultry-processing plant', *MBMH*, 20 (1961): pp. 30–3; J. M. S. Dixon and F. E. Pooley, 'Salmonellae in two turkey processing factories', *MBMH*, 21 (1962): pp. 138–41.

[92] Enid Vernon, 'Food poisoning and *Salmonella* infection in England and Wales, 1967', *PH*, 83 (1968–69): p. 214.

[93] Andrew B. Semple et al., 'Outbreak of food poisoning caused by Salmonella Virchow in spit-roasted chicken', *British Medical Journal* (1968), iv: pp. 801–3; W. J. Elwood et al., 'An outbreak of salmonellosis Virchow food poisoning amongst hospital staff', *MO*, 123 (1970): pp. 273–8.

[94] Sojka et al., 'Incidence of salmonella infection', p. 282.

appeared to derive from animal feedstuffs.[95] By 1970, *Salmonella* infection had become indigenous to British poultry meat production, and now constituted an on-going risk to human health.

FEEDSTUFFS AND FERTILIZERS

The explosion of veterinary interest in the epidemiology of *Salmonella* after 1945 carried two associated concerns. First, the dramatic expansion in the number of serotypes identified as present in Britain, and the fact that these were being isolated both from food animals and humans, suggested a direct link between the two; second, the question of where and how these serotypes were entering the country. As noted in Chapter 7, up to 1939 just 14 *Salmonella* serotypes had been identified as indigenous to Britain and the appearance of new serotypes was first associated with war-time imports of American spray-dried egg, which was eaten by both humans and animals (being incorporated into poultry mashes, for example). These introductions continued after the war and escalated with the end of rationing in 1953. By 1967, some 100 serotypes were afflicting British people every year.[96] For the most part these newly introduced serotypes were not an animal health hazard—they rarely produced clinical disease in cattle or poultry—but subclinical infections resulted in healthy animal carriers whose milk, meat, or eggs, on entering the human food chain, could lead to food-poisoning outbreaks and apparently sporadic incidents.

If the first breach in Britain's internal *Salmonella* ecology came with the war-time imports of dried egg, other products were instrumental in widening the breach. Organic fertilizers and animal feedstuffs were under suspicion as the source for this unprecedented bacterial invasion by the later 1950s. Concern over industrial practices relating to fertilizers and feedstuffs was first raised in Britain by J. H. C. Walker, Director of the PHLS facility at Maidstone, in 1957.[97] Walker's initial focus was on organic fertilizers, both human (sludge) and animal (bone, horn, hoof, 'meat', blood, and fish). These, he noted, were widely advertised and recommended by experts, and were used on a large scale in both agriculture and horticulture. The infection of animals and vegetables by means of these products could lead indirectly to human infections.[98] Walker's analyses showed that 40 per cent of 123 samples of organic fertilizer contained *Salmonella*, with bone-meal samples rating at 70 per cent. In all, 34 different serotypes were identified, almost all of which had been found to infect humans, animals, and poultry in Britain.

[95] Enid Vernon and H. E. Tillett, 'Food poisoning and Salmonella infections in England and Wales, 1969–1972', *PH*, 88 (1974): p. 234.

[96] Taylor, 'Salmonellosis II', p. 148.

[97] J. H. C. Walker, 'Organic fertilisers as a source of salmonella infection', *Lancet*, 1957, ii: p. 283. Walker noted that a literature search on this topic had turned up just one previous reference in a German journal from 1956. The Kauffmann–Edwards correspondence on this topic (Chapter 7) dates from April 1958.

[98] Walker, 'Organic fertilisers', p. 283.

The three most commonly found—*Salmonella* seftenberg, *Salmonella* taksony, and *Salmonella* anatum—were all high on the list of isolations from human cases.[99] Observing that bone-meal was much more widely used than any of the other products, Walker drew attention to its use in animal feedstuffs, and reported that *Salmonella* had also been isolated from turkey starter meal and fish-meal.[100]

Walker's paper was published in the *Lancet*, indicating the significance of his findings for human health. Given medical familiarity with the 'amazing and disquieting' increase in the number of human *Salmonella* infections since the war, Walker's article attracted attention.[101] Two years later, Irish investigators were warning that 'the only place to break the chain of infection is by attempting to break the animal cycle' through the bacteriological control of feedstuffs.[102] The warning was the more pertinent because the feedstuffs trade was undergoing rapid expansion following the end of rationing, the freeing up of the import trade, and the new emphasis on modernization and increased production in agriculture. Until the 1920s British farmers largely relied on oil cake, a by-product of the oil milling industry, as a supplementary feedstuff for cattle. The mills were situated in the main British ports, and oil was extracted from imported seeds such as groundnuts, copra, linseed, and cottonseed for manufacturing soap, margarine, and edible oils. The residues, rich in protein and carbohydrates, were usually marketed as 'slab cake', to be mixed with cereal feedstuffs on the farm: before World War I British farmers mixed virtually all their own feed.[103]

In the inter-war period, however, ideas deriving from the 'newer knowledge of nutrition' were introduced into animal husbandry, and millers began appointing nutritionists to their staff, and developed the concept of balanced rations.[104] Animal nutritionists formulated rations and introduced chemical testing to monitor the quality both of raw materials and of the finished compound feeds. It quickly became standard practice to add small quantities of animal protein to these formulas, generally up to 10 per cent of a given product.[105] The earliest attempts to provide British farmers with scientifically based diets by means of protein concentrates for blending with cereals were made in 1921, and by 1939 animal nutritionists were discussing the use of white fish-meal, meat-meal, 'carcas [*sic*] meal' (meat and bone-meal), and dried blood to provide protein and minerals in supplements for young stock, milk production mixtures, and poultry feeds.[106]

99 Walker, 'Organic fertilisers', p. 284. 100 Walker, 'Organic fertilisers', p. 284.

101 Editorial, 'Food infection hazards', *MO*, 102 (1959), p. 258.

102 Newell et al., 'Salmonellosis in Northern Ireland', p. 103.

103 D. B. Bellis, 'The role of commercial companies in modern farm husbandry', *Vet Rec*, 75 (1963): p. 1291.

104 On the newer knowledge of nutrition see Celia Petty, 'Primary research and public health: The prioritization of nutrition research in inter-war Britain', in *Historical Perspectives on the Role of the MRC: Essays in the History of the Medical Research Council of the United Kingdom*, edited by Joan Austoker and Linda Bryder (1989), pp. 83–108; Celia Petty, 'The impact of the newer knowledge of nutrition: Nutrition science and nutrition policy, 1900–1939' (PhD dissertation, London University, 1989).

105 Bellis, 'Commercial companies', p. 1291.

106 James C. B. Ellis, *The Feeding of Farm Live Stock* (1937), chapter 7, and Stephen J. Watson, *Feeding of Livestock* (1949), chapter 7.

In the years after the war, as they waited for de-rationing, the feed companies planned ahead and looked to America to develop new ranges of scientifically designed products that were more effective and economical in use.[107] Farmers increasingly bought in compound feeds rather than mixing their own; in 1953, compound feed sales amounted to 5,500,000 tons a year and constituted half of all concentrated feeds; by 1963 the figures stood at 9,500,000 tons and 60 per cent.[108] The industry itself remained something of a mixture. There were some 1,200 compounders by 1963, ranging from small country firms selling feeds locally to large firms with national markets. The largest dozen companies sold nearly 70 per cent of all compound feed.[109]

The rising importance of the feedstuffs industry was already a veterinary concern by the early 1950s.[110] The industry did not employ vets to give them advice and their technical field advisers, who dealt with the farmers on nutrition-related issues, were frequently perceived to trespass on veterinary territory. Not only did they give advice on feeding, economic production, and related questions of general animal management and disease control, but they also advised on antibiotics and drug regimes, and performed simple surgical interventions such as castration and de-budding. The costs of this service, being rolled into the price of feed, appeared free to the farmer, unlike the services of the veterinary surgeon.[111] The issues between the veterinarians and the feedstuffs industry came to a head in the mid-1960s, when public health concerns over the content of animal feeds became increasingly vociferous.[112] At issue now was not just the transmission of animal *Salmonella* infections to humans, but the biological consequences of the now almost universal practice of adding antibiotics to animal feedstuffs. Although a tripartite discussion committee was set up in 1966 between the industry, the British Veterinary Association, and the National Agricultural Advisory Service, tensions between industry and the profession continued into the 1970s.[113]

Through these years, the PHLS played a central role both in evaluating the importance of the animal feedstuffs issue for human health and in alerting the wider scientific community to the question of antibiotic use in animal health.[114] E. S. Andersen, Director of the PHLS Enteric Reference Laboratory 1954–78 and subsequently Director of the whole PHLS organization, is remembered above

[107] H. C. H. Graves, 'Structures and modes of operation in the feeding-stuffs industry', *Vet Rec*, 78 (1966): p. 833.

[108] Bellis, 'Commercial companies', p. 1291.

[109] Bellis, 'Commercial companies', p. 1295.

[110] A. J. Wright, in discussion following Bellis, 'Commercial companies', p. 1298.

[111] J. B. Johnson, in discussion following Bellis, 'Commercial companies', p. 1297.

[112] On relations between the veterinarians and the Associated Feed Stuffs industry see Bellis, 'Commercial companies', pp. 1295–1300; 'Joint Conference of the Animal Feedingstuffs Trade Association and the British Veterinary Association', *Vet Rec*, 78 (1966): pp. 868–74; A. M. E. Carmichael, 'Liaison between the nutritional adviser and the practising veterinary surgeon', *Vet Rec*, 79 (1966): pp. 9–15.

[113] A. Steele-Bodger, 'Investigating outbreaks of disease allegedly due to feeding-stuffs', *Vet Rec*, 86 (1970): p. 166.

[114] On this issue, see Robert Bud, *Penicillin: Triumph and Tragedy* (2006), chapter 8.

all for his role in drawing attention to the antibiotic issue,[115] but he also played a significant role regarding salmonellosis. Under Andersen, the PHLS established successive investigatory committees on *Salmonella* which reported in 1959, 1961, and 1972.[116] These investigations confirmed that *Salmonella* were indeed present in many of the raw ingredients used in preparing animal feeds, but that their numbers were greatly reduced in the finished feeds, especially when these had been pelleted (the feed being exposed to high temperatures in the process of pelleting). Nonetheless, the 1961 Committee noted the need for further research into the epidemiological significance of its findings, and into the importance of animal feeds as a source of *Salmonella* capable of causing food poisoning in humans.[117] Despite a general consensus that infected feedstuffs were not a major hazard to the animals themselves,[118] their role in causing subclinical infections that permitted *Salmonella* to enter the human food chain continued to exercise the public health and veterinary communities.[119] While the large compounders did begin to monitor their raw materials and reject those shown by bacteriological tests to be contaminated with *Salmonella*, the medium-sized and smaller firms, especially numerous in the north-west of England, generally had no facilities for such control measures.[120] Moreover, into the 1970s, more than half British pig-fattening units continued to mix their own feed. These farms were in no position to test the raw materials, and contaminated feedstuffs rejected by the big companies were known to find their way on to the pig-fattening units.[121] As late as 1978, Kenneth Blaxter, Director of the Rowett Institute, was still calling for the control of plants processing fish and bone-meals.[122]

The on-going investigations into methods of husbandry changed perceptions of the *Salmonella* problem over time. As indicated, E. S. Anderson moved during the 1960s from emphasizing the role of chicks and calves to view bovines as the main source of human infection (Chapter 5). The investigations of J. A. Lee and colleagues in the early 1970s returned the emphasis to pigs and poultry. They pointed to seven serotypes as principally implicated in the doubling of human *Salmonella* incidents between 1966 and 1971: *enteritidis*, panama, stanley, virchow, agona, S4,12:d:-, and indiana. 'Strong evidence exists', they observed, 'that these

[115] Bernard Dixon, 'E. S. Anderson', *The Independent,* 23 March 2006: <http://www.independent.co.uk/news/news/obituaries/e-s-anderson-470974>, accessed 29 June 2014; Bud, *Penicillin*, pp. 176–83.

[116] PHLS Report, 'Salmonella organisms in animal feeding stuffs and fertilisers', *MBMH*, 18 (1959): pp. 26–35; PHLS Working Party Report, 'Salmonella organisms in animal feeding stuffs', *MBMH*, 20 (1961): pp. 73–85; PHLS Working Group et al., 'Salmonellas in pig and animal feeding stuffs in England and Wales and in Denmark', *Jnl Hyg*, 70 (1972): pp. 127–40.

[117] Working Party Report, 1961, p. 84.

[118] Reviews of the Progress of Dairy Science: E. A. Gibson, 'Diseases of dairy cattle. Salmonella infection in cattle', *Journal of Dairy Research*, 32 (1965): p. 117.

[119] McCoy, 'Trends', p. 280.

[120] H. C. Dawkins and L. Robertson, 'Salmonella in animal feeding stuffs', *MBMH*, 26 (1967): p. 221.

[121] J. A. Lee et al., 'Salmonellas in pig farms and in abattoirs', *Jnl Hyg*, 70 (1972): p. 149.

[122] News and Reports, British Veterinary Association Congress, 'Nutrition and animal disease', *Vet Rec*, 103 (1978): p. 324.

serotypes have a path of infection from animal feedingstuffs to the pig and poultry animal reservoirs to pork and poultry foods to man.'[123] While beef consumption had remained stable, consumption of both pork and poultry had increased substantially: pork by 20 per cent and poultry by 49 per cent. Cattle feeds, they pointed out, contained mainly vegetable protein, while pig and poultry rations consisted of animal protein, of types known to be contaminated with *Salmonella*.[124]

Recognition of *Salmonella* reservoirs in domestic food animals provided no easy solution to the problems of human infection. If, in Joan Taylor's words, 'detailed pernickety bacteriology' had permitted an understanding of 'some of the factors affecting the individual, the contacts, the herd and the world of living creatures', it offered no more than understanding.[125] The detection and eradication of healthy animal carriers was not an economic proposition.[126] Where the discovery of pathways of infection in the years to 1940 offered the opportunity of barring them by appropriate sanitary measures, the problem of reservoirs offered no obvious precautionary measure. Lee emphasized the importance of studying and controlling the primary animal reservoirs, and obliquely indicated that legislation to require the sterilization of feed ingredients of animal origin, such as existed in Denmark, was desirable.[127] Once carcass contamination had taken place, he considered, it became difficult to break the chain of infection to humans.[128] J. H. McCoy, of the Public Health Laboratory, Hull, while suggesting prevention by non-introduction of carrier animals and the use of clean feedstuffs, pointed to the need for preventive measures in the slaughterhouse and the kitchen.[129] If animal reservoirs of *Salmonella* infection remained highly problematic, there were preventive measures that could be practised effectively further along the line of food production. As with the healthy human carrier, in the final event, British public health professionals chose public education in preference to radical action damaging to personal freedoms or economic interests.

[123] Lee et al., 'Human salmonellosis', p. 185. [124] Lee et al., 'Human salmonellosis', p. 192.
[125] Taylor, 'Salmonellosis II', p. 147. [126] McCoy, 'Trends', p. 280.
[127] For the Danish position see PHLS Working Group et al., 'Salmonellas', pp. 127–40.
[128] Lee et al., 'Human salmonellosis', pp. 193–4. [129] McCoy, 'Trends', p. 280.

9

Ghastly Kitchens—the Borgia Tradition

The identification of slaughterhouse and kitchen as sites of preventive intervention for food poisoning may have been made in response to difficulties perceived in countering the problems in field and farm, but it carried a core truth. Careless or doubtful slaughterhouse practice and deficiencies in kitchen hygiene remain key agents in food poisoning into the twenty-first century. In translating foods of animal origin from field or water source to fork, necessary alchemy takes place in a series of sites that may be described as kitchens. The great French physiologist Claude Bernard notoriously described his search for the origins of life as being through 'a long and ghastly kitchen'.[1] Bernard was referring to live animal experimentation, but the concept of the ghastly kitchen works well as a descriptor of sites of *Salmonella* infection. From the composition and mixing of high-protein animal feeds to the procedures of the abattoir and poultry packing station, to the practices of butchers and of commercial and domestic food preparation, the kitchen broadly defined was and is the critical site for the dissemination of *Salmonella* to both humans and animals.[2] In each of these sites, the perpetuation of food infections is nearly always due to negligence on the part of a human being. In 1958, the journal *Public Health* referred to this simply as 'the Borgia tradition'—a popular cultural reference to the supposed habit of the notorious fifteenth-century Italian Borgia princes of administering poison to their enemies in food served at glorious banquets.[3]

FOOD HANDLING

From the earliest days of epidemiological concern with food poisoning in the 1880s, food handling and preparation were identified as problem areas. Although Edward Ballard's reports on the outbreak at Welbeck, and on the 14 incidents identified to 1889, reflect his continuing belief in miasmatic influences, the specific circumstances of cooking and kitchen environment played a critical part in his understanding of these outbreaks (Chapter 4). He noted in 1890 that the conditions in which food was prepared and stored were key 'to the knowledge we want':

[1] Claude Bernard, *Introduction to the Study of Experimental Medicine*, translated Henry C. Greene (1949): p. 15.

[2] J. F. Gracey et al., *Meat Hygiene*, 10th edn (1999): p. 328.

[3] Editorial, 'The Borgia Tradition', *Public Health*, 72 (1958): p. 162.

observation suggested that the cause lay in 'an infectiveness of the place where these things were done, in association with uncleanliness of air, of soil, or of surface'.[4] The one significant precaution, he advised, was '*cleanliness*' (italics in original). He then set out the necessary preventive measures to be adopted in kitchens, 'and above all in pantries and places where food is stored in hotels, public refreshment rooms, or pastry-cooks' premises, and in private houses'. Such measures, he emphasized, were the business not just of the 'conservators of public health', but of 'every master or mistress of a family'.[5] Responsibility for household health and hygiene was not, in Ballard's eyes, a gendered one.

One persistent theme running through the early reports of food poisoning incidents was the role of foods prepared outside the home. We are accustomed to thinking of takeaways and ready-prepared supermarket meals as recent phenomena, but the use of bought-in prepared foods by ordinary working people dates from the sixteenth century.[6] John Walton has hymned the rise of fish and chips as a convenience food in the early twentieth century,[7] but hot baked meats and meat pies were equally ubiquitous. The Nottingham outbreak of February 1881 was caused by hot baked pork sold from a 'cook shop' which supplied corned beef, potted meats, and pies and pastries made on the premises. Hot pork was mostly sold in the evenings, the largest sales being on Friday and Saturday nights. As described by Ballard, 'This hot pork customarily stands in the window of the shop upon a tinned disk having a well for gravy, which dish again rests upon a metal vessel containing water kept boiling by a gas arrangement beneath it'. To modern eyes, this appears an excellent arrangement for the fostering of food poisoning bacteria. At the time of Ballard's unannounced visit, the shop itself was scrupulously clean, but the cellar where the 'various processes of the trade' were carried out was not.[8]

Although Ballard drew no critical conclusions about popular eating habits, others did. Harold Ashton, MOH for Chadderton, observed astringently following the 1898 veal pie poisonings that 'as long as people—especially working people—will buy such ready-made articles as meat pies, fried fish *et hoc genus omne*, for supper, instead of going to the trouble of cooking something at home, they will run a certain amount of risk'. For Ashton, there was a direct correlation between the consumption of such foods and food-poisoning outbreaks, acute indigestion, and diarrhoea.[9] William Savage, similarly, drew attention in 1909 to the 'enormous alteration in the food habits of the people' then taking place, whose striking feature

[4] Edward Ballard, 'A summary review of 14 instances reported since 1879 . . . ', Medical Officer's Annual Report, Local Government Board, 1890, British Parliamentary Papers, 1890–91, xxxiv, Appendix 21, p. 258.

[5] Ballard, 'Summary review', p. 258.

[6] Sara Pennell, 'Great quantities of gooseberry pie and baked clod of beef: Victualing and eating out in early modern London', in *Londinopolis: Essays in the Cultural and Social History of Early Modern London,* edited by Paul Griffith and Mark Jenner (2000): p. 234.

[7] John K. Walton, *Fish and Chips and the British Working Class, 1870–1940* (1992).

[8] Edward Ballard, 'On a series of cases of acute specific disease . . . ', MOAR LGB, BPP, 1881, xlvi, Appendix A no 6, p. 779.

[9] Harold Ashton, 'An outbreak of food poisoning at Chadderton', *PH,* 11 (1898–9): p. 233.

was the 'very extensive quantity' of prepared and semi-prepared foods now eaten.[10] Henry Mayhew's investigations in the 1840s show that mid-Victorian London had a vibrant street food culture, but rising real wages later in the century, combined with still cramped and overcrowded housing conditions and limited cooking facilities, probably encouraged working people in urban areas to adopt new eating habits. It was observed in the late 1930s that it was common to consume food prepared outside the home in industrial areas, especially where many women worked.[11] An element of class may lie behind these observations by medical professionals, who also noted the adverse effects of popular celebrations at holiday times. An outbreak of 'Gaertner-like' food poisoning due to pork pies at Leeds in May 1915, for example, began on the Saturday of Whitsun weekend, and was embedded in a much more extensive occurrence of minor food poisoning independent of the major outbreak. 'It may be', observed MOH William Angus, 'that the Whitsuntide holiday-making led to an abnormally large consumption of prepared food prone to cause digestive disturbance'.[12]

Early twentieth-century public health authorities had little power to regulate sanitary conditions in the food trades, apart from confiscation of foods deemed by adulteration or putrescence to be dangerous to health, conditions which were often difficult to identify.[13] In the context of the Leeds outbreak, William Angus called for statutory powers for supervision of all places where food was prepared for human consumption, and for powers to make and enforce regulations regarding cleanliness of premises, utensils, and workers, and for food poisoning to be made notifiable.[14] Yet he admitted that even with such regulation there would still be problems; 'it is impossible to ensure constant cleanliness by compulsion', he noted, 'till there is a real love of cleanliness for its own sake, we shall get dirty food'. He drew an unlovely picture of contemporary bakers' premises. 'Why', he wondered, 'do bakers when at work wear the dirtiest and untidiest of clothes?' Only the other day, he continued, he had been assured by the manager of a large provisions firm that they had no time in his business for keeping their premises clean.[15] If the British public seemed indifferent to intrinsic infection in their meat and milk, British producers were either ignorant of the requirements for hygienic food preparation, or discounted them in the interests of profits and economic production.[16] Cost, convenience, lack of control, and little fear of prosecution all discouraged change, and if structures of public health control and inspection existed in the big towns, they rarely did so in small towns and rural areas.

[10] William G. Savage, 'Administrative measures for the protection of the food supply', *Journal of the Royal Institute of Public Health*, 17 (1909): p. 681.

[11] V. T. Thierens, 'The control of food and its preparation', *Journal of the Royal Sanitary Institute,* 57 (1936–7): p. 572.

[12] William Angus, 'Notes on an outbreak of food poisoning', *Journal of the Sanitary Institute*, 37 (1916): p. 15.

[13] Notes and Comments, 'Dirt in food', *Medical Officer* 28 (1922): pp. 191–2; Thierens, 'The control of food': p. 572.

[14] Angus, 'Notes': p. 15.

[15] Angus, 'Notes': p. 15; See also William G. Savage, *Food and the Public Health* (1919), p. 56.

[16] William G. Savage, *Food Poisoning and Food Infections* (1920), p. 5.

Several areas of concern emerged during the 1920s. The dangers inherent in the butchers' practice of making meat pies with savoury jelly fillings, and other products, in premises where slaughtering took place were repeatedly emphasized.[17] More generally, the preparation and serving of food and drink in public places was a matter of persistent concern. In the early 1900s, MOH J. T. C. Nash narrowly avoided dismissal after drawing critical attention to the way in which food was prepared in some Southend eateries.[18] Such criticism had become less contentious by 1920, and in the inter-war years MOHs began attempting to improve conditions. The Birmingham health authorities, for example, surveyed and classified 145 eating establishments according to cleanliness, while the Manchester authorities took action through the agency of the Licensing Board against the general public house practice of cleaning glasses by dipping them in dirty water.[19] Dr McClure, Manchester's Assistant Medical Officer, drew attention to deficiencies in catering practice under four heads: utensils (failure to sterilize); personal cleanliness (lack of 'ordinary cleanly habits'); structure (grossly insanitary kitchen surroundings); and dust and flies (contamination by 'almost universal').[20] McClure also noted that 'the custom of washing the hands after opening the bowel is generally disregarded' and the habit of putting fingers into nose and mouth while serving food commonly observed.[21] The journal *Medical Officer* was even more forthright:[22]

> The habits of the waiter who presides over the cold buffet at the restaurant luncheon are seldom above suspicion: he dismembers the cold chicken with his unclean hands, he uses his dirty fingers when he might employ a fork, with his grimy nails he arranges our galantine upon a plate. In moments when business is slack, he sucks his fingers, picks his nose, scratches himself, and so prepares again for his task of serving the next customer.

Personal observation plainly leant the edge of disgust to such commentaries.

The articulation of such revulsion at intimate personal habits was a novel feature of post-1918 public health commentaries. Whereas mid-nineteenth-century disgust was primarily olfactory, based in the idea that dirt and bad smells caused disease, the last decade of the century marked the beginning of a transition towards the acceptance of germ theory in which smell, while still offensive, no longer caused disease.[23] Instead, realization not only of the faecal–oral route for typhoid

[17] See for example K. F. Peckham, 'An outbreak of pork pie poisoning at Derby', *Journal of Hygiene*, 22 (1923–4): pp. 75–6; Notes and Comments, 'Lincoln food poisoning outbreak', *MO*, 45 (1931): p. 24.

[18] Editorial, 'Hotel and restaurant kitchens', *MO*, 24 (1920): p. 259.

[19] Editorial, 'Kitchens', p, 259; Anon, 'Dirty drinking and eating utensils', *MO*, 29 (1923): pp. 19–20.

[20] W. St C. McClure, 'The importance of cleanliness in the preparation and distribution of food', *Jnl San Inst*, 44 (1923–4): pp. 315–18; see also Notes and Comments, 'Dirt in food'.

[21] McClure, 'Importance': p. 317.

[22] Notes and Comments, 'Dirt in food', p. 191.

[23] Peter Stallybrass and Allon White, *The Politics and Poetics of Transgression* (1986), chapter 3; David S. Barnes, 'Confronting sensory crisis in the Great Stinks of London and Paris', in *Filth. Dirt, Disgust, and Modern Life* (2005), edited by William A. Cohen and Ryan Johnson; David S. Barnes, *The Great Stink of Paris and the Nineteenth-century Struggle against Filth and Germs* (2006).

transmission, but also of the respiratory transmission of diseases like tuberculosis, diphtheria, influenza, and colds, translated into disgust at contamination not only with dirt and faeces, but also with other excretory products, such as mucus and spittle.[24] The fact that diphtheria, like typhoid, was conveyed by healthy carriers also fed into this realization. During the first two decades of the twentieth century, and possibly reinforced by the experiences of war and influenza, these ideas, and disgust at the secretions associated with them, became engrained in the public health community.

Concerns around food poisoning and the insanitary habits of many food handlers brought calls for the registration and licensing of premises where food was prepared and dispensed from *c.*1920.[25] Milk shops already operated subject to registration and licensing, and so it was asked why 'sausage shops, fish and chip bars and stately restaurants' were not?[26] Political interests, however, worked against the passing of any such ordinances, either at local or national level. The food supply sector was too vast and powerful for any such intervention to be risked. Local authorities had enough trouble trying to insist that retailers stopped displaying food uncovered in windows or on the street, and make use of glass coverings or glass-fronted cabinets instead.[27] The costs associated with the introduction of such precautions, as with the pasteurization of milk, were regarded as 'disturbing' the industries concerned.[28] Parliament and people, protested Captain G. S. Elliston at a meeting of the Royal Sanitary Institute in 1936, were more interested in national and individual prosperity than in national and individual health.[29]

There was some consensus, however, that the British public was largely indifferent to issues of clean food. The Assistant MOH for Manchester charitably remarked in 1924 that 'people generally' had not realized the significance of the fact that 'much of the food presented to them is unclean'.[30] At much the same time, Charles Porter, MOH for Marylebone, observed that in the matter of food production and protection, 'we are of the progressive nations, perhaps the most neglectful'.[31] The British, he argued, exhibited 'a serious want of appreciation of what actually food may mean so far as . . . personal hygiene is concerned'. Although renowned for their sanitary fastidiousness, his compatriots displayed no such sensitivity where food hygiene was concerned.[32] Medical officers and sanitary inspectors had painfully detailed knowledge of the negligent and unsavoury habits

[24] My Danish grandmother, born in 1896, always as a child and young woman drank from cups as close to the handle as possible when using public crockery in an attempt to avoid infection with tuberculosis.

[25] Notes and Comments, 'Registration of food premises', *MO*, 36 (1926): p. 246; H. Dart, 'The food trades: Registration, licensing and notification', *PH*, 49 (1936): pp. 281–7; see also Notes and Comments, 'Dirt in food'; McClure, 'Importance'; Thierens, 'Control of food'.

[26] Editorial, 'Clean food', *MO*, 35 (1926): p. 129.

[27] C. S. Thomson, 'The Meat Regulations', letter, *MO*, 33 (1925): pp. 295–6; G. E. Body, 'The contamination of foodstuffs when exposed for sale', *Jnl Roy San Inst*, 49 (1928–9): pp. 507–9.

[28] Discussion, *Jnl Roy San Inst*, 57 (1936–7): p. 579.

[29] Discussion, p. 579. [30] McClure, 'Importance', p. 315.

[31] Charles Porter, 'Cleanliness in food handling: Impressions of American methods', *Jnl San Inst*, 44 (1924–5): p. 280.

[32] Charles Porter, 'The public and food hygiene', *Jnl San Inst*, 44 (1924–5): pp. 427, 429.

widespread in the food industries, but 'even the man in the street', he observed, would rather not know the details of what they had seen.[33] There was little help or guidance from the Ministry of Health. Trying experiences over meat regulation may have engendered a defeatist approach here: as Chief Medical Officer, George Newman argued that although it would be easy to prescribe rules of conduct to prevent food poisoning, it would be very difficult to ensure that they were consistently followed.[34]

The theme of public indifference was resurrected in the late 1940s, when standards were perceived to have slipped under the stresses of war. The MOH for Penzance noted in 1950: 'we are a nation of dirty feeders'. Echoing Porter a quarter of a century previously, he reflected that the lack of care given to the transport, offering for sale, and preparation of food for the public 'consorts ill with this country's reputation as the pioneer of modern Public Health'.[35] Eight years later, the editor of *Public Health* opined that 'the British public . . . do not care about food. They shovel into their mouths, without discrimination, almost any ill-cooked, slovenly-served mess of indifferent ingredients that a caterer cares to insult them with'. As a result, catering staff generally had no incentive to take pride in their work.[36] Lest these dyspeptic male observations be viewed as deriving from adverse experiences with the lower ends of the food trades, we find Mary Adams, deputy Chair of the Consumers' Association and of the Women's Group on Public Welfare, asking in 1966, 'How come we all profess food hygiene but do not practice it?'[37] The continuous rise in food-poisoning notifications in these years justified these observations.

Against this background, concerned MOH and their local authorities struggled to clean up the nation's kitchens. Efforts were made in a number of directions, as in urging the installation of glass protection for foods, and encouraging the wrapping of bread,[38] and the proper sterilization of pub and restaurant glasses. Dr Gordon Lilico organized a demonstration of the latter for the licensed victuallers and restaurant owners of West Hartlepool in 1925, but was defeated by poor attendance and a 'mainly hostile' attitude. The publicans argued that the process took too long; the glasses were too slow to cool and beer put into warm glasses lost its head. They admitted that greasy mouths and moustaches also turned the beer flat, but would not agree that hot water was necessary to remove the grease from the glass.[39] The practice of displaying food wares uncovered on the street or on inside counters was very general, and continued to be so into the 1950s (and beyond), to the

33 Porter, 'The public', p. 428.

34 Chief Medical Officer's Annual Report (CMOAR), (1929), p. 213.

35 Notes of the Week, 'Food hygiene', *MO*, 83 (1950): p. 30.

36 Editorial, 'Borgia tradition', p. 162.

37 Report, 'Food hygiene—a new approach?', *MO*, 115 (1966): p. 63.

38 Notes of the Week, 'Hygienic distribution of bread', *MO*, 30 (1923): p. 188; Notes and Comments, 'The hygienic wrapping of bread', *MO*, 33 (1925): pp. 176, 179.

39 Notes of the Week, 'Unclean glasses in bars and restaurants', *MO*, 33 (1925): p. 90.

surprise of foreign visitors in whose own countries this practice had been ended.[40] The Public Health Act 1925 had empowered health authorities to inspect rooms where food was prepared for sale, but seems to have had low priority with both authorities and the public.[41] The growing public health anxiety about food poisoning did, however, result in preventive measures being put into place with the Food and Drugs Act 1938, which also introduced notification of food poisoning cases. Section 13 of the Act set out a number of specific requirements for premises where food and drink were manufactured and sold, relating to ventilation, sanitation, cleanliness of machinery and utensils, provision for washing facilities for staff, and cleanliness of staff persons. With the outbreak of war in 1939, however, the attention of local authorities turned to more urgent matters, amid competing duties and manpower shortages.[42] Problems with the washing of glasses, crockery, and cutlery persisted through the years of war and rationing.[43]

The war also brought significant changes in the ways in which Britons were fed and catered for. As workplace canteens became common, and British Restaurants sprang up in towns and cities across the country, the population was exposed to mass catering as never before. Food shortages and rationing also took their toll in the adoption of practices which favoured pathogenic bacteria. Pre-cooking and reheating of meat and made-up dishes became standard practice in many outlets, as did the recycling or consumption of left-overs, which had never been practised before the war. Many of these practices persisted through the days of rationing and beyond. Eating out became an established habit—it was calculated in 1951 that there was one catering establishment for every 210 persons in Great Britain, which 'week in week out' provided every member of the population with two full meals, three light snacks, and six drinks.[44] There was a far greater consumption of meat foods prepared in bulk in commercial establishments and widely distributed, with the result that specific infection led to much more extensive outbreaks than those derived from old-fashioned, shop-made preparations. 1953, for example, saw a very extensive outbreak of *Salmonella bovis morbificans* in West Lancashire (1,149 cases and five deaths), resulting from meat pies all made in one bakery using meat from several butchers.[45] The journal *Public Health* referred in 1958 to the 'widespread and growing practice in the name of economy' of cooking, cooling, and slicing joints of meat when cold, then reheating them to lukewarm to serve—a practice which offered ample opportunity for contamination (and indeed for the multiplication of any pathogenic bacteria if not cooked enough)—noting also that the public did not have to accept food so treated. Reheated meat was easily recognized by the flavour; the public had only to complain.[46] While the accuracy of food

[40] W. A. Lethem, 'Food hygiene', *Monthly Bulletin of the Ministry of Health*, 6 (1947): pp. 53–4. See also C. E. Sanderson, 'The supervision of food supplies'. *Jnl Roy San Inst*, 61 (1940–1): pp. 75–6.

[41] Lethem, 'Food hygiene', p. 53.

[42] Lethem, 'Food hygiene', p. 54.

[43] I. Hutchinson, 'Food utensil bacteriology', *BMJ* (1947), i: pp. 134–5.

[44] R. Sutherland, 'Catering hygiene', *MO*, 85 (1951): p. 56.

[45] William G. Savage, 'Problems of salmonella food poisoning', *BMJ* (1956), ii: p. 320.

[46] Editorial, 'Borgia tradition', p. 162; W. R. Martine, 'Food hygiene and the Medical Officer of Health', *PH*, 75 (1960–1): p. 174.

poisoning notification statistics is open to question, the rising curve of notifications was there for all MOHs to see. By 1945 there was a widespread perception in the public health services that standards of food hygiene had declined further under the duress of war.[47] 'We must admit', wrote one observer in 1947, 'that the hygiene of food, always lax in this country, has deteriorated so much that we shall have to start afresh in order to try to secure the necessary reforms'.[48] The evidence also suggested that public health action had not kept up with the revolution in food habits engendered by war and new methods of transport and mass production.[49] Such problems were to persist indefinitely.

BLOOD, GUTS, AND FAECAL CONTAMINATION

In the translation of animal foodstuffs from field to fork, two sites of transition attracted special anxiety from the mid 1950s. The first was the slaughterhouse, long a cause of concern to veterinarians and public health reformers; the second was the poultry packing station, a new phenomenon developed alongside the novel and rapidly expanding broiler chicken industry. Whereas before the 1950s concerns over slaughtering practices had centred on emergency slaughtered creatures entering the food chain through ignorance or dishonest practice, the maturing of microbiology in the inter-war period, and the specialist scientific interest in *Salmonella* food infections which had developed on a worldwide basis in the 1930s, now narrowed attention more specifically to slaughtering practices and their impact on ecologies of infection. The development of large-scale poultry production in America during the inter-war period had led American veterinarians and bacteriologists working in agricultural stations and university departments to develop interests in *Salmonella* well before the American public health community discovered *Salmonella* food poisoning as an issue of concern (Chapter 7).[50] In the post-war era, the British *Salmonella*/food-poisoning community learnt from American research when seeking to resolve microbiological problems in food production. It was, for example, the work done by Mildred Galton and her colleagues in the laboratory of the Florida State Board of Health that illuminated the role played by lairage practices in escalating infection among animals before slaughter.[51] While the new farming methods and livestock feeding practices were instrumental in

[47] Editorial, 'Food-spread disease,' *MO*, 74 (1945): p. 49; Notes and Comments, 'Food pollution,' *MO*, 78 (1947): p. 166.

[48] Notes and Comments, 'Infected food', *MO*, 78 (1947): p. 154.

[49] Savage, 'Food poisoning', p. 323; Notes and Comments, 'Food pollution', *MO*, 74 (1947): p. 166.

[50] See Index of the *Journal of Infectious Diseases*, volumes 1–50 (1904–32), (1935), and subsequent volumes to 1950. The *American Journal of Public Health* published its first survey article on non-typhoid gastro-enteric disease in 1950: Milton Feig, 'Diarrhea, dysentery, food poisoning and gastroenteritis. A study of 926 outbreaks and 49,879 cases reported to the United States Public Health Service (1945–1947)', *AJPH*, 40 (1950): pp. 1372–94.

[51] Mildred M. Galton et al., 'Salmonella in swine, cattle and the environment of abattoirs,' *Journal of Infectious Diseases*, 95 (1954): pp. 236–45.

embedding *Salmonella* infections among British cattle, pigs, and poultry, slaughtering practices and poultry packaging methods created critical sites of transmission for food-poisoning organisms into the human food chain.

Changes in slaughtering practice had already begun this process of transformation during the war. In 1939, the British government took steps to control the meat trades. The introduction of rationing, and the need to curb black market activities, necessitated rigorous slaughterhouse supervision. Slaughtering was concentrated in a few large, strategically placed facilities. From the pre-war figure of some 15,000, the number of slaughterhouses in England and Wales was reduced to 500.[52] These facilities came under the management and control of the Ministry of Food from January 1940 until the end of meat rationing in July 1954. The war-time management of slaughtering was generally considered—by veterinarians at least—to have been a great success, achieving the unheard-of tally of 100 per cent inspection, even if some variable quality was admitted.[53] Evidence on the ground suggests, however, that the centralized system was far from perfect, given the pressures of rationing. At Preston in 1944, 2,655 casualty animals were included in the count at the Municipal Abattoirs, much of their meat making its way into the human food market. As the Acting MOH explained, the scarcity of meat caused by rationing and 'the necessity of conserving as much good as possible for economic reasons' meant that the slaughter of casualties had increased in both volume and importance. Casualty meat was the main source of supply of 'manufacturing meat' (i.e. for commercially produced pies and sausages). Nor was this simply local Preston practice: it was Ministry of Food policy, reflecting war-time demands. Before the war, calves a few days old were not passed for food; now they were, on Ministry instructions, as were animals slightly affected by tuberculosis.[54] Sorting out and examining the carcasses and offal of these casualties was an enormous task, 'the most difficult side of meat inspection as a whole'. It was made no easier by the pressure to maximize available meat supplies which continued for as long as meat rationing remained in place.[55] The situation also gave rise to an extensive black market in meat.[56] Perceptions of the success of the war-time slaughter controls thus depended to some extent on perspective. Veterinary approbation may have had a strong element of professional propriety, while public health personnel were more equivocal.

With the return of peace, the veterinarians were anxious to have the centralized system retained, and the public health authorities, despite long-standing difficulties between the two professions, agreed that a return to the pre-war situation would be unfortunate.[57] Government concern for adequate slaughtering provision in the

[52] H. E. Bywater, 'Public and private slaughter houses in England and Wales', *Veterinary Record*, 60 (1948): p. 219.

[53] R. Blamire, 'Slaughterhouses and the 1958 legislation,' *Roy Soc Hlth Jnl*, 82 (1962): p. 155.

[54] Anon, 'Casualty meat', *MO*, 75 (1946): p. 157.

[55] Notes and Comments, 'Methods and criteria of meat inspection', *MO*, 89 (1953): p. 50.

[56] W. A. Lethem, 'Trading in diseased meat', *MO*, 79 (1948): pp. 274–5.

[57] Editorial, 'The profession and meat control', *Vet Rec*, 58 (1946): p. 107; W. J. Brenner, 'The economic and public health advantages of centralised slaughtering', *Vet Rec*, 58 (1946): pp. 105–6;

run-up to deregulation in 1954, combined with pressure from private interests, ensured otherwise. The policy adopted was one of no restriction on the re-licensing of slaughterhouses that had been in operation before control, unless local authorities considered existing provision sufficient. As a result, some 4,000 more private slaughterhouses came into use when meat came off the ration in July 1954.[58] In some areas local authorities licensed 20 or more, and in many districts meat inspectors were sorely stretched to inspect all meat intended for human consumption.[59] Although Memo 3/Meat, issued at the time of deregulation, asked that arrangements be made where practical for both ante and post-mortem inspection of meat intended for human consumption, this was not always achieved. In 1958, 80 per cent of fresh meat was inspected, post-mortem but not generally ante. Four years later the percentage had reached 90. In Scotland, meanwhile, all meat was now inspected both before and after slaughter.[60]

Against this background, and spurred by Field's 1948 finding that *Salmonella* dublin infection was common in cattle in Wales (Chapter 8), the Public Health Laboratory Service swung into action. In 1955 a report was published of a survey of materials taken from abattoirs in six cities (Birkenhead, Birmingham, Bradford, Newcastle, Nottingham, and Taunton), with a view to ascertaining levels of *Salmonella* dublin in cattle slaughtered for human consumption in England. Incidence appeared to be low, and since dublin was considered much the commonest *Salmonella* infection in British cattle, the PHLS team concluded that contamination of beef products with other *Salmonella* was probably due to contamination after slaughter.[61] In that year, however—the year after the end of rationing—the number of sporadic human *Salmonella* infections showed a striking increase.[62] Since pork was the meat most commonly implicated in British food poisoning outbreaks, as well as that most frequently found infected with *Salmonella*,[63] research now began to focus on the problem of pork.

English researchers began to follow up on the role of the slaughterhouse in the later 1950s. Bradford's public health department investigated the city's abattoir and found that 2.9 per cent of pigs were excreting *Salmonella* on arrival, but after one to seven days in the lairage the percentage increased to 13.5. Just over a third of infections were of *Salmonella* typhimurium (36 per cent); the remainder were

D. L. Hughes, 'Meat inspection and production: An examination of standards', *Roy Soc Hlth Jnl*, 82 (1962): p. 83; Editorial, 'Meat inspection', *MO*, 75 (1946): p. 27.

[58] Blamire, 'Slaughterhouses,' p. 155.

[59] G. G. Critchley, 'Slaughtering and meat inspection: An examination of current problems,' *Roy Soc Hlth Jnl*, 78 (1958): p. 582.

[60] In Parliament, 'Meat (Inspection)', *Vet Rec*, 70 (1958): pp. 131–2; News and Comments, 'In Parliament', *Vet Rec*, 74 (1962): p. 214. For the provisions of Memo 3/Meat, see Notes and Comments, 'Methods and criteria of meat inspection,' *MO*, 89 (1953): p. 50.

[61] Salmonella Sub-Committee of the PHLS, 'Salmonella in carcass meat for human consumption,' *MBMH*, 14 (1955): p. 134.

[62] A Report of the PHLS, 'Food poisoning in England and Wales, 1954', *MBMH*, 14 (1955): pp. 203–16, 203; A Report of the PHLS, 'Food poisoning in England and Wales, 1955', *MBMH*, 15 (1956): p. 263.

[63] V. P. McDonagh and H. G. Smith, 'The significance of the abattoir in salmonella infection in Bradford', *Jnl Hyg*, 56 (1958): p. 271.

Salmonella derby (64 per cent).[64] Follow-up studies of human infection in the city over the same period showed a close relation to the abattoir findings. The abattoir, the team concluded, was the most important source of *Salmonella* infection in the city, and pigs the main animal reservoir of infection.[65] The Bradford study proved a seminal piece of research, easily acceptable perhaps because of the earlier debates over meat. Although a similar study in Coventry showed no such correlation, a further study by a PHLS working party, involving 22 laboratories and 32 abattoirs over 1961 and 1962, confirmed the importance of pigs as a source of human infection, and the frequent similarity of serotype occurrence in abattoirs and human cases in the same area. It also confirmed that pork, beef, and veal (but not lamb) were responsible for both outbreaks and sporadic infections in humans, and that cattle introduced *Salmonella* into the abattoir more frequently than other species.[66] From the late 1950s, the slaughterhouse was identified as a crucial site along the human food chain where *Salmonella* could achieve critical mass.[67]

These bacteriological investigations came at a decisive time in the late 1950s and early 1960s. While public health concerns with indigenous typhoid and paratyphoid infections were fading, the rapidly rising notification figures for food poisoning awoke recognition of their economic implications (in terms of working days lost), cost in human distress, and the fact that the problem was much larger than the notification figures suggested. The concept of food animals as a major source of infection in human food poisoning was new, and produced a shift in the emphasis of research and investigation from human to animal sources of infection.[68] Slaughterhouse practices came in for increased scrutiny. One of the benefits of this realization was elucidation of the chain of infection associated with veal calves, which had caused several serious human outbreaks. Co-operation between PHLS bacteriologists and the veterinary profession, using the new techniques of phage-typing in detailed and wide-ranging bacteriological investigations, confirmed the devastating part played by transport and lairage in spreading infection among the young animals. A classic case was of calves from an Oxfordshire farm, whose meat resulted in some 500 human cases of *Salmonella* typhimurium scattered across ten London boroughs and the south-eastern quadrant of England over four months in the summer of 1958.[69] This outbreak neatly illustrated the observation by one of

[64] McDonagh and Smith, 'Salmonella infection', p. 273.

[65] McDonagh and Smith, 'Salmonella infection', pp. 274–7.

[66] A. Parry Jones et al., 'Salmonella food poisoning and abattoir slaughtered meat', *MBMH*, 20 (1961): pp. 229–33; Report of a Working Party of the PHLS, 'Salmonella in abattoirs, butchers' shops and home-produced meat, and their relation to human infection', *Jnl Hyg*, 62 (1964): pp. 283–302.

[67] John H. McCoy, 'Recent advances in the epidemiology of salmonellosis in man and animals', *The Sanitarian*, 68 (1959): p. 119. See also Anne Hardy, 'John Bull's beef: Meat hygiene and veterinary public health in England in the twentieth century', *Review of Agricultural and Environmental Studies*, 91 (2010): pp. 369–92.

[68] Betty C. Hobbs, 'Contamination of meat supplies', *MBMH*, 24 (1965): p. 123.

[69] E. S. Anderson et al., 'An outbreak of human infection due to Salmonella Typhimurium Phage-type 20a', *Lancet* (1961), i: pp. 854–8.

the PHLS team that 'the chain of infection from animals to man is often long and devious'.[70]

Legislative regulation of the meat industry had moved forward somewhat meanwhile. The Interdepartmental Committee on Slaughterhouses, which had been guiding government policy since 1953, published its final report in July 1955.[71] It was clear that much needed to be done in modernizing premises, and the Committee recommended that the number of provincial slaughterhouses should be allowed to decrease and that all should conform to certain minimum standards respecting facilities for humane slaughtering, adequate performance of meat inspection, the hygienic processing of meat, and the health and safety of workers. All existing slaughterhouses should in time be brought up to these minimum standards. With a few minor changes, these recommendations were enacted in the Slaughterhouses Act, 1958.[72] By the end of 1960, the new regulations had been effective in reducing the number of slaughterhouses to some 3,800, down from the 4,500 of the immediate post-control period, and the indications were that another 1,000 or more would close within a few years, being mostly small operations unable for various reasons to reach the required standards. At the same time there was a trend towards the construction of new, modern abattoirs under both private and local authority ownership.[73]

There were observers for whom the 100 per cent war-time inspection record remained the ideal. David Hughes, Professor of Veterinary Pathology at Liverpool University, was such a case. For Hughes, the post-war abandonment of control had been 'disastrous'. He believed that effective inspection and the attainment of civilized standards in meat processing could only be achieved by concentrating slaughtering.[74] Hughes drew critical attention to specific slaughterhouse practices. He condemned the use of the wiping cloth, used for cleaning newly slaughtered carcasses—'that hygienic horror'—which in many instances simply replaced obvious blood and dirt with a 'rich and varied biological suspension'. Would not paper towels be preferable? They were already used to clean udders prior to milking. Another target was the slaughterman's knives and steels, which existing regulations required be sterilized at the end of each working day. Surely each man should have two sets of tools, for use on alternate carcasses and sterilized in between? He also suggested automatic flushing water points around walls to keep floors relatively clean. Clean protective clothing was also an issue: 'Some slaughtermen's garb can only be described as unspeakable.'[75]

Hughes' critique was clearly influenced by the *Salmonella* problem, and reflected a shift in ideas about food safety. He argued that inspection was too focused on

[70] N. S. Galbraith, 'Studies of human salmonellosis in relation to infection in animals', *Vet Rec*, 73 (1961): pp. 1296–7.

[71] Blamire, 'Slaughterhouses', 155.

[72] Blamire, 'Slaughterhouses', pp. 155–6.

[73] Blamire, 'Slaughterhouses', p. 157.

[74] David L. Hughes, 'Meat inspection and production: An examination of standards', *Roy Soc Hlth Jnl*, 82 (1962): p. 83.

[75] Hughes, 'Meat inspection', p. 84.

gross lesions, now decreasingly relevant with the (then) decline in bovine tuberculosis. The rise in food poisoning incidents necessitated the implementation of an effective back-up laboratory structure, since *Salmonella* infections generally did not result in pathological lesions. Current laboratory provision was, he observed, of a 'low order', even at the largest British abattoirs, and few were equipped to carry out even simple and routine laboratory tests. 'Until laboratory services are readily available for all doubtful cases', Hughes emphasized, the meat inspection services would not meet modern requirements.[76] Changing patterns of animal disease meant that laboratory methods must be 'a regular feature of the inspection system', and labs must be properly staffed by veterinarians trained in laboratory procedure and with adequate technical staff.[77] Finally Hughes stressed the need for research into the whole process of slaughtering, dressing, and inspection: 'An industry as complex as the meat industry, dependent on a biological product as its starting material, which is subject to extrinsic and intrinsic contamination, should be relying heavily on research into all its aspects'.[78] Nor was Hughes alone in his concerns. The veterinary superintendent of Dundee's markets and slaughterhouses concluded on similar grounds that a complete reform of the existing meat supply system was required.[79] Fifteen years later, the British Association for the Advancement of Science report on *Salmonella* was still indicating insanitary abattoir practices and the absence of the laboratory facilities needed for effective meat inspection.[80] Little had changed since the 1890s.

In the early 1960s, the walls of the slaughterhouse became permeable. The new microbiology and new technologies in construction meant that meat hygiene became reconceptualized as a process beginning with the live animal in the closing weeks of its life and continuing until the finished product reached the consumer.[81] In this process, the environment of the abattoir came to be seen as a crucial site in the infection and contamination of meat animals alive and dead. The concerns of the early 1960s were only the beginning of a long haul. Despite repeated revisions of meat hygiene regulations, and increasingly acrimonious debates regarding necessary reforms ahead of Britain joining the European Economic Community and meeting the higher EEC meat hygiene standards, the meat industry continued to fall short of public health expectations. A report published in 1975 concluded that the industry had failed to apply existing scientific knowledge, and that 'many inadequacies' remained in the entire process of transport, lairage, slaughter of animals, and subsequent handling of meat.[82] The situation, it seemed, was not so different from that at the end of the nineteenth century, and while improvements

[76] Hughes, 'Meat inspection', p. 85. [77] Hughes, 'Meat inspection', p. 85.

[78] Hughes, 'Meat inspection', pp. 85–6.

[79] A. Spruell, 'Practical slaughterhouses and clean meat production', *Roy Soc Hlth Jnl*, 82 (1962): p. 266. See also Notes and Comments, 'Meat hygiene', *MO*, 108 (1962): p. 352; W. R. Cockrill, 'International problems and practices in meat hygiene', *Vet Rec*, 75 (1963): pp. 875–83.

[80] British Association for the Advancement of Science (BAAS), *Salmonella. The Food Poisoner* (1977), pp. 31–2.

[81] Cockrill, 'International problems', p. 882.

[82] Second Report of the Board of the Joint Consultative Organisation for Research and Development in Agriculture and Food, 1975; see News and Reports, 'JCO hits at inadequacies in transport and slaughter of animals', *Vet Rec*, 98 (1976): p. 124.

did follow the BSE crisis of the 1990s, the European horsemeat scandal of 2013 indicated that continuing problems in the management and regulation of slaughterhouses were not simply an issue for Britain.

PACKING POULTRY

As concerns about slaughterhouse practices came to a head in the early 1960s, the first intimations of trouble in the poultry sector emerged. Although the risks of *Salmonella* infection from table poultry and eggs were considered around 1950, informed discussants appeared then to deem risks as minimal.[83] R. F. Gordon thought the eradication of 'such ubiquitous organisms' as *Salmonella* from poultry 'impractical'; it was the industry's responsibility to retain public confidence in their products, since there appeared to be no sanitary legislation regarding egg-packing stations. Gordon thought the problem of *Salmonella* in poultry meat was 'less acute' than that in eggs, since surface contamination of the body was mainly due to unsanitary handling.[84] Despite the concern over eggs, shell hen eggs were not found to be vehicles for *Salmonella*, and between 1952 and 1958 only one *Salmonella* outbreak in Britain was definitely associated with eating poultry.[85] At the same time, the general lack of concern for risks to human health from *Salmonella*-infected poultry was illustrated by the first incident in which humans in Britain were infected with *Salmonella typhimurium* after contact with diseased poultry. An extensive outbreak of the infection on a large Wiltshire turkey farm in 1955 not only killed a great many young poults but also caused illness in the farmer and his wife. The episode was investigated by PHLS staff, but at the end of the season the breeding flock on the farm was slaughtered, and the carcasses sold for human consumption.[86]

It was only in 1960 that concern over the public health implications of salmonellosis in the broiler industry took centre stage, with the publication of an article by J. H. C. Walker, Director of the MRC's Public Health Laboratory at Maidstone. Walker's initiative was stimulated partly by the immense increase in broiler production that had taken place and was projected to take place, and partly by the example of America. Intensive poultry farming having been established there before World War II, the results were becoming clear for public health personnel to see. American poultry was now regarded as the largest natural reservoir of

[83] A. Bernstein, 'Salmonella infection of hen eggs', *MBMH*, 11 (1952): p. 67; W. P. Blount, 'The public health aspect of poultry disease', *Roy San Inst Jnl*, 69 (1949): pp. 361–2; R. F. Gordon, in discussion following Blount's paper, *Roy San Inst Jnl*, 69 (1949): pp. 366–7, 369.

[84] Gordon, 'Discussion', p. 369.

[85] J. H. C. Walker, 'The broiler industry—transmission of salmonella infection', *Roy Soc Hlth Jnl*, 80 (1960): p. 142.

[86] M. S. Pereira and J. D. Blaxland, 'Salmonella typhimurium infection in man contracted from turkeys', *MBMH*, 14 (1955): p. 53. I have come across just one previous British reference to a poultry-borne outbreak, that occurring in the Northampton police force in March 1939. This was caused by *Salmonella typhimurium* in a New York dressed turkey imported from Hungary: S. Rowland, 'An outbreak of food poisoning', *MO*, 62 (1939): pp. 199–200.

Salmonella infection in the world, and by 1960 30 per cent of outbreaks of human salmonellosis and 40 per cent of cases in the USA were associated with poultry.[87] The American example thus provided both a point of comparison and a warning of likely future developments in the British industry. Walker was particularly concerned by the emergence of antibiotic-resistant *Salmonella* infections resulting from the medical management of poultry flocks—a phenomenon recently demonstrated in America, and confirmed by experimental work at England's Houghton Poultry Research Station.[88] More immediately, however, Walker drew attention to unhygienic practices in British broiler houses and poultry packing plants. The former might contain up to 15,000 or more 'highly susceptible' young birds, in conditions which would facilitate the spread of infection if introduced by carriers.[89]

Practices in the poultry packing stations, many of which used the latest American machinery and techniques, potentially compounded any problems of infection present in the flocks. Once de-feathered and eviscerated, the birds were treated in one of three ways, rapid cooling being essential to production of a high-quality product. In modern plants carcasses might be cooled in tanks of slush ice, after which they were packed and immediately frozen, or they were thrown into tanks of water after de-feathering and eviscerated later. Although chlorinated water was used in all these processes, the tanks in particular carried risks of infection from faecal contamination and discharges from the sinuses. At one well-conducted plant, tank water was only changed once a day. In a third type of operation, of a more traditional kind, the birds were killed and dressed in 'disused cowsheds, stables and dirty outhouses'. The conditions here, Walker noted wryly, 'leave much to be desired'.[90] Further concerns centred on the use of antibiotics in the cooling water, and on refrigeration and distribution practices. The overriding impression was of a production process fraught with risk to the consumer. Although Walker assessed the risk as 'probably not great', he noted that the incidence of *Salmonella* infection in chickens appeared to be increasing, and warned that in Denmark *Salmonella* new to the country, derived from imported feedstuffs, were being found quickly to transfer into poultry and humans. In the safeguarding of poultry meat supplies from infection, the highest standards of processing and sanitation were needed.[91]

The pathways of infection from birds to humans were quickly clear. Uncooked poultry, possibly contaminated in processing, needed careful handling and proper cooking to avert danger. Ready-cooked, spit-roasted chicken was a hazard, as the birds were not always properly cooked. Raw chicken portions were not always kept refrigerated by retailers, and (in the early 1960s) many homes did not possess a refrigerator, so bacterial multiplication could reach dangerous levels if whole birds were kept too long before cooking.[92] Hazards generated in processing plant and

[87] Walker, 'Broiler industry', p. 142.
[88] Walker, 'Broiler industry', pp. 142–3.
[89] Walker, 'Broiler industry', p. 143.
[90] Walker, 'Broiler industry', p. 143.
[91] Walker, 'Broiler industry', p. 144.
[92] Walker, 'Broiler industry', p. 144. See also Anon, 'Frozen poultry: Health hazards', *Roy Soc Hlth Jnl*, 89 (1969): pp. 52, 96; D. Roberts, 'Observations on procedures for thawing and spit-roasting frozen dressed chickens, and post-cooking care and storage: with particular references to food-poisoning bacteria', *Jnl Hyg*, 70 (1972): 565–88.

domestic kitchen were compounded by practices in butchers' shops. Investigating an outbreak of *Salmonella* saint paul in West Sussex in 1960, PHLS staff found that 11 out of 13 incidents were caused by various cooked meats bought at the local butcher's, and eaten without further cooking. It transpired that locally sourced ducks were supplied to the butcher plucked but not drawn (New York dressed), and were eviscerated by the butcher's staff in the room where the cooked meats were prepared. The practice of eviscerating poultry in retail shops was said to be common across England and Wales; the lack of evidence for association between poultry and human salmonellosis, it was concluded, might partly be due to a failure to appreciate such indirect means of transmission.[93]

Despite these findings, and increasing international research into the microbiology of avian salmonellosis, preventive measures were not systematically implemented. Science was not strong enough to combat market forces. The broiler industry had grown too vast, too rapidly, and the logistics of sanitary policing and regulation of this now important industry were daunting.[94] In the early 1960s, poultry escaped any regular form of inspection except under local bye-laws in some of the larger cities; little changed in the following decade. In 1971, the part played by poultry products in initiating outbreaks of food poisoning was still being emphasized: carcass contamination during evisceration, undercooking, spit roasting, and the re-contamination of cooked birds all remained problematic.[95] Six years later the report of the British Association for the Advancement of Science's Study Group on *Salmonella* focused exclusively on the abattoir and the poultry processing plant as critical sites for the entry of *Salmonella* into the human food chain.[96]

In both the broiler and the meat industries, laboratory science was the means of alerting and sharpening public health concerns in the years after 1940. Just as microbiology had highlighted the environmental issues around *Salmonella* infections in poultry and animals, so it played a critical part in the identification of slaughterhouse and packing station as crucial sites for the onward spread of infection into the human food chain. At one remove, the butcher's shop continued to cause local concern, as a place where the hazards generated in the natural environment and in the processes of slaughter were compounded and passed on to the consumer. The worries about British standards of cooking and eating, aggravated by the experience of war, added to these anxieties. These concerns were not allayed with time. Salmonellosis, the PHLS specialist Enid Vernon noted towards the end of the 1960s, existed as an 'intractable' problem in public health.[97] The continuing peril of butchers' practices was brought home again by the 1996 *E. coli* outbreak at Wishaw in Scotland.[98]

[93] N. S. Galbraith et al., 'An outbreak of human salmonellosis due to salmonella saint-paul associated with infection in poultry', *MBMH*, 21 (1962): p. 214.

[94] Leading Article, 'Avoiding anomalies in poultry meat inspection', *Vet Rec*, 73 (1974): p. 405.

[95] W. A. Watson, 'Salmonella infection and meat hygiene', *Vet Rec*, 96 (1975): p. 351.

[96] BAAS, *Salmonella*, pp. 31–2.

[97] Enid Vernon, 'Food poisoning and *Salmonella* infections in England and Wales, 1967', *PH*, 83 (1968–9): p. 205.

[98] See Hugh Pennington, *When Food Kills. BSE, E coli and Disaster Science* (2003), pp. 1–24.

FILTH, FOOD, AND FINGERS

The prevention of food poisoning, the American commentator Henry Bauer observed in 1973, centres on 'the five fs': faeces, fingers, flies, food, and filth, and the only way to prevent human salmonellosis is to break the chain of events which allows faecal material to get into food.[99] The creation of human disgust around flies, filth, and food was established in developed countries by the 1920s (Chapter 3), but convincing individual humans that their own fingers are a hygiene risk proved much more difficult. While abattoir and poultry plant were demonstrated as critical sites for the onward transmission of infection, the fact remained that proper kitchen hygiene, whether domestic or commercial—the washing of hands, the prevention of cross-contamination between foods such as raw and sliced meats, and the thorough cooking and correct storage of raw and cooked foodstuffs—constituted a crucial last preventive bastion against human infection. In the years after 1945, concern over kitchen and personal hygiene practices never disappeared. The MOH for Witham Urban District, recounting an outbreak caused by tinned meat sliced and distributed from a butcher's shop, observed that 'advice about washing the hands after visiting the w.c. is often repeated but rarely heeded'. If this elementary precaution were practised in food shops and private houses, the risks of food poisoning would be negligible.[100] The worries about war-induced standards and rising food poisoning notifications were compounded by serious typhoid outbreaks at Aberystwyth and in the Halifax area in 1946.[101]

Typhoid being now a rarity, the professional response was swift. In January 1947, the Medical Research Council (MRC) set up a Food Hygiene Unit to investigate outbreaks and to conduct research and educational work on food-borne infections and food sanitation.[102] In October, the Central Council for Health Education (CCHE), which had been established by the Society of Medical Officers of Health 20 years previously, organized a day conference on food and drink infections. The conference was addressed by the Council's President, Lord Woolton (the least unpopular of the war-time food ministers), William Savage, and Graham Wilson. Woolton was recorded as particularly urging the attendant Press to tell the general public that hand-washing after using the toilet would greatly reduce the number of food-poisoning outbreaks.[103] This was the general message—as one observer noted, 'if every newspaper had published "Everybody should wash their hands after visiting the water closet", they would have covered the main outcome of the day'.[104] Not unusually, the Press, like the public, failed to

[99] Henry Bauer, 'The growing problem of salmonellosis in modern society', *Medicine*, 52 (1973): p. 29.

[100] F. C. Camps, 'An outbreak of food poisoning due to Salmonella typhimurium', *BMJ* (1946), ii: p. 131.

[101] Editorial, 'Epidemic typhoid', *MO*, 76 (1946): p. 158; Public Health, 'Outbreak of typhoid fever', *Lancet* 1946, ii: pp. 211, 255, 287, 329, 434.

[102] Medical Research Council, Annual Report for the Years 1945–48 (1949): pp. 231–2.

[103] Editorial, 'Food and infection', *PH*, 61 (1947): p. 20.

[104] Notes and Comments, 'Food pollution', *MO*, 78 (1947): p. 166.

take home the message. Newspaper coverage, it was said, showed that 'we are scarcely at the beginning of gaining the bridge of the fourth estate between the advisers of the people and the people themselves'. Systematic training and instruction were needed if the bridge was to be gained, not a series of stunts.[105]

1947 marked the beginning of a period of interest in and activity around the topic of food hygiene education, much of it focused on the training and education of food handlers.[106] In 1948, government launched a national 'clean food' campaign, assisted by a number of bodies, including the PHLS, the CCHE, the Ministries of Food and Health, the Catering Association of Great Britain, and the British Tourist and Holidays Board. Press and Parliament took active interest, and the Ministry of Food led efforts at rousing public attention.[107] Local authorities also showed initiative. The market town of Guildford set about investigating its own food retailers, including dairies and dairy farms, ice-cream makers and retailers, butchers, cooked meat shops, confectioners, general stores, cafes, and restaurants. The outcome was less than satisfactory: 16 of the 48 cafes and restaurants had no sanitary or washing facilities for customers, while the snack bar-type cafes produced food in 'the most unsatisfactory conditions'. As a result, a Guildford Hygienic Food Trades Guild was established through the joint efforts of town council and food trade representatives.[108] A code of practice was put in place for the various types of operation, prospective Guild members were inspected by health officers, and certificates were issued and publicly displayed by traders who met requirements. Other towns followed suit, and at least 65 such guilds were in operation by 1951.[109]

Despite these efforts, the situation continued to be problematic. The wording of existing legislative provision under section 13 of the 1938 Food and Drugs Act was at times opaque in the effort not to appear draconian and so set up hostile reactions. Phrases such as 'as far as may be necessary' and 'suitable and sufficient' did not help the cause of reform. One eminent Guildford trader told the town's chief sanitary inspector, 'Give me the words "suitable and sufficient" in any piece of legislation and I'll win the day every time'.[110] Food handlers' responses to local educational initiatives were mixed. The London borough of Hammersmith found the response satisfactory, but at Southampton classes in food hygiene run for the benefit of the city's 400-plus food trading establishments attracted only 19 people. In Oxford, the response to talks and advice was so unsatisfactory that the city health department introduced on-the-spot tickets for contravention of the bye-laws.[111] Traders could be slow in responding to local government efforts. Of 388 premises in which food was handled or sold in Tunbridge Wells in 1950, 196 were without constant hot

[105] Notes and Comments, 'Food pollution', p. 166.

[106] Richard I. Barr, 'Food hygiene. The arousal of public awareness', *Roy Soc Hth Jnl*, 98 (1978): p. 56.

[107] Barr, 'Arousal', p. 56.

[108] Editorial, 'Guildford's initiative in food hygiene', *PH*, 61 (1947): p. 52.

[109] Barr, 'Food hygiene', p. 56.

[110] H. A. Perry, 'Food hygiene. Theory and practice', *Roy Soc Hth Jnl*, 71 (1951): p. 513.

[111] Discussion following J. G. Molner, 'Food hygiene', *Roy Soc Hth Jnl*, 76 (1956): pp. 374–5.

water for food-handling purposes. Just 66 had complied with the regulations by the end of the year, although many were said to have ordered the necessary equipment.[112] Other authorities noted that elderly people were unenthusiastic about regulations and admonitions.[113]

Given these problems, legislation came to be viewed as 'sheer necessity'.[114] It came in 1954, with the Food and Drugs Amendment Act. Immediately translated into the consolidatory Food and Drugs Act 1955, this legislation imposed food hygiene regulations, although a proposal for the compulsory registration of catering establishments with local authorities was dropped under pressure from vested interests.[115] Nonetheless, the Food Hygiene Regulations 1955 were regarded as revolutionary: responsibility had been at last been placed on each individual handler of food.[116] Clubs, canteens, school kitchens, and civic restaurants were included in the provisions, and unsanitary premises were for the first time banned. Requirements for compliance included constant hot water; adequate and utilized lighting; wash basins, nail brushes, soap, and clean towels for staff; and first aid equipment.[117] A decade later, the journal *Medical Officer* praised the 'tremendous impetus' the Act had given to food hygiene implementation. Significantly, the journal pointed out that the Act had been framed in light of the findings in epidemiology, microbiology, and biochemistry which had 'thrown so much light on the nature of the problem since the war years'.[118] In achieving compliance with the new regulations, food handlers had to understand the basic principles of food hygiene; once that was done, the task of compliance was relatively easy. While lack of enthusiasm for the new practices continued to be noted among food handlers, the sociologist Richard Barr, looking back from the vantage point of 1978, considered that public awareness of the need for hygienic food processing and preparation 'probably' remained at a higher level than before 1940.[119] In 1966, however, *Medical Officer*, while admitting that there were problems in the domestic arena that were less straightforward than those in the catering industry, remained critical of the general public, which had not been obliged to put its own house in order.[120] And despite Barr's contention, food-poisoning notifications continued remorselessly to rise into the 1990s.

Threads of concern about food hygiene continued to surface in the public health literature. The 1964 Aberdeen typhoid outbreak (caused by contaminated corned beef) provoked another spike in attention to methods of food handling.[121]

[112] Notes of the Week, 'Clean food propaganda', *MO*, 86 (1951): p. 154.

[113] Notes, 'Propaganda', p. 154.

[114] Martine, 'Food hygiene', p. 170.

[115] Barr, 'Food hygiene', p. 57. For unenthusiastic food handlers see Notes of the Week, 'Reluctant food handlers', *MO*, 95 (1956): p. 196; Discussion following Molner, 'Food hygiene', pp. 370–6, 374–5; L. H. Vale, 'Food hygiene. What progress?', *Roy Soc Hth Jnl*, 77 (1957): p. 436; Martine, 'Food hygiene', pp. 171–4.

[116] Martine, 'Food hygiene', p. 170.

[117] Martine, 'Food hygiene', pp. 170–1.

[118] Notes and Comments, 'The re-teaching of the principles of food hygiene', *MO*, 115 (1966): p. 206.

[119] Barr, 'Food hygiene', p. 57.

[120] Notes and Comments, 'Re-teaching', p. 206.

[121] For this outbreak see David Smith et al., *Food Poisoning, Policy and Politics: Corned Beef and Typhoid in Britain in the 1960s* (2005).

The Committee of Inquiry into the outbreak focused on deficiencies in the hygienic training of food handlers, and suggested that the Ministry of Health's Food Hygiene Advisory Council should investigate. It pointed out that there had been a more marked decline in general outbreaks of food poisoning than in sporadic and family cases, recommended that codes of practice be drawn up for both commercial and domestic food handlers, and called for the production of more educational films. While commending these suggestions, *Medical Officer* observed tartly that what was needed was 'new stuff—not more and more of the present material'.[122] The truth of this remark was borne out by Mary Adams JP, deputy Chair of the Consumers' Association and of the Women's group on Public Welfare, who, at the CCHE's second conference on food hygiene in 1966, declared that most people considered the subject of food hygiene 'boring'.[123] Although Adams' declaration met with protest from the floor, the Ministry of Health's food hygiene advisory officer admitted that food hygiene education had achieved least success with the general public.[124]

The rising trend in food poisoning cases, and changing patterns of distribution in the years after 1970, underscored continuing failures in the food hygiene education project. Curiously, this failure occurred against the backdrop of a cultural revolution in other aspects of personal hygiene that had begun with the inter-war emphasis on light, colour, space, and healthy outdoor exercise, and was reinforced, via film and television in the 1950s, by the American preoccupation with domestic and personal cleanliness.[125] Considerations of hand-washing were (and are) perhaps too mundane when compared to the pleasures of clean clothes, shower gels, liquid soap, and the security of intimate personal freshness offered by deodorant and mouthwash. Reviewing the entire subject of commercial food hygiene in 1978, Barrie Sheard, an environmental health officer with 25 years' service in local government, concluded that 'we must all have taken the wrong road' since 1954. There had been too much emphasis on 'face value' standards of hygiene, construction, and inspection techniques, and a core neglect of education in personal hygiene.[126] Sheard's gaze encompassed the broad picture of food production, including farming practices. *Salmonella* infection went uncontrolled on farms and in breeding herds; a new law was needed to require the heat treatment of all animal feeding stuffs to kill off pathogenic bacteria; and the British practice of feeding poultry and livestock with infected food must be stopped. Unpublished PHLS reports, he claimed, detailed widespread environmental distribution of *Salmonella* and other pathogenic bacteria not only in the 'expected places' of 'sewage, effluent, river, estuary and sea water, poultry farm, packing station' but also in the unexpected places of food factory, shop, canteen, and kitchen.[127] A full 30 years after the public health effort at national food hygiene education had begun, there was little

122 Notes and Comments, 'Re-teaching', p. 206.
123 Anon, 'Food hygiene. A new approach', *MO*, 115 (1966): p. 62.
124 Anon, 'Food hygiene', p. 63.
125 See Virginia Smith, *Clean. A History of Personal Hygiene and Purity* (2007), pp. 307–40.
126 L. Barrie Sheard, 'Inspection of food and food premises', *Roy Soc Hlth Jnl*, 98 (1978): pp. 62, 65.
127 Sheard, 'Inspection', p. 63.

suggestion in the food poisoning statistics or in microbiological and epidemiological investigations that it had achieved any degree of success. Despite the revolutions in human environmental sanitation and intimate personal cleanliness, at least three of the five fs, it seemed, remained as interconnected as ever. The optimistic deflection of responsibility towards slaughterhouse and kitchen, as envisaged by John McCoy (Chapter 8) just three years earlier, seemed,[128] in the light of Sheard's conclusions, delusory.

[128] J. H. McCoy, 'Trends in salmonella food poisoning in England and Wales, 1941–72', *Jnl Hyg*, 74 (1975): p. 280.

Conclusion

In the 1970s the microbiological landscape of food infections in Britain began to change. While *Salmonella* continued to play a prominent role, improving laboratory techniques began to reveal a new complex of bacterial, viral, and protozoan causes of gastro-enteritis.[1] *Campylobacter* was first identified in 1977, and in the following decade *Clostridium difficile,* rotavirus, norovirus, and *Cryptospiridium* were added to the list.[2] *E. coli*, once regarded as a harmless inhabitant of animal intestines, became an issue with the emergence of the virulent 0157 strain in 1982.[3] By the 1980s the laboratory investigation of faecal samples relating to outbreaks and sporadic cases was increasingly complicated, requiring the use of a wide range of techniques including 12 different liquid or solid culture media incubated at three different incubator temperatures; light microscopy of stained and unstained preparations; electron microscopy; and either tissue culture or latex agglutination for detecting bacterial toxins.[4] Notifications of food-poisoning incidents meanwhile rose steadily. Reported *Campylobacter* infections have outstripped *Salmonella* every year since 1981, while *Clostridium perfringens* (a major cause of industrial outbreaks) and giardiasis appeared to be on the increase in the 1980s.[5] Salmonellosis can involve serious complications, whereas *Campylobacter* is generally regarded as milder, although serious complications are not unknown.[6] But while *Salmonella* is in individual cases a greater danger to individuals, and a greater expense to the state in terms of illness, lost hours of work, and costs of treatment, the sheer number of cases of *Campylobacter* infections—460,000 a year in Britain at the most recent estimate, against some 10,000 *Salmonella*—makes this bacterium the most expensive in terms of social and economic costs.

Meanwhile, the first indication of antibiotic resistance in *Salmonella* came in 1975, when E. S. Anderson drew attention to typhoid's increasing resistance to

[1] G. C. Turner et al., 'Investigating gastroenteritis: The Merseyside experience 1983–1987', *Public Health*, 102 (1988): p. 428.

[2] Turner et al., 'Investigating gastroenteritis'; M. B. Skirrrow, '*Campylobacter enteritis*: A "new" disease', *BMJ* (1977), ii: pp. 9–11.

[3] L. W. Riley et al., 'Hemorrhagic colitis associated with a rare *Escherichia coli* serotype', *New England Journal of Medicine,* 308 (1983): pp. 681–5; Hugh Pennington, *When Food Kills: BSE, E. coli and Disaster Science* (2003), pp. 96–7.

[4] Turner et al., 'Investigating gastroenteritis': p. 428.

[5] CMOAR 1985: 51. N. S. Galbraith et al., 'The changing pattern of food borne diseases in England and Wales', *PH,* 101 (1987): p. 325.

[6] Galbraith et al., 'Changing pattern', pp. 324–5. Ros Stanwell-Smith, personal communication, 20 September 2013.

chloramphenicol, the broad-spectrum antibiotic which had marked a revolution in typhoid treatment when it was introduced in 1949.[7] More worryingly, a multi-drug-resistant (MDR) strain of *Salmonella typhimurium*—DT104—emerged in cattle in England and Wales in 1988. It was soon found in poultry, pigs, sheep, and horses, and, being resistant, proved difficult to control, quickly entering the human food chain. By the early 1990s, the emergence of MDR strains of *Salmonella typhimurium* was threatening to become a serious public health problem: between 1990 and 1996, notified human cases of DT104 rose from 500 to 3,500 a year.[8] During 1990s, MDR *Salmonella typhimurium* and DT104 became a global problem, although primarily in Europe and North America.[9] By the 2000s, however, MDR enteric fever infection was raising serious concerns elsewhere, notably in India.[10]

Within this increasingly complex picture, the pathways of foodborne infection in Britain remained much the same as those identified and discussed in Chapters 1–4 and Chapter 7. Outbreaks caused by sewage-contaminated shell-fish, raw milk, meat products (pâté, pies), creamed coconut, and liquid egg all featured in the CMO's reports in the 1980s—suggesting remarkable consistency in vehicles of infection, failure in control, and failure of education. In 1987 21 outbreaks of viral gastro-enteritis (2,000 plus cases) were traced to cockles between May and October, provoking an urgent review of cockle-processing methods.[11] In May 1987, evidence that 60 per cent of British frozen poultry was infected with *Salmonella* raised questions over whether eggs too would be infected, as was suggested by large egg-borne outbreaks in Spain and America.[12] In the following year *Salmonella enteritidis* PT4 associated with eggs and egg products overtook *Salmonella typhimurium* as the principal cause of human salmonellosis, and warnings began to be issued to the general public.[13] It was against this background that Edwina Currie, then a junior government minister, made her notorious observation to Independent Television News on 3 December 1988 that 'most of the egg production in this country . . . is infected with *Salmonella*', so generating a public panic to out-rival that over oysters in 1902–3.[14]

[7] E. S. Anderson, 'The problem and implications of chloramphenicol resistance in the typhoid bacillus', *Journal of Hygiene*, 74 (1975): pp. 289–99.

[8] WHO Fact Sheet no 139, Salmonella (non-typhoidal): <http://www.who.int/mediacentre/factsheets/fs139/en/>, accessed 29 June 2014.

[9] M. Helms et al., 'International *Salmonella* Typhimurium DT104 infections, 1992–2001', *Emerging Infectious Diseases,* 11 (2005): p. 859.

[10] S. Kumar et al., 'Rising prevalence of enteric fever due to multidrug-resistant Salmonella: an epidemiological study', *Journal of Medical Microbiology*, 57 (2008): pp. 1247–50.

[11] Chief Medical Officer's Annual Report (CMOAR) 1987: pp. 107–8.

[12] Christopher G. Forshner, 'The British government, mad cows and rotten eggs: Decision–making under uncertainty and risk as it occurs in the real world' (M Phil dissertation, Oxford University, 1993), p. 66.

[13] CMOAR, 1988: pp. 8–9, 137–8; Forshner, 'British government', p. 67. See also Editor's Diary, 'One threat after another', *Poultry World*, September 1988: p. 9.

[14] See *Poultry World*, December 1988: p. 2.

At the same time as this disaster was brewing, concerns were growing around bovine spongiform encephalopathy—a new disease of dairy cattle, first identified in November 1986—and its possible transmission to humans through the food chain.[15] The BSE epidemic was perhaps the ultimate reflection of the anxiety expressed by Philip Edwards in 1958 regarding the recycling of animal parts in high-protein feeds, even though that had been expressly directed at the seeding of *Salmonella* through food animal populations (Chapter 6). The BSE epidemic is thought possibly to have occurred following a random gene mutation in a bovine whose carcass had made it into the protein feed manufactory. In the universal scheme of things, however, *Salmonella typhimurium* DT104, also generated by high-protein feed, proved an infinitely more potent problem than BSE has done to date. While great alarm attended the identification of a new human infection, New Variant Creutzfeldt–Jakob Disease (NvCJD), in 1996, as of January 2012 just 176 cases had been diagnosed in Britain, of which 80 per cent had occurred before 2005.[16] By contrast, MDR *Salmonella typhimurium* DT104 was an international problem of more or less significance locally by 2000.[17]

While the pathways of infection through the food chain described in Part I continue to exist and are now known to carry pathogens other than *Salmonella*, the scientific communities and networks engaged in the study of these various organisms have expanded accordingly. The global nature of this scientific enterprise is reflected in the range of papers published in, for example, *Epidemiology and Infection*, the modern continuation of the *Journal of Hygiene*. Nor has *Salmonella* science stood still: the breakthroughs made in the 1940s have been extended and developed with new microbiological methods. During the 1980s, for example, epidemiologists and students of pathogenesis adopted interdisciplinary approaches to the typing of micro-organisms using a wide variety of techniques originating in immunology, biochemistry, and genetics: an interdisciplinary practice referred to as 'molecular epidemiology'.[18] A survey of these typing systems conducted in 1993 concluded that molecular techniques provided 'a powerful set of new tools that augment both patient management and epidemiological investigation'.[19] Pulse-field gel electrophoresis was being used in epidemiological investigation by the mid-1990s, and by 2000 multiple genotyping methods had begun to clarify links between particular serotypes, their animal hosts, and human infections.[20] The investigation of *Salmonella* serotypes has continued, and new methods applied to their elucidation. In 1996, K. A. Lampell and colleagues at the US Food and Drugs Administration published their polymerase chain reaction assay for detecting *Salmonella enteritidis*—'specific, reproducible and less time consuming than the

[15] See <webarchive.nationalarchives.gov.uk/200607 1514 1954/bseinquiry.gov.uk/>.

[16] <http://www.food.gov.uk/policy-advice/bse/what/#.UhYo1Y9qRlk>, accessed 22 August 2013.

[17] Helms et al., 'International *Salmonella* Typhimurium DT104', pp. 859–67.

[18] J. N. Maslow et al., 'Molecular epidemiology: Application of contemporary techniques to the typing of micro organisms', *Clinical Infectious Disease,* 17 (1993): p. 153.

[19] Maslow et al., 'Molecular epidemiology', p. 161.

[20] D. C. Old et al., 'Grouping of *Salmonella enterica* serotype Montevideo strains by ribotyping and IS200 profiling', *Epidemiology and Infection,* 124 (2000): pp. 380–1.

standard bacteriological methods'.[21] Their research was a direct response to the emergence of *Salmonella enteritidis* PT4 as the dominant serotype not just in America, but also in Britain, Finland, Norway, Sweden, and Canada.[22] It was this upsurge in *enteritidis* that concerned England's CMO in the late 1980s. As a result, vaccination for egg-laying hens was introduced in 1997, and resulted in significantly reduced isolations of *Salmonella enteritidis* PT4 from human cases.[23] These developments illustrate the limitations of science and technology: pathogen evolution drives a continuing search for new methods of identification and control.

Despite the widening canvas of food infections from the late 1970s, *Salmonella* outbreaks played a major role in spurring public health inquiries and interventions.[24] The 1984 Stanley Royd outbreak generated the committee of enquiry into the future development of public health, whose report was published in 1988, while the *Salmonella* in eggs affair of 1988 also played a role in generating the Food Safety Act and the Advisory Committee on the Microbiological Safety of Food in 1990.[25] The impact of such very visible episodes was illustrated later in the decade. During the 1990s pressure began to build for reform of the Ministry of Agriculture Fisheries and Food (MAFF) and for the creation of an independent Food Standards and Safety Executive.[26] Further epidemic outbreaks precipitated follow up on these demands. The Food Standards Agency (FSA) was set up in 2000 following a major outbreak of *E.* coli 0157 resulting from poor butcher's shop hygiene in Scotland. The recreation of MAFF as the Department for Environment, Food and Rural Affairs (DEFRA) in June 2001 followed the perceived failure of MAFF to deal with the foot and mouth disease outbreak of 2000–1—an outbreak which developed from cases first identified in a slaughterhouse.[27] Foot and mouth rarely affects humans, and does not travel through the human food chain, but the impact on the farming community, and public outrage and dismay at Britain's slaughter-and-burn policy for affected animals and proximate herds, made news headlines for months.

These public health-oriented reforms have as yet provided no answer to the problems presented by a global food market and engrained 'dodgy' practices in certain key food industries, notably the meat production trades, discussed in Chapters 7 and 8. Among various examples of imperfect food safety practices in the recent past are a series of British *Salmonella* outbreaks associated with imported Spanish eggs between 2002 and 2011, and a nationwide American outbreak in 2012 linked to a raw tuna product prepared in India.[28] In 2009, a major American

[21] K. A. Lampell et al., 'Specific detection of *Salmonella enterica* serotype Enteritidis using the polymerase chain reaction', *Epi and Inf,* 116 (1996): p. 137.

[22] Lampell et al., 'Specific detection', p. 137.

[23] T. A. Cogan and T. J. Humphrey, 'The rise and fall of *Salmonella* Enteritidis in the UK', *Journal of Applied Microbiology*, 94 (2003): pp. 1148–98.

[24] S. Palmer et al., 'The role of outbreaks in developing food safety policy: Population based surveillance of *Salmonella* outbreaks in Wales 1986–98', *Epi and Inf,* 125 (2000): pp. 467–72.

[25] Palmer et al., 'The role of outbreaks'.

[26] Tim Lang, 'Food policy and public health', *PH*, 106 (1992): p. 123.

[27] See Judith Cook, *The Year of the Pyres* (2001); Abigail Woods, *A Manufactured Plague. The History of Foot-and-Mouth Disease in Britain* (2004).

[28] <http://www.cdc.gov/salmonella/outbreaks.html>.

outbreak due to contaminated peanut butter put the Peanut Corporation of America into liquidation.[29] In February 2013 four former officials of the now defunct company were indicted on charges of conspiracy, fraud, and introduction of adulterated food into interstate commerce with intent to defraud or mislead.[30] In 2011, Germany suffered the world's worst ever *E. coli* outbreak, with 48 deaths, 857 cases with severe complications, and 3,078 cases in total, when organic bean sprouts became contaminated. Germany's initial attempt to blame Spanish cucumbers caused a Europe-wide food panic.[31] In October 2012 Canada made its largest ever meat recall following the import of some 1,134 million kilograms of boneless American beef contaminated with *E. coli* 0157.[32] Chicken contaminated with multiple *Salmonella* strains, seven of which were MDR, infected several hundred people in 20 American states between March and October 2013.[33] The European horsemeat scandal, which broke in January 2013 and whose revelations carried on for months, demonstrated only too clearly the continuing structural problems of slaughterhouse supervision and the tracking of food products in both national and international markets.[34] Although horsemeat itself is harmless, the scale of the fraud revealed, and the unwitting involvement of several household food brands, provoked general outrage. More broadly, however, evaluations of national food safety performance show that population size, the degree of internationalization in local food trades, and the nature of agencies responsible for food safety and the meat industries may all affect different countries' ability to achieve safe food supplies.[35] The notable success of the Scandinavian countries in controlling *Salmonella* illustrates this point, with Denmark also in recent years achieving increasing success with *Campylobacter*.[36] The frequency of *Salmonella* infections has, however,

[29] See <http://www.dailymail.co.uk/news/article-2017350/Health-warning-Spanish-eggs-blamed-136-cases-salmonella-UK.html>, accessed 22 July 2011; 'U.S indicts peanut processors in 2009 salmonella outbreak': <http://www.reuters.com/article/2013/02/21/us-usa-crime-salmonella-idUSBRE91KOWI20130221>, accessed 22 July 2011.

[30] <http://www.bloomberg.com/news/2013-02-21/peanut-corp-of-america-executives-indicted-over-salmonella-1-.html>, accessed 5 September 2013.

[31] 'German tests link bean sprouts to deadly E.coli': <http://www.bbc.co.uk/news/world-europe-13725953>, accessed 29 June 2014; '2011 Germany E. coli 0104H deadly outbreak': <http://www.wikipedia.org/wiki/211_Germany_E._coli_0104:H4_outbreak>, accessed 29 June 2014.

[32] <http://www.cbc.ca/news/canada/better-ways-to-monitor-cand-s-meat-industry-1.>.

[33] 'Continuing Salmonella Outbreaks': http://www.nytimes.com/2013/10/19/opinion/continuing-salmonella-outbreaks.html?nl+todaysheadlines&emc+edit_th_20131019&_r=0>, accessed 29 June 1014.

[34] See eg 'Dutch uncover large scale meat fraud', <http://www.bbc.co.uk/news/world-europe-22098763>, accessed 11 August 2013.

[35] <http://www.bbc.co.uk/news/world-europe-22098763>: Dutch meat fraud.

[36] See eg H. C. Wegner et al., 'Salmonella control programs in Denmark', *Emerging Infectious Diseases*, 9 (2003): pp. 774–80; B. Martin, 'Why is Denmark better than the USA–with chickens and eggs and Salmonella?', *Food Poison Journal.com*, posted 18 August 2010; S. Stevens, 'Knocking out Salmonella in Denmark', *Food Safety Counsel.com*, posted 7 July 2012; S. Jore, 'Surveillance of Salmonella in Norway', Norwegian Veterinary Institute, <http://www.vetinst.no/eng/Highlights/Surveillance-of-Salmonella-in-Norway>, posted 2 July 2008; 'How many are infected with campylobacter?', <http://www.foedevarestyrelsen.dk/english/Food/Campylobacter/Page/How-many-are-infected-with-campylobacter.aspx>, accessed 29 June 2014.

declined in both Britain and Europe since 2006—a development attributed to European poultry control programmes.[37]

Britain's position with regard to controlling the hygiene of food production has historically been more complex than that of the Scandinavian countries. As a rapidly industrializing and urbanizing nation with a strong ethos of entrepreneurial freedom, Victorian Britain instituted regulation of the food industries in relation to fraud. Britain was the first country to enact legislation against food adulteration (in 1872), but apart from provisions under the Nuisances Removal Acts allowing confiscation and prosecution where foods could be deemed to constitute a 'nuisance or injury to health', there was little provision for sanitary food production. With the commercialization of food production and distribution, local authorities all but lost such control as they had been able to maintain when such production was local, and invested instead in meat and milk inspection, related to concerns around tuberculosis but leaving other problems unaddressed. The identification of bacterial food poisoning was beyond the remit of local authority public analysts. Existing legislation was concerned with the nature and substance of food articles, but other than for water and milk, nothing was done to regulate the bacterial condition of foodstuffs.[38] The public health movement had succeeded where, and for as long as, problems were local and locally contained. Where central government was unwilling to take a lead, however, they remained powerless. In the area of food production, twentieth-century health reformers came up against a second tier of opponents: economic interests, in many cases independent of local authority pressure and largely immune to—or uncaring of—public health interventions. Where foodstuffs crossed administrative boundaries, as between town and country or between countries, intervention became more complex. The economic interests involved in meat and milk production, in food production and processing, and in the catering trades, and the interlinking of these interests, presented a much broader and more intractable problem. While England had been at the vanguard in attempting to safeguard its people's food supply against adulteration, it was noted in 1945 that it now stood last in protecting it from contamination.[39]

Health officers had been complaining about the indifference to 'food-fouling' displayed by the legislature since the 1920s, and just before World War II, W. A. Lethem of the Ministry of Health noted the 'national indifference [to] interfering with trade rights and vested interests'.[40] Given the dissenting medical opinions expressed in inter-war debates over pasteurization, some leeway might be suggested for the legislature, but it was also clear that significant economic interests were at stake for agriculture and the dairy industry in the perilous economic

[37] <http://www.efsa.europa.eu/en/efsajournal/doc/2597.pdf>.

[38] Notes of the Week, 'Hygiene and foodstuffs', *Medical Officer*, 76 (1946): p. 155.

[39] Editorial, 'Food-spread disease', *MO*, 74 (1945): p. 49.

[40] W. A. Lethem, 'Slaughterhouse practice at home and abroad: The comparison between the systems of different countries, the methods of meat inspection and the practice of humane killing', *Journal of the Sanitary Institute*, 58 (1937–38): pp. 562–72. See also Charles Porter, 'The public and food hygiene', *MO*, 46 (1925–26): p. 427.

conditions of the 1930s—and the agricultural lobby was very strong.[41] Vested interests in the food industries were also integrated into the wider national and international economy: Britain had, for example, a valuable export trade in stud animals—bulls, rams, and stallions—for much of the twentieth century. Economic pressures and legislative indifference continued after World War II. In the face of EU directives and practice elsewhere in Europe, veterinary ante-mortem inspection of livestock before slaughter was not enforced in England until the impact of the BSE crisis forced the issue in 1995.[42] Despite accumulating evidence of *Salmonella* food poisoning caused by poultry meat, for example, no action was taken to introduce controls on production before imminent incorporation into the European Economic Community system generated the Poultry Meat (Hygiene) Regulations, 1976.[43] Although controls are now being exercised, problems in the hygienic production of poultry meat have persisted into the twenty-first century.[44]

Economic interests and legislative equivocation threw the British public health community back on the last-resort position: education. From the 1920s, repeated attempts were being made to educate food handlers and the general public, if not front-line industrial producers, in the clean handling and preparation of foods for human consumption. Here again, the problems proved intractable. Charles Porter, Medical Officer of Health (MOH) for Marylebone and a keen student of American public health practice, lamented in 1926 that although it was generally thought that the 'sanitary conscience' of the British people had been completely awakened, 'the portion of that apparatus concerned with food has remained to a large extent unaffected'.[45] Beyond fraud and food controls, one theme runs through the modern history of food infections: the importance of personal hygiene and the simple practice of hand-washing—after using the toilet, before and after preparing food, before eating. Since the 1960s, the importance of properly cooking poultry and meat—of 'food education'—has become another preventive strand. Food risks inherent in the production process may be averted by practice in the home. The British were slow and reluctant to be converted to these truths, as Chapter 9 demonstrates, and to some extent remain so.[46] Problems of poverty, of water and soap supplies, and of government indifference compound difficulties in large parts of the world. The initiative of an annual Global Hand Washing day (15 October), inaugurated in 2008 and aimed at school-children, is admirable, but in relation to

[41] Major Quentin Gurney, 'Veterinary medicine and agriculture from a farmer's point of view', *Journal of State Medicine*, 42 (1934): pp. 435–7.

[42] J. Longstreeth et al., 'Veterinary involvement in meat hygiene', *Veterinary Record* (*Vet. Rec.*), 139 (1996): p. 528.

[43] D. L. Haxby, 'Poultry production: From backyard to batteries', *Vet Rec*, 110 (1982): p. 605.

[44] M. Heyndrikx et al., 'Routes for salmonella contamination of poultry meat: Epidemiological study from hatchery to slaughterhouse', *Epi and Inf*, 129 (2002): pp. 253–65. The Food Standard Agency's Food Safety Week 2014 focused on the domestic handling of raw chicken in preventing campylobacter infections: <http://www.food.gov.uk/news=updates/campaigns/campylobacter/fsw-2014/#.U7E15UCufWI>, accessed 29 June 2014.

[45] Porter, 'The public', p. 427. His enthusiasm for American practice can be studied in Charles Porter, 'Cleanliness in food handling: Impressions of American methods', *Journal of the Sanitary Institute*, 45 (1924–25): pp. 280–9.

[46] Richard Slack, 'Forgetting hygiene', *PH*, 114 (2000): p. 307.

FERG's estimates of the global burden of enteric infections (see Introduction) may seem like a triumph of hope.[47] As one concerned gathering noted in 2000, 'there is little point in showing the correct methods if the tools—soap, running water and ways to dry hands—are not available'.[48] And in Britain, even at that date, many schools did not provide 'a satisfactory environment for children to learn and practice the basic social skill'.[49] As recently as October 2012, Sir Liam Donaldson, former English CMO, expressed the view that changing human habits presents the greatest public health challenge, and that hand-washing is one of the most difficult issues to address.[50] Since 2006, the Food Standards Agency has run a National Food Safety Week in the month of June. Ahead of the 2013 Week, an Agency survey found that 80 per cent of people questioned practised one or more food behaviours that put them at risk of food poisoning.[51]

British neglect of personal hygiene has often been contrasted with that of other western nations, notably America and the Scandinavian countries.[52] Aware of its own shortcomings in hygiene education, the British public health community of the inter-war period looked constantly to America in this respect, expressing the greatest admiration for American skills at educating the general public in personal cleanliness and other public health concerns.[53] Why have the British been so impervious to messages about personal hygiene? It may be that old British proverbs such as 'You have to eat a peck of dirt before you die' have inured generations of Britons to eating dirty food.[54] Or it may be, as with Britain's Industrial Revolution, that the learning curve undergone by the pioneering society undermined flexibility and ability to adapt to later ideas.[55] Britain's first sanitary revolution took place between 1840 and 1880 and involved the building of sanitary infrastructure and the education of the British people in the use of drains, sewers, water closets, clean piped water, and routines of daily behaviour that would break what Schoenwald called 'man's self-indulgent unboundedness'.[56] In the era before modern germ

[47] See <http://www.who.int/gpsc/events/2008/15_10_08/en/>.

[48] Slack, 'Forgetting', p. 307. [49] Slack, 'Forgetting', p. 307.

[50] Sir Liam Donaldson, interviewed on *Today*, BBC Radio 4, 5 October 2012.

[51] See <http://www.food.gov.uk/news-updates/campaigns/kitchen-check/#.U6_phkCufWI>, accessed 29 June 2014.

[52] See e.g. G. S. Elliston, in discussion following V. T. Thierens, 'The control of food and its preparation', *Journal of the Royal Sanitary Institute*, 57 (1936–37): p. 579; Thomas Stuttaford, ''Americans come clean on how to avoid tummy trouble', *The Times*, 28 January 1999, p. 11. For the American adoption of personal hygiene see Suellen Hoy, *Chasing Dirt: The American Pursuit of Cleanliness* (1995); Nancy Tomes, *The Gospel of Germs: Men, Women and the Microbe in American Life* (1998).

[53] Editorial, 'Health teaching in the United States', *MO*, 24 (1920): p. 18.

[54] First recorded in Jonathan Swift, *Polite Conversation* (1738), i: 48, it also occurs in Flora Thompson's 1939 memoir of rural England, and elsewhere. See Flora Thompson, *Lark Rise to Candleford* (Penguin edition, 2008), p. 116; *Oxford Dictionary of Proverbs* (2004).

[55] This view of British industry post 1850 is broad-brush and arguable: see the discussion in David Edgerton, *Science, Technology and Britain's Industrial 'Decline'* (1996): pp. 15–23. S. N. Broadberry, *The Productivity Race: British Manufacturing in International Perspective* (1997), p. 4, notes that European manufacturers economised on use of resources and machinery.

[56] Richard Schoenwald, 'Training urban man: A hypothesis about the sanitary movement', in H. J. Dyos and Michael Wolff, eds, *The Victorian City: Images and Realities* (1973), vol 2: pp. 675, 677.

theory became widely accepted, those routines did not include hand-washing. Even after germ theories came on the scene, the English resisted the siren call of hygiene. Ridiculing in 1910 an American author who saw woes unnumbered in unwashed hands and urged that natural functions should be conducted only 'under full aseptic ritual', a *Lancet* commentator exclaimed in exasperation: 'That dirty hands carry disease and death is a truism, but are we therefore to spend all our time washing our hands?'[57] Moving with the times proved no easier with personal hygiene than it had with the 'make do and mend' mentality in British industry.

The British public health community has continued to wrestle with the unhygienic legacy of the first sanitary revolution into the twenty-first century. Modern studies have suggested a greater British vulnerability to food poisoning compared to other nationals. In 1959, it was noted that the standards of hygienists differed in Britain and America and that it was 'chastening to note' that in America, with a population nearly four times that of England and Wales, the total number of recorded food infections in 1955 was 9,633, and 11,133 in 1956. In England and Wales the estimated number in 1957 was 15,100.[58] In 2003, it was reported that the British were more likely than any other nation to suffer from travellers' diarrhoea, a finding that the authors were at loss to explain, although Britain's only consultant in travel medicine believed that lack of personal hygiene was to blame.[59]

In other western countries, Britain's sanitary revolution set an example which began to be followed essentially after germ theories had begun to be taken seriously, and a 'gospel of germs' in Nancy Tomes's phrase was incorporated into the primary process. The United States really began to create a sanitary infrastructure only in the first decades of the twentieth century at a point when the dictates of personal hygiene were already being engrained in its peoples.[60] A reverse model of Britain's sanitary revolution—personal hygiene plus infrastructure—was thus present in the American hygiene education process. As a result, Americans, both private individuals and public health professionals, took the lessons of the healthy disease carriers to heart in a way that escaped the British. Similar patterns can be suggested for Germany and Scandinavia.[61] The lessons of microbiology by contrast failed to become engrained in the British national psyche, because sanitary training had

[57] Annotation, 'Sanitary superstition', *Lancet* (1910), i: p. 398.

[58] Notes and Comments, 'Food infections in the United States', *MO*, 101 (1959): p. 3. See also Notes and Comments, 'Epidemiology of salmonellosis', *MO*, 111 (1964): p. 237. These reports doubtfully reflect reality. The British surveillance system was considerably more comprehensive than others into the 1980s and beyond, and was considered to detect more cases than most other countries. Ros Stanwell-Smith, personal communication, 20 September 2013.

[59] B. Rowlands, 'Clean hands may prevent Delhi belly', *The Times* 8 July 2003, T2: p. 17.

[60] Martin Melosi, *The Sanitary City: Urban Infrastructure in America from Colonial Times to the Present* (2000), pp. 137–8, 144–5. See also John Duffy, *The Sanitarians. A History of American Public Health* (1990): pp. 201–2.

[61] See e.g. H-Net review, 'Cleanliness is next to Germanness': <http://www.h-net.org/reviews/showpdf.php?id=13074>; <http://www.naaf.no/en/inneklima/Useful-facts-on-cleaning/>, accessed 5 September 2013; William Hubbard, personal communication, 5 September 2013. See also George Newman, *Bacteria, especially as they are Related to the Economy of Nature, to Industrial Processes and to the Public Health* (1899): p. xii.

already been achieved according to an older model. Food infections are, however, now a major problem in America, with annual cases estimated at one per six persons, or 48 million nationwide.[62] Modern industry and migration may reconfigure national sanitary cultures and food safety.

The impact of microbiology on the story of the lesser *Salmonella* was by no means as successful in preventive terms as in the case of typhoid. Rather, microbiology offered scientific insights into the hidden lives of these bacteria, into their habits and habitats, their preference for human and animal guts and excreta, their ability to multiply in temperate nutrients, their means of travel in numerous varieties of foodstuffs, their efficiency in infiltrating food processing systems and in returning to the environment of their preferred habitats. The complicated relationship between human and animal salmonellosis makes the understanding and controlling of pathways of infection a continuing project.[63] The vast industry of microbiological enterprise that grew up around *Salmonella* in the twentieth century contributed to knowledge through the identification of organisms, elucidation of outbreaks, and the tracking of infections, but offered little specific in terms of preventive measures beyond the obvious that hygienic behaviours should be observed at all points in the human and animal food chains, and, ideally, by every responsible human individual.[64] Science has its limitations: it does not always connect to popular practice and public health benefits.

The current world situation with regard to foodborne infections remains, as FERG's investigations show, a matter of profound concern. Food safety legislation and the preventive vaccination of poultry in selected instances are of limited value, and food safety education has yet to prove effective in population terms. A recent report shows that the incidence of human *Salmonella* infections in the EU fell by almost nine per cent in 2010 while *Campylobacter* infections rose by seven per cent, with Britain's figures for both reflecting the EU trend.[65] In global terms, however, the picture remains worrying. In 2013 it was estimated that over 94 million people globally fall ill every year with *Salmonella* infections.[66] On the plus side, microbiology has elucidated key aspects of the origins of *Salmonella* and how it causes disease.[67] On the down side, there has been an enormous increase in antibiotic resistance among *Salmonella typhi* serotypes and MDR *Salmonella* is increasingly a serious public health concern in large parts of the world. Both travel widely through

62 <http://www.cdc.gov/foodborneburden/>, accessed 5 September 2013.

63 See for example BBC News, 'Animals "not the source of drug-resistant salmonella"', <http://www.bbc.co.uk/news/health-24063383>, accessed 13 September 2013.

64 This approach has now been adopted by the Food Standards Agency in the effort to control *Campylobacter* infections: <http://www.food.gov.uk/news-updates/news/2013/aug/campylobacter>, accessed 13 September 2013.

65 European Food Safety Authority, Summary Report, *Trends and Sources of Zoonoses, Zoonotic Agents and Food-borne Outbreaks in 2010*: <http://www.efsa.europa.eu/en/efsajournal/doc/2597.pdf>, pp. 24, 113.

66 BBC News, 'Animals'.

67 H. L. Andrews-Polymenis et al., 'Taming the elephant: *Salmonella* biology, pathogenesis, and prevention', *Infection and Immunity*, 78 (2010): pp. 2357–60; C. Kidgell et al., '*Salmonella typhi*, the causative agent of typhoid is approximately 50,000 years old', *Infection, Genetics and Evolution*, 2 (2002): pp. 39–45.

the food chain.[68] Lastly, highly invasive forms of *Salmonella typhimurium* have recently been documented in Africa.[69] Their emergence has been closely linked in time to the current HIV epidemic: the inference is that a large reservoir of immunosuppressed humans with HIV and antibiotic treatment may have created new ecological niches for these *Salmonella* serotypes.[70] The prospect that HIV provides the opportunity for new pathogens to invade humanity is frightening, but this development offers yet one further illustration of the opportunistic character of these infinitely adaptable organisms, for whom social and economic developments in the twentieth century proved remarkably advantageous. Despite all modern advances in scientific knowledge and medical treatment, the *Salmonellas* are still very much with us and remain capable of spreading discomfort, misery, and even death. Locally named and globally distributed, *Salmonella* serotypes adapt happily into new ecological niches. They are resourceful and resilient; they do not respect human boundaries. As long as there is animal life on earth, the *Salmonella* family has a future.

[68] Helms et al., 'DT104 infections'; S. Le Hello et al., 'Highly drug-resistant *Salmonella enterica* serotype Kentucky ST 198-X: a microbiological study', *Lancet Infectious Diseases*, 13 (2013): pp. 672–9.

[69] M. A. Gordon and S. M. Graham, 'Invasive salmonellosis in Malawi', *Journal of Infection in Developing Countries*, 2 (2008): pp. 438–42.

[70] C. K. Okoro et al., 'Intracontinental spread of human invasive *Salmonella* Typhimurium pathovariants in sub-Saharan Africa', *Nature Genetics*, 44 (2012): pp. 1215–21, published online 30 September 2012.

Select Bibliography

PRINTED PRIMARY SOURCES

Reports

Advisory Committee on the Microbiological Safety of Food, *Report on Salmonella in Eggs* (London: HMSO, 1993).

Chief Medical Officer's Report, Ministry of Health, England and Wales, 1920–90.

Medical Officer's Annual Reports, London County Council, 1895–1913.

BRITISH PARLIAMENTARY PAPERS

Reports of the Medical Officer, Local Government Board, 1880–1919.

Royal Commission on Sewage Disposal, Fourth Report, 1904.

JOURNALS AND NEWSPAPERS

American Journal of Hygiene.

American Journal of Public Health.

Biographical Memoirs of Fellows of the Royal Society.

British Medical Bulletin.

British Medical Journal.

Epidemiology and Infection.

Fish Trades Gazette.

International Bulletin of the Bacteriological Nomenclature Committee.

Journal of Hygiene.

Journal of Infectious Diseases.

Journal of the Royal Army Medical Corps.

Journal of the (Royal) Sanitary Institute.

Journal of Pathology and Bacteriology.

Journal of State Medicine.

Lancet.

Meat Trades Journal.

Medical Officer.

Medical Research Council Special Report Series.

Monthly Bulletin of the Ministry of Health and (Emergency) Public Health. Laboratory Service.

Munk's Roll of the Royal College of Physicians.

Obituary Notices of Fellows of the Royal Society.

Poultry World.

Proceedings of the Royal Society of Medicine.

Public Health.

Reports on Public Health and Medical Subjects/Matters.

Royal Society of Health Journal.

Transactions of the Epidemiological Society.

Transactions of the Pathological Society.

Veterinary Journal.

Veterinary Record.

CONTEMPORARY ARTICLES AND MONOGRAPHS

Journal articles of special importance only have been included as separate items in the bibliography.

Austen, Edward E., *The House Fly as a Danger to Health and How to Deal with it* (London: British Museum, 1913).

Bertram, James G., *The Harvest of the Sea, a Contribution to the Natural and Economic History of the British Food Fishes* (London: 1865).

Blount, W. F., 'Public health aspects of the poultry industry', *Royal Sanitary Institute Journal*, 69 (1949): pp. 359–71.

Bradley, William H., 'The control of typhoid fever', *Public Health*, 62 (1949): pp. 159–63.

British Association for the Advancement of Science, *Salmonella. The Food Poisoner* (London: BAAS, 1977).

Brooks, R. St John, ed., *Second International Congress for Microbiology, London 25 July–1 August 1936; Report of Proceedings* (London: International Society for Microbiology, 1937).

Caldwell, Mary E. and Ryerson, Dwight L., 'Salmonellosis in certain reptiles', *Journal of Infectious Diseases*, 65 (1930): pp. 242–5.

Centers for Disease Control, *An Atlas of Salmonella in the United States 1968–1998* (2001), CD-Rom version.

Cockburn, William C. et al., *Food Poisoning* (London, Royal Society of Health, 1962).

Cogan, A. and Humphrey, T. J., 'The rise and fall of *Salmonella* Enteritidis in the UK', *Journal of Applied Microbiology*, 94 (2003): pp. 114S–19S.

Cooper, T. V., 'A case of fever due to infection with bacillus oranienburg', *Monthly Bulletin of the Emergency Public Health Laboratory Service*, 3 (1944): pp. 39–40.

Durham, Herbert E., 'The present knowledge of outbreaks due to meat poisoning', *British Medical Journal*, ii (1898): pp. 1797–801.

Durham, Herbert E., 'On infections by unsound meat, more especially with regard to the *bacillus enteritidis* (Gaertner)', *Transactions of the Pathological Society*, 50 (1899): pp. 262–8.

Editorial, 'The Borgia Tradition', *Public Health*, 72 (1958): p. 162.

European Food Safety Authority, *European Union Summary Report on Trends in Zoonoses*: <http://www.efsa.europa.eu/en/efsa/efsajournal/doc/3547.pdf>

Felix, Arthur, 'Laboratory control of the enteric fevers', *British Medical Bulletin*, 7 (1951): pp. 153–62.

Field, H. I., 'A survey of bovine salmonellosis in Mid and West Wales', *Veterinary Journal*, 104 (1948): pp. 251–66, 294–304, 324–39.

Galton, Mildred M. et al., 'Salmonella in swine, cattle and the environment of abattoirs', *Journal of Infectious Diseases*, 95 (1954): pp. 236–45.

Graham-Smith, George Stuart, *Flies in Relation to Disease. Non-blood Sucking Flies* (Cambridge: Cambridge University Press, 1913).

Greenwood M., *Epidemics and Crowd Diseases* (London: Williams and Norgate, 1935).

Hamilton-Lawrence, Julius, *Imperishable Fresh Fish (Report upon the Fish Markets, Fish Trade Abuses, Fish Frauds and Adulterations and Fish Supply of the Metropolis)*, 2nd edn (London: P. S. King & Son, 1890).

Herdman, William A. and Boyce, Rubert, *Oysters and Disease*, Lancashire Sea Fisheries Memoir no 1 (London: G. Philip & Son, 1899).

Hewitt, Charles G., *House Flies and How They Spread Disease* (Cambridge: Cambridge University Press, 1912).
Hughes, David L., 'Meat inspection and production: An examination of standards', *Royal Society of Health Journal*, 82 (1962): pp. 83–6.
Joint Meeting, 'Discussion on salmonella infections', *Proceedings of the Royal Society of Medicine*, 33(1) (1940): pp. 351–70.
Kauffmann, Fritz, *Erlebte bakteriologie. Zur geschichte der salmonalla-und Escherichia-forschung* (Copenhagen: Munksgaard, 1967).
Kauffmann, Fritz, *Erinnerungen eines bakteriologen* (Copenhagen: Munksgaard, 1969).
Kauffmann, Fritz, *Serological Diagnosis of Salmonella Species: Kauffmann–White Schema* (Copenhagen: Munksgaard, 1972).
Klein, Edward E., *Report of Experiments and Observations on the Vitality of the Bacillus of Typhoid and of Sewage Microbes in Oysters and Other Fish* (London: Worshipful Company of Fishmongers, 1905).
Lane-Claypon, Janet, *Milk and its Hygienic Relations* (London: Medical Research Council, 1916).
Lethem, W. A., 'Food hygiene', *Monthly Bulletin of the Ministry of Health*, 6 (1947): pp. 53–4.
Lethem, W. A., 'Trading in diseased meat', *Medical Officer*, 79 (1948): pp. 274–5.
Madsen, Thorvald, *Statens Seruminstitut: Institutets Udvikling 1902–1940* (Copenhagen: Bianco Lunos Bogtrykkeri, 1940).
McCoy, John H., 'Trends in salmonella food poisoning in England and Wales 1941–72', *Journal of Hygiene*, 74 (1975): pp. 271–82.
Nuttall, George F. H., 'The part played by insects, arachnids and myriapods in the propagation of infective diseases of men and animals', *British Medical Journal*, ii (1899): pp. 642–4.
Nuttall, George F. H., 'On the role of insects, arachnids and myriapods as carriers in the spread of bacterial and parasitic diseases of man and animals', *Johns Hopkins Hospital Reports*, 8 (1900): pp. 1–154.
Peters, Owen H., *Observations on the Natural History of Epidemic Diarrhoea* (Cambridge: Cambridge University Press, 1911).
Reed, Walter et al., *Abstract of report on the origin and spread of typhoid fever in U.S. military camps during the Spanish War of 1898* (Washington: Adjutant-General's Office, 1900).
Royal College of Veterinary Surgeons, *Registers and Directory* (London: Royal College of Veterinary Surgeons, 1967).
Savage, William G., 'Bacterial food poisoning and food infections', *Reports on Public Health and Medical Matters*, Local Government Board, no 77 (1913).
Savage, William, G., *Food and the Public Health* (London: Cassell and Co, 1919).
Savage, William G., *Food Poisoning and Food Infections* (Cambridge: Cambridge University Press, 1920).
Savage, William G., 'Problems of salmonella food poisoning', *British Medical Journal*, ii (1956): pp. 320–3.
Savage, William G. and Bruce White, Philip, 'Food poisoning: A study of 100 recent outbreaks', Medical Research Council, *Special Report Series*, 92 (1925).
Scott, William M., 'Les empoissonnements par les oeufs de cane contenant de bacilles pathogènes', *Bulletin Office Internationale de Santé*, 5 (1933): pp. 828–33.
Sheard, L. Barrie, 'Inspection of food and food premises', *Royal Society of Health Journal*, 98 (1978): pp. 62–5.

Société Internationale de Microbiologie, *Premier Congrès Internationale de Microbiologie* (Paris: International Society for Microbiology, 1930).

Symposium, 'Epidemiology of Salmonellosis', *Public Health Reports* (Washington: US Marine Hospital Service, 1963), 78(12) (1963): pp. 1065–86.

Taylor, Joan, 'The Salmonella Reference Laboratory', *British Medical Bulletin,* 7 (1951): pp. 163–6.

Third International Congress for Microbiology, New York, September 2–9, 1939: *Report of Proceedings* (New York: International Society for Microbiology, 1939).

van Oye, Eugène ed., *The World Problem of Salmonellosis* (The Hague: W. Junk, 1964).

Walker, J. H. C., 'Organic fertilisers as a source of salmonella infection', *Lancet*, ii (1957): pp. 283–4.

Walker, J. H. C., 'The broiler industry–transmission of salmonella infection', *Royal Society of Health Journal,* 80 (1960): pp. 142–4.

WHO Expert Committee on Salmonella Control, *Report* (Geneva: World Health Organisation, 1988).

Wilson, Graham Selby, *The Pasteurisation of Milk* (London: Edward Arnold & Co, 1942).

Wilson, Graham Selby, 'The Public Health Laboratory Service', *British Medical Journal,* i (1948): pp. 677–82.

Wilson, Graham Selby et al., 'The bacteriology of spray-dried egg, with particular reference to food poisoning', Medical Research Council *Special Report Series* no 260 (London: H.M. Stationery Office, 1947): 'Appendix by the Ministry of Food on practical problems presented by the bacteriology of spray-dried egg'.

Wilson, Graham Selby and Milne, Ashley A., eds. *Topley and Wilson's Principles of Bacteriology and Immunity* (London: Edward Arnold, 3rd edn, 1946; 4th edn, 1955; 5th edn, 1964).

SECONDARY PRINTED SOURCES AND ARTICLES

Amsterdamska, Olga, 'Medical and biological constraints: Early research on variation in bacteriology', *Social Studies of Science,* 17 (1987): pp. 657–87.

Amsterdamska, Olga, 'Standardising epidemics: Infection, inheritance and environment in prewar experimental epidemiology', in *Heredity and Infection: The History of Disease Transmission*, edited by Jean-Paul Gaudillière and Ilana Löwy (London: Routledge, 2001).

Amsterdamska, Olga, Demarcating epidemiology', *Science, Technology and Human Values,* 30 (2005): pp. 17–51.

Atkins, Peter J., 'The pasteurisation of England: the science, culture and health implications of milk processing, 1900–1950', in *Food, Science, Policy and Regulation in the Twentieth Century*, edited by David F Smith and Jim Phillips (London: Routledge, 2000).

Atkins, Peter J., 'The Glasgow case: Meat, disease and regulation, 1885–1924', *Agricultural History Review*, 52 (2004): pp. 161–82.

Atkins, Peter J., *Liquid Materialities: A History of Milk, Science and the Law* (Farnham: Ashgate, 2010).

Barnes, David S., 'Confronting sensory crisis in the Great Stinks of London and Paris', in *Filth: Dirt, Disgust, and Modern Life*, edited by William A. Cohen and Ryan Johnson (Minneapolis and London: University of Minnesota Press, 2005).

Barnes, David S., *The Great Stink of Paris and the Nineteenth-century Struggle against Filth and Germs* (Baltimore: Johns Hopkins University Press, 2006).
Barr, Richard I., 'Food hygiene. The arousal of public awareness', *Royal Society of Health Journal*, 98 (1978): pp. 55–7.
Bonner, Thomas N., *American Doctors and German Universities. A Chapter in International Relations* (Lincoln: Nebraska University Press, 1963).
Brand, Jeanne, *Doctors and the State: The British Medical Profession and Government Action in Public Health* (Baltimore: Johns Hopkins University Press, 1965).
Brown, Jonathan, *Agriculture in England: A Survey of Farming, 1870–1944* (Manchester: Manchester University Press, 1987).
Bud, Robert, *Penicillin: Triumph and Tragedy* (Oxford: Oxford University Press, 2006).
Burnett, John, *Plenty and Want: A Social History of Food in England from1815 to the Present Day*, 3rd edn (London: Routledge, 1989).
Chick, Harriette et al., *War on Disease. A History of the Lister Institute* (London: Deutsch, 1971).
Clark, John F. M., 'Sowing the seeds of economic entomology: houseflies and the emergence of medical entomology in Britain', in *Insects and Illnesses: Contributions to the History of Medical Entomology*, edited by Mario Coluzzi et al., *Parassitologia*, 50 (2008): pp. 321–8.
Clark, John F. M., *Bugs and the Victorians* (New Haven and London: Yale University Press, 2009).
Cogan, A. and Humphrey T. J., 'The rise and fall of *Salmonella* Enteritidis in the UK', *Journal of Applied Microbiology*, 94 (2003): pp. 114S–19S.
Collier, Leslie H., *The Lister Institute and Preventive Medicine. A Concise History* (London: Lister Institute of Preventive Medicine, 2000).
Cunningham, Andrew, 'Transforming plague: The laboratory and the identity of infectious disease', in *The Laboratory Revolution in Medicine*, edited by Andrew Cunningham and Perry Williams (Cambridge: Cambridge University Press, 1992), pp. 209–44.
Curtis, Valerie and Biran, Adam, 'Dirt, disgust, and disease: is hygiene in our genes?', *Perspectives in Biology and Medicine*, 44 (2002): pp. 17–31.
Dewberry, Elliott B., *Food Poisoning. Foodborne Infection and Intoxication. Nature, History and Causation; Measure for Prevention ad Control*, 4th edn (London: Leonard Hill, 1959).
Dolman, Claude E. and Wolfe, Richard J., *Suppressing the Diseases of Animals and Man. Theobald Smith, Microbiologist* (Boston: Boston Medical Library, 2003).
Doyle, Michael P. and Cliver, Dean O., 'Epidemiology of salmonellosis', in *Foodborne Diseases*, edited by Dean O. Cliver (San Diego and London: Academic Press, 1990).
Durie, Alastair, 'Medicine health and economic development: Promoting spa and seaside resorts in Scotland c 1750–1830', *Medical History*, 47 (2003): pp. 195–216.
Etheridge, Elizabeth W., *Sentinel for Health: A History of the Centers for Disease Control* (Berkeley: California University Press, 1992).
Foster, William H., *A History of Medical Bacteriology* (London: Heinemann Medical, 1970).
French, Michael and Phillips, Jim, *Cheated Not Poisoned? Food Regulation in the United Kingdom, 1875–1938* (Manchester: Manchester University Press, 2000).
Godley, Andrew C. and Williams, Bridget, 'The chicken, the factory farm and the supermarket: The emergence of the modern poultry industry in Britain', in *Food Chains: From Farmyard to Shopping Cart*, edited by Warren Belasco and Roger Horowitz (Philadelphia: University of Philadelphia Press, 2009), pp. 47–61.

Godley, Andrew C. and Williams, Bridget, 'Demarcating luxury and the contentious "invention of the technological chicken" in Britain', *Business History Review*, 83 (2009): pp. 267–90.

Hamlin, Christopher, *What Becomes of Pollution: Adversary Science and the Controversy on the Self-Pollution of Rivers in Britain 1750–1914* (New York: Garland, 1987).

Hamlin, Christopher, *A Science of Impurity: Water Analysis in Nineteenth Century Britain* (Bristol: Hilger, 1990).

Hardy, Anne, 'Food, hygiene and the laboratory: A short history of food poisoning in Britain, circa 1850–1950', *Social History of Medicine*, 12 (1999): pp. 293–311.

Hardy, Anne, 'Animals, disease and man: Making connections', *Perspectives in Biology and Medicine*, 46 (2002): pp. 200–15.

Hardy, Anne, 'Exorcising Molly Malone: typhoid and shellfish consumption in urban Britain 1860–1960', *History Workshop Journal*, 55 (2003): pp. 73–90.

Hardy, Anne, 'Professional advantage and public health: British veterinarians and state veterinary services', 1865–1939, *Twentieth Century British History*, 14 (2003): pp. 1–23.

Hardy, Anne, 'John Bull's beef: Meat hygiene and veterinary public health in England in the twentieth century', *Review of Agricultural and Environmental Studies*, 91 (2010): pp. 369–92.

Hardy, Anne, 'Scientific strategy and ad hoc response: The problem of typhoid in America and England, c. 1910–50', *Journal of the History of Medicine and Allied Sciences*, 69 (2014): pp. 1–37.

Hassan, John, *A History of Water in Modern England and Wales* (Manchester: Manchester University Press, 1998).

Hassan, John, *The Seaside, Health and Environment in England and Wales since 1800* (Aldershot: Ashgate, 2003).

Howard, Leland O., 'A fifty year sketch history of medical entomology', *Smithsonian Report for 1921* (1923): pp. 565–86.

Howard, Leland O., 'A history of applied entomology', *Smithsonian Miscellaneous Collections*, 84 (1930): whole issue.

Huber, Valeska, 'The unification of the globe by disease? The International Sanitary Conferences on cholera, 1851–1894', *Historical Journal*, 49 (2006): pp. 453–76.

Kaukianen, Yrjo, 'Growth, diversification and globalisation: Main trends in international shipping since 1850', in *International Merchant Shipping in the Nineteenth and Twentieth Centuries: The Comparative Dimension*, edited by Lewis R. Fischer and Even Langes (St John's Newfoundland: International Maritime Economic History Association, 2008).

Kettle, D. S., *Medical and Veterinary Entomology*, 2nd edn (Wallingford: C.A.B. International, 1995).

Kohler, Robert E., *Landscapes and Labscapes: Exploring the Lab-Field Border in Biology* (Chicago: Chicago University Press, 2002).

Koolmees Peter A., et al., 'The traditional responsibility of veterinarians in meat production and meat inspection', in *Veterinary Aspects of Meat Production, Processing and Inspection. An Update of Recent Developments in Europe*, edited by Frans J. Smulders (Utrecht: ECCEAMST, 1999), pp. 7–30.

Kupferberg, Eric, *A History of the International Union of Microbiological Societies (1927–1990)*, (1993): <http://www.iums.org/index.php/homepage/history>.

Lambert, Royston, *Sir John Simon (1816–1904) and English Social Administration* (Bristol: McGibbon and Kee, 1965).

Leonards, Chris and Randeraal, Nico, 'Transnational experts and social reform, 1840–1900', *International Review of Social History*, lv (2010): pp. 213–39.

Levitz, Judith Walzer, 'Typhoid Mary fights back'. Bacteriological theory and practice in early twentieth century public health', *Isis*, 83 (1992): pp. 608–29.

Levitz, Judith Walzer, *Typhoid Mary: Captive to the Public's Health* (Boston: Beacon Press, 1996).

Livingstone, David N., *Putting Science in its Place: Geographies of Scientific Knowledge* (Chicago and London: Chicago University Press, 2003).

Livingstone, David N. and Withers, C. J., eds, *Geographies of Nineteenth-Century Science* (Chicago and London: Chicago University Press, 2011).

Martin, John, *The Development of Modern Agriculture: British Farming since 1931* (Basingstoke: Macmillan, 2000).

McLeod, Roy M., 'The frustration of state medicine, 1880–1899', *Medical History*, 11 (1967): pp. 15–40.

Mølbak, Kare et al., 'Salmonella infections', in *Foodborne Infections and Intoxications*, edited by Hans P. Reimann and Dean O. Cliver (London: Elsevier, 2006).

Morgan, Nigel, 'Infant mortality, flies, and horses in later-nineteenth-century towns: A case study of Preston', *Continuity and Change*, 17 (2002): pp. 97–132.

Neild, Robert, *The English, the French and the Oyster* (London: Quiller Press, 1995).

Old, D. C. and Threlfall, E J., 'Salmonella', in *Topley and Wilson's Microbiology and Microbial Infections*, 9th edn, edited by Leslie Collier et al. (London: Arnold, 1998).

Otter, Chris, 'Civilizing slaughter: The development of the British public abattoir, 1850–1910', in *Meat, Modernity and the Rise of the Slaughterhouse*, edited by Paula Young Lee (Hanover and London: University Press of New England, 2008), pp. 89–106.

Peluffo, C. A., 'Hormaeche Estenio (1892–1964)': <http://www.smu.org.uy/dpmc/hmed/historia/articulos/hormaeche>.

Pennell, Sara, 'Great quantities of gooseberry pie and baked clod of beef: Victualing and eating out in early modern London', in *Londinopolis: Essays in the Cultural and Social History of Early Modern London*, edited by Paul Griffith and Mark Jenner (Manchester: Manchester University Press, 2000).

Pennington, Hugh, *When Food Kills. BSE, E. coli and Disaster Science* (Oxford: Oxford University Press, 2003).

Perren, Richard, *The Meat Trade in Britain, 1840–1914* (London: Routledge and Kegan Paul, 1978).

Perren, Richard, *Agriculture in Depression* (Cambridge: Cambridge University Press, 1995).

Perren, Richard, 'Filth and profit, disease and health: Public and private impediments to slaughterhouse reform in Victorian Britain', in *Meat, Modernity and the Rise of the Slaughterhouse*, edited by Paula Young Lee (Hanover and London: University Press of New England, 2008): pp. 127–50.

Petty, Celia, 'Primary research and public health: The prioritization of nutrition research in inter-war Britain', in *Historical Perspectives on the Role of the MRC: Essays in the History of the Medical Research Council of the United Kingdom*, edited by Joan Austoker and Linda Bryder (Oxford: Oxford University Press, 1989).

Petty, Celia, 'The impact of the newer knowledge of nutrition: Nutrition science and nutrition policy, 1900–1939' (PhD dissertation, London University, 1989).

Phillips, Jim and French, Michael, 'State regulation and the hazards of milk, 1900–1939', *Social History of Medicine*, 12 (1999): pp. 371–88.

Richardson, Nigel, *Typhoid at Uppingham: Analysis of a Victorian Town and School in Crisis 1875–1877* (London: Chatto and Pickering, 2008).

Rogers, Naomi, 'Germs with legs: flies, disease and the new public health', *Bulletin of the History of Medicine*, 63 (1989): pp. 599–617.

Schleifer, Karl-Heinz, 'The International Union of Microbiological Societies, IUMS', *Research in Microbiology*, 159 (2008): pp. 45–8: <http://www.iums.org/index.php/homepage/history>.

Schwarz, Maxime, *How the Cows Turned Mad: Unlocking the Mysteries of Mad Cow Disease* (Berkeley and Los Angeles: University of California Press, 2003).

Secord, James A., 'Knowledge in transit', *Isis*, 95 (2004): pp. 654–72.

Shoenwald, Richard L., 'Training urban man. A hypothesis about the sanitary movement', in *The Victorian City: Images and Realities*, edited by H J Dyos and Michael Wolff (London: Routledge and Kegan Paul, 1973), vol 2, pp. 669–92.

Smith, David and Diack, H. Lesley, with Hugh T. Pennington and Elizabeth M. Russell, *Food Poisoning, Policy and Politics: Corned Beef and Typhoid in Britain in the 1960s* (Woodbridge: Boydell Press, 2005).

Smith, Virginia, *Clean. A History of Personal Hygiene and Purity* (Oxford: Oxford University Press, 2007).

Stark, James F., *The Making of Modern Anthrax, 1875–1920: Uniting Local, National, and Global Histories of Disease* (London: Pickering and Chatto, 2013).

Steere-Williams, Jacob, 'The perfect food and the filth disease: Milk-borne typhoid and epidemiological practice in late Victorian Britain', *Journal of the History of Medicine and Allied Sciences*, 65 (2010): pp. 514–45.

Strick, James, 'Evolution of microbiology as seen in the textbooks of Edwin O Jordan and William H Park', *Yale Journal of Biology and Medicine*, 72 (1999): pp. 321–8.

Stuttaford, Thomas, 'Americans come clean on how to avoid tummy trouble', *The Times*, 28 January 1999, p. 11.

Trentmann, Frank, 'Bread, milk and democracy: Consumption and citizenship in twentieth century Britain', in *The Politics of Consumption, Material Culture and Citizenship*, edited by Martin Daunton and Matthew Hilton (Oxford: Oxford University Press, 2001).

Vernon, Keith, 'Pus, sewage, beer and milk: microbiology in Britain, 1870-1940', *History of Science*, 28 (1990): pp. 289–325.

Vernon, Keith, 'Desperately seeking status: Evolutionary Systematics and the taxonomists' search for respectability 1940–60', *British Journal for the History of Science*, 26 (1993): pp. 207–27.

Waddington, Keir, '"Unfit for human consumption": tuberculosis and the problem of infected meat in late Victorian Britain', *Bulletin of the History of Medicine*, 77 (2003): pp. 636–61.

Waddington, Keir, *The Bovine Scourge. Meat Tuberculosis and Public Health, 1850–1914* (Woodbridge: Boydell and Brewer, 2006).

Waddington, Keir, 'The dangerous sausage: Diet, meat and disease in Victorian and Edwardian Britain', *Cultural and Social History*, 81 (2011): pp. 51–71.

Wall, Rosemary, *Bacteria in Britain, 1880–1939* (London: Pickering and Chatto, 2013).

Walton, John K., *The English Seaside Resort: A Social History 1750–1914* (Leicester: Leicester University Press, 1983).

Walton, John K., *Fish and Chips and the British Working Class, 1870–1940* (Leicester: Leicester University Press, 1992).

Welshman, John, 'The Medical Officer of Health in England, 1900–1974: Watchdog or lapdog?', *Journal of Public Health*, 19 (1997): pp. 443–50.

Welshman, John, *Municipal Medicine: Public Health in Twentieth Century Britain* (Oxford: Peter Lang, 2000).

Williams, Robert E. O., *Microbiology for the Public Health. The Evolution of the Public Health Laboratory Service, 1939–1980* (London: Public Health Laboratory Service, 1985).

Woods, Abigail, 'A historical synopsis of animal diseases and public policy in twentieth century Britain', *Philosophical Transactions of the Royal Society*, series B, 366 (2011), doi: 10.1098/rstb.2010.0388.

Woods, Abigail and Matthews, Stephen, '"Little if at all removed from the illiterate farrier or cow-leech". The English veterinary surgeon c 1860–1885 and the campaign for veterinary reform', *Medical History* 54 (2010): pp. 29–54.

Worboys, Michael, *Spreading Germs: Disease Theories and Medical Practice in Britain, 1865–1900* (Cambridge: Cambridge University Press, 2000).

Worboys, Michael, 'Was there a bacteriological revolution in late-nineteenth-century medicine?', *Studies in the History and Philosophy of Biology and Biomedical Sciences*, 38 (2007): pp. 20–42.

Index